Tumors and Cysts of the Jaws

AFIP Atlas
of
Tumor Pathology

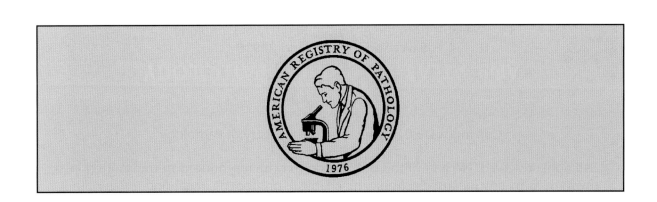

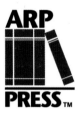

ARP PRESS

Silver Spring, Maryland

Editorial Director: Mirlinda Q. Caton
Production Editor: Dian S. Thomas
Editorial Assistant: Magdalena C. Silva
Editorial Assistant: Alana N. Black
Copyeditor: Audrey Kahn

Available from the American Registry of Pathology
Silver Spring, Maryland 20910
www.arppress.org
ISBN 1-933477-23-7
978-1-933477-23-7

AFIP ATLAS OF TUMOR PATHOLOGY

Fourth Series
Fascicle 16

TUMORS AND
CYSTS OF THE JAWS

by

Robert A. Robinson, MD, PhD
Professor, Department of Pathology
Carver College of Medicine
University of Iowa, Iowa City, Iowa

Steven D. Vincent, DDS, MS
Professor and Head
Department of Oral Pathology, Radiology, and Medicine
College of Dentistry
University of Iowa, Iowa City, Iowa

Published by the
American Registry of Pathology
Silver Spring, Maryland
2012

AFIP ATLAS OF TUMOR PATHOLOGY

EDITORS' NOTE

The Atlas of Tumor Pathology has a long and distinguished history. It was first conceived at a cancer research meeting held in St. Louis in September 1947 as an attempt to standardize the nomenclature of neoplastic diseases. The first series was sponsored by the National Academy of Sciences-National Research Council. The organization of this Sisyphean effort was entrusted to the Subcommittee on Oncology of the Committee on Pathology, and Dr. Arthur Purdy Stout was the first editor-in-chief. Many of the illustrations were provided by the Medical Illustration Service of the Armed Forces Institute of Pathology (AFIP), the type was set by the Government Printing Office, and the final printing was done at the Armed Forces Institute of Pathology (hence the colloquial appellation "AFIP Fascicles"). The American Registry of Pathology (ARP) purchased the Fascicles from the Government Printing Office and sold them virtually at cost. Over a period of 20 years, approximately 15,000 copies each of nearly 40 Fascicles were produced. The worldwide impact of these publications over the years has largely surpassed the original goal. They quickly became among the most influential publications on tumor pathology, primarily because of their overall high quality, but also because their low cost made them easily accessible the world over to pathologists and other students of oncology.

Upon completion of the first series, the National Academy of Sciences-National Research Council handed further pursuit of the project over to the newly created Universities Associated for Research and Education in Pathology (UAREP). A second series was started, generously supported by grants from the AFIP, the National Cancer Institute, and the American Cancer Society. Dr. Harlan I. Firminger became the editor-in-chief and was succeeded by Dr. William H. Hartmann. The second series' Fascicles were produced as bound volumes instead of loose leaflets. They featured a more comprehensive coverage of the subjects, to the extent that the Fascicles could no longer be regarded as "atlases" but rather as monographs describing and illustrating in detail the tumors and tumor-like conditions of the various organs and systems.

Once the second series was completed, with a success that matched that of the first, ARP, UAREP, and AFIP decided to embark on a third series. Dr. Juan Rosai was appointed as editor-in-chief, and Dr. Leslie H. Sobin became associate editor. A distinguished Editorial Advisory Board was also convened, and these outstanding pathologists and educators played a major role in the success of this series, the first publication of which appeared in 1991 and the last (number 32) in 2003.

The same organizational framework applies to the current fourth series, but with UAREP and AFIP no longer functiong, ARP will now be the responsible organization. New features include a hardbound cover, illustrations almost exclusively in color, and an accompanying electronic version of each Fascicle. There is also an increased emphasis (wherever appropriate) on the cytopathologic (intraoperative, exfoliative, and/or fine needle aspiration) and molecular features that are important in diagnosis and prognosis. What does not change from the three previous series, however, is the goal of providing the practicing pathologist with thorough, concise, and up-to-date information on the nomenclature and classification; epidemiologic, clinical, and pathogenetic features; and, most importantly, guidance in the diagnosis of the tumors and tumorlike lesions of all major organ systems and body sites.

As in the third series, a continuous attempt is made to correlate, whenever possible, the nomenclature used in the Fascicles with that proposed by the World Health Organization's Classification of Tumors, as well as to ensure a consistency of style throughout. Close cooperation between the various authors and their respective liaisons from the Editorial Board will continue to be emphasized in order to minimize unnecessary repetition and discrepancies in the text and illustrations.

Particular thanks are due to the members of the Editorial Advisory Board, the reviewers (at least two for each Fascicle), the editorial and production staff, and—first and foremost—the individual Fascicle authors for their ongoing efforts to ensure that this series is a worthy successor to the previous three.

Steven G. Silverberg, MD
Ronald A. DeLellis, MD
William A. Gardner, MD
Leslie H. Sobin, MD

ACKNOWLEDGMENTS

As authors of the fourth series Fascicle *Tumors and Cysts of the Jaws*, we recognize that nomenclature for cysts and neoplasms of the jaws is dynamic, as demonstrated by the evolving schemes based on previously unrecognized microscopic, clinical, radiographic and therapeutic features. This edition is not an attempt to promote one nomenclature scheme versus another, but simply to present the best information available for each lesion discussed using the most current World Health Organization classification system.

While this edition continues in the American Registry of Pathology tradition of providing the most current diagnostic information available for the practicing pathologist, we recognize that in some cases, surgeons will consult with pathologists regarding therapeutic management. Hence, information regarding peer-reviewed treatment protocols for many tumors and cysts is included in each section.

We also recognize that our responsibility as authors for this edition is a privilege and an honor, especially given the stature of the third series authors, Drs. James J. Sciubba, John E. Fantasia, and Leonard B. Kahn. Their work in the previous edition has been a vital resource for anatomic pathologists everywhere.

We would like to thank other mentors and colleagues who have patiently guided our development over the years including Drs. Gilbert E. Lilly, Harold L. Hammond, Bruce F. Barker, Charles L. Dunlap, Michael W. Finkelstein, John W. Hellstein, David C. Dahlin, K. Krishnan Unni, Louis H. Weiland, Charles E. Platz, and Frank A. Mitros.

Finally, we are deeply grateful to our families, Marita Gutierrez-Robinson, and Paula, Aaron and Aurora Vincent, without whom our professional and personal lives would be substantially diminished.

Robert A. Robinson, MD, PhD
Steven D. Vincent, DDS, MS

CONTENTS

1 DEVELOPMENT OF THE JAWS

ODONTOGENESIS

Similar to tumors of other organ systems, odontogenic neoplasms and cysts often recapitulate the tissues seen in various stages of embryogenesis. A basic understanding of the embryology of odontogenesis is essential for pathologists to understand the features of many lesions that occur in the jaws of children and adults.

All ectodermal organs, including hair, teeth, and exocrine glands, develop as a result of complex interactions between the primitive epithelium and mesenchyme (1). Tooth germs exhibit many features that are morphologically and molecularly similar to these other epithelial appendages (2). The pharyngeal (branchial) apparatus consists of a series of paired structures, including arches, pouches, grooves, and membranes, that are numbered in a cranial to caudal direction. The first branchial arch forms the mandible and maxilla (3). The arch is surfaced by ectoderm that covers mesoderm and neural crest ectomesenchyme. Neural crest cells are central to the process of mammalian tooth development in heterodonts (4). They are the only source of mesenchyme able to sustain tooth development, and give rise not only to most of the dental tissues, but also to the periodontal tissues that hold teeth in position.

DEVELOPMENT OF THE TOOTH AND SUPPORTING TISSUES

At about 6 weeks' gestation, tooth development begins as 20 separate invaginations of ectoderm, termed buds, from the dental lamina. Signaling molecules secreted by the oral epithelium establish cellular fields which form specific teeth. The critical information to model tooth shape resides in the neural crest–derived mesenchyme. Neural crest cells ultimately differentiate into highly specialized cell types to produce mature dental organs (5). The enamel organs that eventually form the crowns of each deciduous and permanent tooth develop through three identifiable stages: bud, cap, and bell (fig. 1-1).

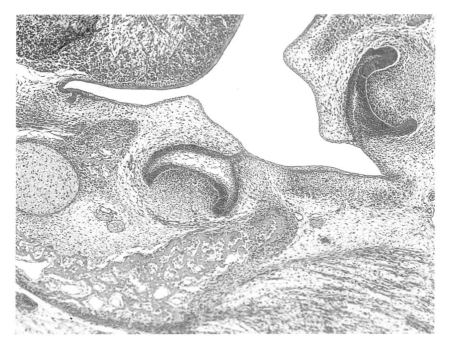

Figure 1-1

ODONTOGENESIS: CAP STAGE

The early enamel organ is attached to the epithelial surface of the primitive stoma by the dental lamina.

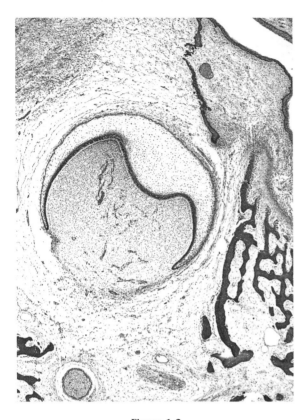

Figure 1-2

ODONTOGENESIS: BELL STAGE

The inner and outer enamel epithelium and induced dental papillae are no longer connected to the surface by the dental lamina.

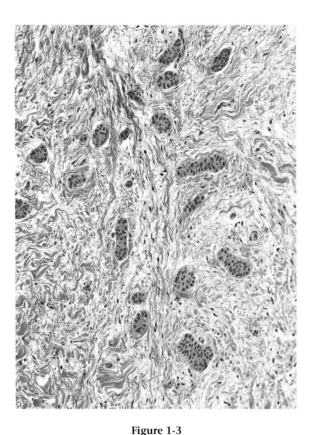

Figure 1-3

ODONTOGENESIS

Epithelial rests of Serres persist in the connective tissue following the degeneration of the dental lamina.

Each dental lamina proliferates apically, eventually taking on a bell shape (fig. 1-2). At this time, the connection between the overlying stomodeum and the forming enamel organ fragments into small epithelial islands referred to as the epithelial rests of Serres (fig. 1-3). The enamel organ consists of three cell layers: inner enamel epithelium, stellate reticulum, and outer enamel epithelium, and forms a cap over the dental papillae. Together, the enamel organ and a dental papilla are referred to as the tooth germ.

The bell stage is notable for cellular histo-differentiation, morphologic alteration, and early mineralization. Cells of the enamel organ directly adjacent to the dental papillae, termed the inner enamel epithelium, transform into columnar ameloblasts. Through a subsequent process of induction, the ameloblasts cause cells in the periphery of the dental papillae to differentiate into columnar odontoblasts. At this

point only a basement membrane separates the ameloblasts from the odontoblasts.

With the apposition of predentin by the odontoblasts, the enamel organ begins to show a fourth cell layer, termed the stratum intermedium, directly adjacent to the ameloblasts (fig 1-4). Once the stratum intermedium forms, ameloblasts become more columnar and the nuclei move away from the basement membrane, a process called reverse nuclear polarization (figs. 1-5,1-6). Most other columnar secretory cells have nuclei located near the basement membrane and secrete their product at the opposite end of the cell, usually into a duct lumen. The presence of nuclei that are polarized away from the basement membrane is a feature of a variety of odontogenic tumors.

The terminal differentiation of odontoblasts is controlled by the inner enamel epithelium and occurs according to a tooth-specific pattern.

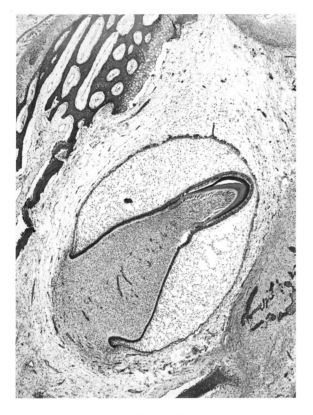

Figure 1-4

ODONTOGENESIS

Early mineralization is seen at the interface of the inner enamel epithelium and the dental papillae.

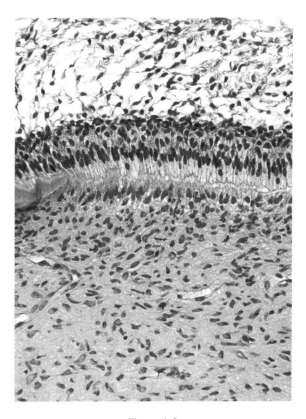

Figure 1-5

ODONTOGENESIS

Early tooth mineralization is characterized, from bottom to top, by basophilic dental papillae, columnar odontoblasts, tall columnar ameloblasts with polarized nuclei and vesiculated cytoplasm, stratum intermedium, and stellate reticulum.

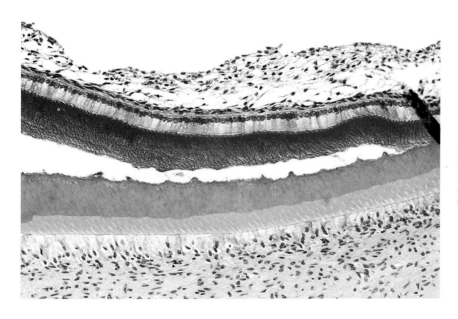

Figure 1-6

ODONTOGENESIS

Columnar odontoblasts adjacent to the dental papillae at the bottom lay down predentin matrix and tall columnar ameloblasts at the top produce enamel matrix.

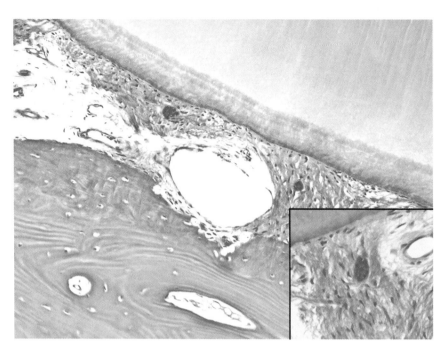

Figure 1-7

EPITHELIAL RESTS OF MALASSEZ

Epithelial rests, remnants of the Hertwig epithelial root sheath, persist in the periodontal ligament which attaches the tooth root cementum to the surrounding cortical bone. Inset shows rest of Malassez at higher power.

During the cap-bell transition, cells from the inner enamel epithelium segregate to form single or multiple cusps (6). When crown formation is completed, the enamel organ degenerates into a thin layer of cuboidal or squamous cells, referred to as the reduced enamel epithelium. Like the rests of Serres, the reduced enamel epithelium retains the potential to form odontogenic cysts and tumors.

Tooth root formation continues through the apposition of dentin tubules, which are eventually sheathed in cementum, necessary for attachment to bone via Sharpey fibers of the periodontal ligament. For the apposition of root dentin to occur, the odontoblasts require an induction effect from cells of the enamel organ. The enamel epithelium forms a collar of cells known as Hertwig epithelial root sheath, which proliferates apically and induces the differentiation of odontoblasts. As it proliferates through the forming jaw bone, the root sheath apically leaves behind residual epithelial islands known as rests of Malassez (fig. 1-7). These rests persist in the periodontal ligament and provide an additional source of odontogenic epithelium capable of forming cysts and tumors. Even though they appear inactive microscopically, experimental evidence has shown that the rests of Malassez continue to have low levels of mitotic activity, indicating that cellular

proliferation is responsible for the formation and enlargement of cysts and neoplasms under certain physiologic conditions (7).

Dentin that is not covered by enamel is covered by cementum which is a form of modified osteoid produced by cementoblasts that are indistinguishable from osteoblasts. The cementum is attached via Sharpey fibers through the periodontal ligament to a thin layer of cortical bone termed the lamina dura.

Because the mineralized tooth constitutes the hardest substance in humans and is resistant to the natural forces of decomposition after death, the features of tooth development also play an instrumental role in forensic identification, and in the evolutionary classification of our hominid ancestors (8).

While normal tooth development usually ends by about age 21, the potential for the development of reactive, cystic, or neoplastic lesions of the jaws persists in the remnants of odontogenesis that are left behind. In addition to the reduced enamel epithelium and unnamed rests often found in the tooth follicle, as well as the rests of Serres or Malassez, the original basal epithelium, which in the adult is represented by the gingiva and alveolar mucosa, retains the capability to form odontogenic tissue. This capability is supported by the formation of peripheral odontogenic tumors, such as the ameloblastomas that appear to bud directly from the basal cells of the gingiva.

RECENT ADVANCES

While the process of odontogenesis has been characterized for decades, recent research has shed more light on this process at the molecular level. More than 300 genes have so far been associated with tooth development. Most of these genes are associated with signaling pathways mediating cellular communication between epithelial and mesenchymal tissues (9). Recently, micro-RNA pathways have emerged as important regulators of various aspects of embryonic development including odontogenesis (10).

Restriction of the signaling peptide encoded by the sonic hedgehog gene in localized thickenings of oral epithelium has been shown to play a crucial role during the initiation of odontogenesis (11). While the sonic hedgehog gene helps regulate tooth growth and helps to determine the shape of the tooth, signaling is not essential for differentiation of ameloblasts or odontoblasts (12).

Members of the *Msx* homeobox gene family are expressed at sites of epithelial-mesenchymal interaction during tooth formation. *Msx1*-deficient mice exhibit an arrest in tooth development at the bud stage, while *Msx2*-deficient mice exhibit defects in later stages of tooth development. (13).

Nestin, one of the intermediate filaments constituting the cytoskeleton, is a marker of neural stem cells or progenitor cells. Nestin is also involved in the differentiation of odontogenic ectomesenchyme to odontoblasts and in the formation of mesenchymal tissues in odontogenic tumors (14).

The genetic causes of most cases of abnormal enamel development, such as amelogenesis imperfecta, are associated with mutations in enamel matrix specific genes. Recent evidence, however, has shown that mutations in genes involved in pH regulation may affect enamel structure as well (15).

New treatments for systemic disease also effect tooth development. The use of oral and intravenous bisphosphonates in young children with diseases such as osteogenesis imperfecta inhibits tooth formation and eruption, and has induced several types of dental abnormalities, which may be attributed to altered osteoclastic activities (16).

By combining the knowledge of molecular regulation of tooth development with the recent breakthroughs in stem cell research, tooth regeneration may someday be possible (17). The transfer of embryonic tooth primordia into the adult jaw has resulted in the formation of tooth structures, indicating that embryonic primordia can continue to develop in an adult environment (18).

REFERENCES

1. Pispa J, Thesleff I. Mechanisms of ectodermal organogenesis. Dev Biol 2003;262:195-205.
2. Miletich I, Sharpe PT. Normal and abnormal dental development. Hum Mol Genet 2003;12 Spec No 1:R69-73.
3. Nanci A. Ten Cate's oral histology: development, structure and function, 7th ed. St. Louis: Mosby Elsevier; 2008.
4. Jarvinen E, Tummers M, Thesleff I. The role of the dental lamina in mammalian tooth replacement. J Exp Zool B Mol Dev Evol 2009;312B:281-291.
5. Miletich I, Sharpe PT. Neural crest contribution to mammalian tooth formation. Birth Defects Res C Embryo Today 2004;72:200-212.
6. Lisi S, Peterkova R, Peterka M, Vonesch JL, Ruch JV, Lesot H. Tooth morphogenesis and pattern of odontoblast differentiation. Connect Tissue Res 2003;44(Suppl 1):167-170.
7. Cerri PS, Goncalves Jde S, Sasso-Cerri E. Area of rests of Malassez in young and adult rat molars: evidences in the formation of large rests. Anat Rec (Hoboken) 2009;292:285-291.
8. Bermudez de Castro JM, Martinon-Torres M, Prado L, et al. New immature hominin fossil from European Lower Pleistocene shows the earliest evidence of a modern human dental development pattern. Proc Natl Acad Sci U S A 2010;107:11739-11744.
9. Thesleff I. The genetic basis of tooth development and dental defects. Am J Med Genet A 2006;140:2530-2535.
10. Michon F, Tummers M, Kyyronen M, Frilander MJ, Thesleff I. Tooth morphogenesis and ameloblast differentiation are regulated by micro-RNAs. Dev Biol 2010;340:355-368.
11. Cobourne MT, Miletich I, Sharpe PT. Restriction of sonic hedgehog signalling during early tooth development. Development 2004;131:2875-2885.
12. Dassule HR, Lewis P, Bei M, Maas R, McMahon AP. Sonic hedgehog regulates growth and morphogenesis of the tooth. Development 2000;127:4775-4785.
13. Maas R, Bei M. The genetic control of early tooth development. Crit Rev Oral Biol Med 1997;8:4-39.
14. Fujita S, Hideshima K, Ikeda T. Nestin expression in odontoblasts and odontogenic ectomesenchymal tissue of odontogenic tumours. J Clin Pathol 2006;59:240-245.
15. Lacruz RS, Nanci A, Kurtz I, Wright JT, Paine ML. Regulation of pH during amelogenesis. Calcif Tissue Int 2010;86:91-103.
16. Hiraga T, Ninomiya T, Hosoya A, Nakamura H. Administration of the bisphosphonate zoledronic acid during tooth development inhibits tooth eruption and formation and induces dental abnormalities in rats. Calcif Tissue Int 2010;86:502-510.
17. Thesleff I. Developmental biology and building a tooth. Quintessence Int 2003;34:613-620.
18. Ohazama A, Modino SA, Miletich I, Sharpe PT. Stem-cell-based tissue engineering of murine teeth. J Dent Res 2004;83:518-522.

2 CLASSIFICATION OF ODONTOGENIC TUMORS AND CYSTS

EARLY REPORTS AND CLASSIFICATION SYSTEMS

In 1746, Pierre Fauchard (1) provided the first published description of an odontogenic tumor, which was an odontoma. A maxillary cementoblastoma was described in the American Journal of Dental Science in 1839 (2). This journal was the official publication of the first American Dental Association and at that time the only dental journal recognized by the American Medical Association. Another odontoma was reported in 1847 (3).

In 1869, the French physician Pierre Paul Broca (4) proposed several tumor classification systems, including one for odontogenic tumors. He used the term odontome for any tumor arising from the dental formative tissues.

In 1888, Sir John Bland-Sutton (5) formulated the first modern classification system for odontogenic tumors, which was based on the cells of tooth germ origin. Bland-Sutton included odontogenic cysts in his classification, but the term odontoma remained the common designation for any tumor of odontogenic origin.

In 1914, Gabell et al. (6) further modified Bland-Sutton's classification. Their system recognized three groups of odontomes: 1) the epithelial odontomes, which included multilocular or nonneoplastic cysts; 2) the composite odontomes, comprising those lesions derived from both epithelium and mesenchyme; and 3) connective tissue odontomes thought to arise from dental mesenchyme. The multilocular cysts became the adamantinoma or adamantoblastoma, terms used until Ivy and Churchill in 1930 introduced the term ameloblastoma (14). The connective tissue odontomes became fibromas or cementomas. The composite lesions, consisting of both epithelial and mesenchymal elements, retained their original designation as odontomes, or odontomas.

The Thoma and Goldman classification, published in 1946, formed the nucleus of the classification adopted by the American Academy of Oral Pathology in 1952 (7). The term odontoma was truncated to designate only those lesions consisting of both epithelial and mesenchymal elements. They utilized the classification system shown in Table 2-1.

The Pindborg and Clausen classification (8), slightly modified by Gorlin et al. in 1961 (9), was at the time viewed as a major step forward, and played an important role in the World Health Organization (WHO) publication *Histological Typing of Odontogenic Tumours* in 1971 (10). This system was the first to include developmental cysts of odontogenic origin.

Twenty-one years later, in 1992, a second WHO edition appeared (11) followed by a third in 2002 (12), which included advances in odontogenic tissue interaction during tumor development, immunohistochemistry, and molecular biology. The latest WHO classification was published in 2005 (Table 2-2) (13). An outstanding review of the evolution of odontogenic tumor and cyst classification was authored by Philipsen and Reichart in 2006 (14).

Table 2-1

THOMA-GOLDMAN CLASSIFICATION OF ODONTOGENIC TUMORS

I. Epithelial Tumors
    1. adamantoblastoma
    2. enameloma

II. Mesenchymal Tumors
    1. odontogenic fibroma
    2. dentinoma
    3. cementoma

III. Odontogenic Mixed Tumors
    1. soft odontoma epithelium and mesoderm
    2. soft and calcified odontoma, adamantoblastoma arising in conjunction with a forming or completely formed odontoma
    3. completely formed odontoma with enamel, dentin, pulp, cementum, and periodontal membrane
       a. compound (many small teeth)
       b. complex (irregular tooth formation)

7

Table 2-2

CLASSIFICATION OF ODONTOGENIC HEAD AND NECK TUMORS, WHO 2005[a]

Benign Tumors

Odontogenic epithelium with mature stroma without odontogenic ectomesenchyme

Ameloblastoma, solid/multicystic

Ameloblastoma, extraosseous/peripheral

Ameloblastoma, desmoplastic

Ameloblastoma, unicystic

Squamous odontogenic tumor

Calcifying epithelial odontogenic tumor

Adenomatoid odontogenic tumor

Keratocystic odontogenic tumor

Odontogenic epithelium with ectomesenchyme with or without hard tissue

Ameloblastic fibroma

Ameloblastic fibrodentinoma

Ameloblastic fibro-odontoma

Odontoma

Complex

Compound

Odontoameloblastoma

Calcifying cystic odontogenic tumor

Dentinogenic ghost cell tumor

Mesenchyme and/or ectomesenchyme with or without odontogenic epithelium

Odontogenic fibroma

Odontogenic myxoma/myxofibroma

Cementoblastoma

Bone-related disease

Ossifying fibroma

Fibrous dysplasia

Osseous dysplasias

Central giant cell lesion (granuloma)

Cherubism

Aneurysmal bone cyst

Simple bone cyst

Other Tumors

Melanotic neuroectodermal tumor of infancy

Malignant Tumors

Odontogenic carcinomas

Malignant (metastasizing) ameloblastoma

Ameloblastic carcinoma (primary)

Ameloblastic carcinoma (secondary, dedifferentiated intraosseous)

Ameloblastoma carcinoma (secondary, dedifferentiated peripheral)

Primary intraosseous squamous cell carcinoma

Primary intraosseous squamous cell carcinoma derived from keratocystic odontogenic tumor

Primary intraosseous squamous cell carcinoma derived from odontogenic cysts

Clear cell odontogenic carcinoma

Ghost cell odontogenic carcinoma

Odontogenic sarcomas

Ameloblastic fibrosarcoma

Ameloblastic fibrodentinoma and fibro-odontosarcoma

[a]Modified from WHO histologic classification table in Barnes L, Eveson JW, Reichart P, Sidransky D, eds. World Health Organization classification of tumours. Pathology and genetics of head and neck tumours. Lyon: IARC Press; 2005:284.

REFERENCES

1. Fauchard P. Le chirugien dentiste,ou traite des dents. Tome 1-2 Paris: Pierre Jean Mariette; 1746.
2. Rodrigues BA. Case of exostosis of the upper jaw. Am J Dent Sci 1839;1:88-89.
3. Harris CA. Miscellaneous notes. Am J Dent Sci 1847;8:106-112.
4. Broca P. Traite des tumeurs. P. Asselin, Librare de la Faculte de Medicine 1869;2.
5. Bland-Sutton J. Odontomes. Trans Odont Soc (Lond) 1888;20:32-87.
6. Gabell DP, James W, Payne JL. The report on odontomes. London: John Bale, Sons & Danielsson, Ltd; 1914.
7. Thoma KH, Goldman HM. Odontogenic tumors. A classification based on observations of epithelial, mesenchymal and mixed varieties. Am J Pathol 1946;22:433-471.
8. Pindborg JJ, Clausen F. Classification of odontogenic tumors. A suggestion. Acta Odontol Scand 1958;16:293-301.
9. Gorlin RJ, Chaudhry AP, Pindborg JJ. The odontogenic tumors: their classification, histopathology and clinical behavior in man and domestic animals. Cancer 1961;14:73-101.
10. Pindborg JJ, Kramer IR, Torloni, H. Histological typing of odontogenic tumors, jaw cysts and allied lesions. Geneva: WHO; 1971.
11. Kramer IR, Pindborg JJ, Shear M. WHO international histological classification of tumours. Histological typing of odontogenic tumours. Berlin: Springer-Verlag; 1992.
12. Philipsen HP, Reichart PA. Revision of the 1992 edition of the WHO histological typing of odontogenic tumours. A suggestion. J Oral Pathol Med 2002;31:253-258.
13. Barnes L, Eveson JW, Reichart P, Sidransky D, eds. World Health Organization classification of tumours. Pathology and genetics of head and neck tumours. Lyon: IARC Press; 2005.
14. Philipsen HP, Reichart PA. Classification of odontogenic tumors. A historical review. J Oral Pathol Med 2006;35:525-529.

3 ODONTOGENIC CYSTS

One of the unique features regarding the pathology of the jaws is the occurrence of a variety of cysts. By definition, a cyst is a pathologic cavity lined by epithelium. The odontogenic tooth-forming apparatus leaves behind a multitude of epithelial cells in the gingival soft tissues and alveolar processes of both the mandible and maxilla. These include cells within the basal cell layer of the gingiva and the reduced enamel epithelium, odontogenic epithelial rests of Serres in the gingival soft tissues and crestal alveolar bone, rests in the tooth follicle, and the rests of Malassez surrounding the roots in the periodontal ligament.

Numerous authors have speculated on the epithelial cells of origin for odontogenic tumors and cysts. Since there are no cytologic or immunohistochemical markers that tie any of these residual odontogenic epithelial tissues to a specific cyst or tumor, the association remains speculative and is most often based entirely on the location of the developing tumor or cyst. Following the 1992 World Health Organization (WHO) reclassification of calcifying epithelial odontogenic cysts as calcifying cystic odontogenic tumors and the 2005 reclassification of odontogenic keratocysts as keratocystic odontogenic tumors, a larger percentage of odontogenic cysts appear similar if not identical microscopically, requiring additional clinical and radiographic information to arrive at a specific diagnosis. A few cysts, including botryoid, orthokeratinizing, and glandular odontogenic cysts, continue to show microscopic features that lead to a specific diagnosis; most other odontogenic cysts have an epithelial lining that by itself is nondiagnostic.

Most classification schemes initially divide odontogenic cysts into two main groups. Cysts that seem to form for no clinical reason are termed *developmental cysts.* These include dentigerous, eruption, lateral periodontal, botryoid, glandular, orthokeratinizing, and primordial cysts.

Although developmental odontogenic cysts are benign growths, many can grow to several centimeters in diameter, causing significant displacement or destruction of the normal jaw anatomy, loss of function, and increased risk of additional conditions including pathologic bone fracture and osteomyelitis. Cyst expansion has been studied for decades and is probably the result of several mechanisms. First and foremost, cyst expansion clearly involves mitotic activity and hyperplasia within the epithelial lining. If the mitotic activity is unregulated and primary, not secondary to other factors such as inflammation, some lesions with a cystic morphology are classified as *cystic neoplasms,* including keratocystic odontogenic tumors and calcifying cystic odontogenic tumors referred to above and in chapter 6 (1–5).

The second group of cysts is initiated in areas of acute and chronic inflammation. These include *periapical,* or *radicular, cysts, residual cysts,* and *buccal bifurcation* and *paradental cysts.* Acute and chronic inflammation leads to the release of mediators that stimulate mitotic activity (6). Inflammation of odontogenic tissues, including the epithelium, commonly occurs as a result of tooth pulp degeneration or periodontitis. When this inflammation involves odontogenic epithelium, such as a rest of Malassez, cellular hyperplasia can lead to the formation of a sphere or cyst as the central cells degenerate, forming a lumen. Following the formation of the central lumen, a variety of factors play a part in the continued expansion of the cyst, including debris accumulation, hydraulic pressure (7–12), epidermal growth factor and transforming growth factor alpha (13), and the activity of succinate, lactate, glutamate, and glucose-6-phosphate dehydrogenase (14).

INFLAMMATORY CYSTS OF THE JAWS

Radicular Cyst (Periapical Cyst)

Definition. *Radicular (periapical) cysts* form when epithelial rests of Malassez, in the periodontal ligament, are stimulated by inflammation of

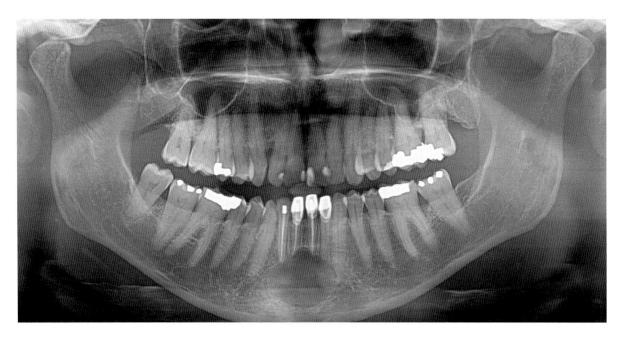

Figure 3-1

RADICULAR CYST

A panoramic radiograph shows a well-circumscribed radiolucency in the anterior mandible associated with the roots of the incisors, which have had endodontic treatment.

an adjacent nonvital tooth. Dental disease that causes inflammation and necrosis of tooth pulp usually spreads to involve the periradicular tissues, including the periodontal ligament, bone, and marrow. Depending on local factors, periradicular inflammation may be acute, forming an abscess; chronic, forming granulation tissue; or a combination of both. Periradicular inflammation stimulates hyperplasia in one or more of these rests, resulting in an epithelial-lined sac. Left untreated, radicular cysts can achieve considerable size and cause significant damage to adjacent structures.

Clinical Features. Radicular cysts, by definition, must be associated with the root of a nonvital primary or permanent tooth. They are most often initially identified radiographically following a complaint of pain. If the cyst is of adequate size, expansion of the adjacent cortical plates may be identified. If the associated inflammatory condition is acute, a draining sinus tract may be present in the oral mucosa overlying the cyst.

Radiographic Features. A radicular cyst presents as a well-demarcated radiolucency associated with the apex of a nonvital tooth (figs.

3-1, 3-2). Some cysts appear on the lateral aspect of the root because of the image angle, or as the result of a lateral pulp canal. The periphery of the radiolucency is usually corticated or sclerotic, an indication of slow expansion, although some lesions associated with acute inflammation have diffuse, poorly defined radiographic margins focally. Most lesions are less than 1 cm in diameter, although if left untreated, radicular cysts can expand to several centimeters causing displacement and/or resorption of bone structures and adjacent teeth. The radiographic features alone are not diagnostic (15). Periapical radiolucencies identical to these cysts are often found microscopically to be the result of acute and chronic abscesses, nonspecific granulation tissue, developmental cysts, and sometimes benign neoplasms.

Microscopic Findings. The cyst lumen is lined by nonkeratinized stratified squamous epithelium that varies from 1 to 2 cell layers in thickness to areas that are hyperplastic with irregular rete ridge formation (figs. 3-3, 3-4). Mucous cell metaplasia may be noted but is not as common as in dentigerous cysts (16). Rushton bodies are found in a variety of odontogenic

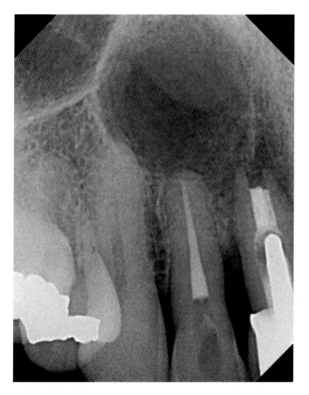

Figure 3-2

RADICULAR CYST

A well-circumscribed radiolucency in the anterior maxilla is associated with the root of the nonvital lateral incisor.

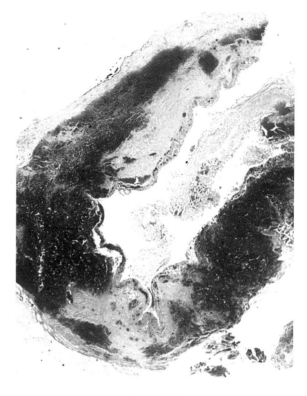

Figure 3-3

RADICULAR CYST

Thick walls of inflamed and hemorrhagic fibrovascular connective tissue surround a central lumen.

cysts including radicular cysts. These entities are described in more detail below with dentigerous cysts. Cholesterol slits, foreign body giant cells, and hemosiderin deposits are common findings. In endodontically treated teeth, foreign material is often identified in the lumen of the cyst or in the surrounding fibrous connective tissue wall. Bacterial colonies may also been seen (17–19).

Immunohistochemical Findings. The epithelium of radicular cysts has a broad range of cytokeratins (20). Langerhans cells in association with T lymphocytes have been identified in periapical inflammatory lesions, including radicular cysts (21). The inflammatory parameters of the host response, including levels of nitric oxide, interleukin (IL)-4, tumor growth factor (TGF)-beta, tumor necrosis factor (TNF)-alpha, and interferon-gamma, are different in radicular cysts and granulomas (22).

Treatment and Prognosis. Radicular cysts are treated with simple enucleation, often accomplished during tooth extraction or fol-

lowing endodontic treatment of the associated nonvital tooth. Specimens should always be evaluated microscopically because, as noted above, periapical radiolucencies associated with nonvital teeth can be caused by a variety of other lesions including but not limited to developmental cysts and benign tumors (23).

Residual Cyst

Definition. Radicular cysts that persist in the jaws, following tooth extraction are termed *residual cysts*. These cysts are indistinguishable microscopically from other nonkeratinizing jaw cysts. They are usually asymptomatic, but the persistence of acute inflammation can result in symptoms (24–26).

Radiographic Features. Residual cysts are either slow growing or static, resulting in a well-demarcated radiolucency with a well-defined, corticated border (fig. 3-5). Similar to radicular cysts, acute inflammation may blur the radiographic margins focally.

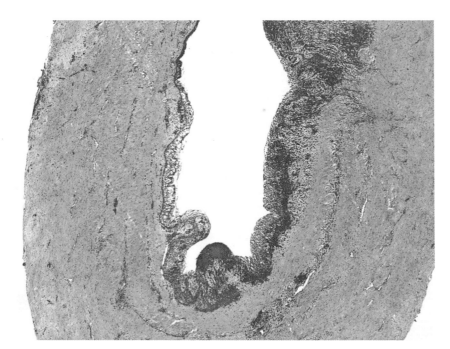

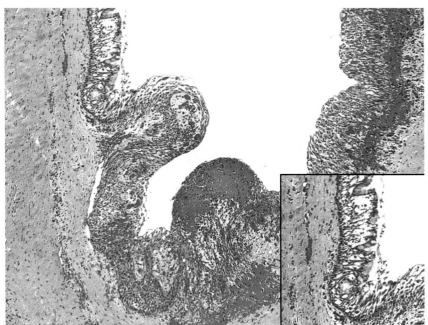

Figure 3-4

RADICULAR CYST

Top: The lumen is lined by hyperplastic, stratified squamous epithelium.

Bottom: A dense infiltrate of lymphocytes, plasma cells, and neutrophils is subjacent to the epithelial lining, within the connective tissue. A focus of mucous goblet cell metaplasia is seen on the left (higher power shown in inset).

Microscopic Findings. The cyst lining is identical microscopically to that of a radicular cyst (fig. 3-6). The nonkeratinizing lining ranges from 1 to 2 cells in thickness to hyperplastic with rete ridge formation. The underlying fibrovascular connective tissue has varying amounts of acute and chronic inflammatory cells.

Treatment and Prognosis. Treatment for these lesions is simple enucleation and persistence or recurrence rates are low (27). As with other cystic lesions of the jaws, the diagnosis cannot be presumed from the clinical and radiographic features alone. Failure to identify these lesions can complicate future jaw surgeries including placement of implants (28). Muglali et al. (29) reported a case of squamous cell carcinoma arising in the wall of a residual cyst.

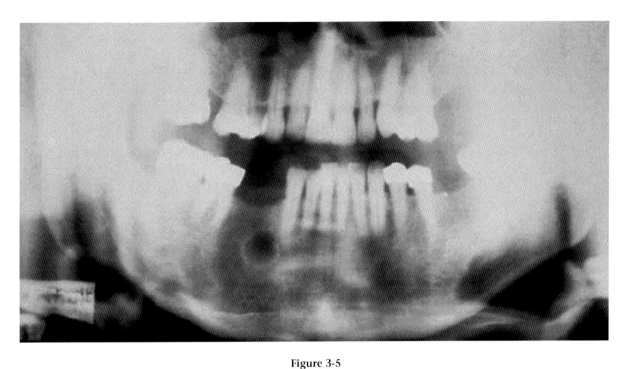

Figure 3-5

RESIDUAL CYST

A well-demarcated, corticated radiolucency is seen in the right mandible at the site of a previous tooth extraction.

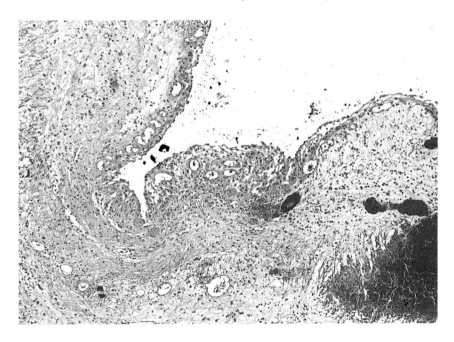

Figure 3-6

RESIDUAL CYST

Inflamed fibrovascular connective tissue surrounds a central lumen lined by hyperplastic stratified squamous epithelium.

Paradental Cyst

Definition. *Paradental cyst* is an inflammatory lesion involving the soft tissues around a partially erupted tooth. A closely related lesion is the buccal bifurcation cyst described below.

The paradental cyst was described by Craig in 1976 (30) as a cyst localized to the distal, buccal or, rarely, mesial aspect of a partially erupted molar. The pathogenesis appears to be stimulation of reduced enamel epithelium,

15

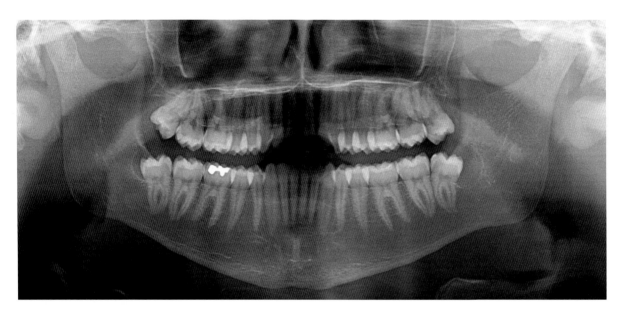

Figure 3-7

PARADENTAL CYST

Bilateral radiolucencies are seen on the distal aspects of both partially erupted mandibular third molars.

odontogenic epithelial rests of Serres in the gingival soft tissues, or rests of Malassez in the coronal aspect of the periodontal ligament. Other terms used include *inflammatory collateral cyst* and *mandibular infected buccal cyst* (31,32).

General Features. In one series, paradental cysts accounted for 3 percent of all odontogenic cysts (33). In a review of 325 odontogenic cysts, Philipsen et al. (34) found 0.9 to 4.7 percent were paradental and the majority occurred distally or distobuccally to vital, permanent mandibular molars. Paradental cysts comprise up to 25 percent of all lesions associated with mandibular third molars and also involve premolars (35,36). Most patients have a history of one or more episodes of pericoronitis (34,37); most patients are under the age of 30 years (34,38).

While the cysts are inflammatory in origin, the vitality of the associated tooth is irrelevant. Most retrospective studies suggest that these cysts are found more often in males, although one study identified a female predominance (37). Colgan et al. (35) proposed a relationship between the site of the cyst and the angle of the impacted tooth: mesially with mesioangularly impacted teeth, buccal with vertically impacted teeth, and distal/distobuccal with distoangular impactions. The cysts are sometimes associated with a developmental enamel projection or ridge extending into the buccal bifurcation (39).

Clinical Features. Most paradental cysts present as a smooth-surfaced, soft tissue enlargement involving the crown of a partially erupted tooth in patients with generalized evidence of periodontal inflammation (40). Some occur in the absence of inflammation (41). The size of the cyst varies from 1 to 2 cm. The cyst is attached to the cementoenamel junction and the coronal third of the root (42).

Radiographic Features. A paradental cyst will present as a well-demarcated radiolucency associated with the crown of a partially erupted molar tooth (fig. 3-7) (39). Since these cysts often involve the alveolar soft tissues, the radiolucency may appear as a cupping-out of the crestal alveolar bone cortex directly adjacent to the tooth crown.

Microscopic Findings. Microscopically, paradental cysts are indistinguishable from other nonkeratinizing inflammatory cysts. The epithelium is most often stratified squamous, varying from thin and atrophic to hyperplastic (fig. 3-8). The cyst lining has been reported to mimic unicystic ameloblastoma, a potential diagnostic pitfall (33). The connective tissue usually shows a dense infiltrate of lymphocytes, plasma cells, macrophages, and

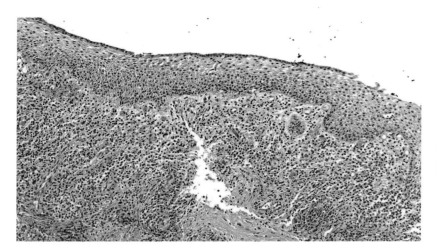

Figure 3-8

PARADENTAL CYST

Nonkeratinized stratified squamous epithelium surfaces fibrovascular connective tissue with a dense infiltrate of lymphocytes, plasma cells, and neutrophils.

neutrophils. Because the cysts have an epithelial lining that is indistinguishable from chronic periodontal pocket inflammation, they are probably underdiagnosed (34,38,43,44).

Treatment and Prognosis. The treatment of choice is conservative excision, with or without extraction of the tooth depending on the clinical circumstance. As is the case with other inflammatory lesions, recurrence is only expected if the source of inflammation persists (45).

Buccal Bifurcation Cyst

Definition and General Features. The *buccal bifurcation cyst* was first described by Stoneman and Worth in 1983 (46). This inflammatory cyst has a specific location, classically the buccal surface of the mandibular first molar and less frequently the mandibular second molar. The age at diagnosis ranged from 5 to 11 years (40,47). Buccal bifurcation cysts must be correctly diagnosed to ensure that the cyst is enucleated without extraction of the associated tooth.

Craig (30) reported the occasional presence of developmental enamel projections near the furcation of some teeth. These projections, however, are not always associated with the formation of cysts and their significance remains unclear (43,48–50).

Clinical Features. There is usually a painless, slowly progressive expansion of gingiva and vestibular mucosa buccal to the furcation of a mandibular first or second permanent molar. The surface mucosa is smooth unless ulcerated by secondary trauma.

Radiographic Features. A well-demarcated, corticated radiolucency involves the furcation

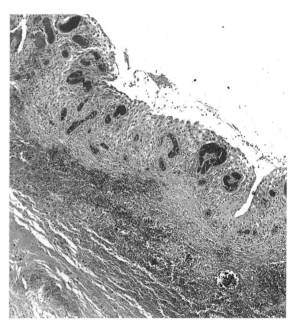

Figure 3-9

BUCCAL BIFURCATION CYST

Hyperplastic, nonkeratinized stratified squamous epithelium lines a wall of fibrovascular connective tissue containing hemorrhage and a mixed inflammatory infiltrate.

and buccal surface of a mandibular permanent molar. Seldom, if ever, should there be evidence of external root resorption.

Microscopic Findings. The microscopic features are identical to those of a radicular (periapical) cyst including an inflamed, often hyperplastic, nonkeratinizing stratified squamous epithelium lining the luminal surface (fig. 3-9). The surrounding fibrovascular connective tissue shows varying degrees of acute and chronic inflammatory cell infiltration that consists of lymphocytes, plasma cells, and neutrophils.

Treatment and Prognosis. Reported treatment options vary from extraction of the involved molar to marsupialization and enucleation of the cyst (51–53). However, Pompura et al. (54) reported the successful treatment of 44 buccal bifurcation cysts by simple enucleation without tooth extraction.

DEVELOPMENTAL CYSTS OF THE JAWS

Dentigerous Cyst

Definition and General Features. *Dentigerous cysts* are nonkeratinizing cysts that develop in association with the crown of an unerupted or impacted primary or permanent tooth. Dentigerous cysts are the most common developmental cysts of the jaws. They most likely develop from residual fragments of epithelium from reduced enamel following odontogenesis (55). Cysts that develop from the reduced enamel epithelium are attached to the tooth crown at the cementoenamel junction and the crown is contained within the cystic lumen. Because the third molars and maxillary canines are the teeth most frequently impacted, they are also the most likely to be associated with dentigerous cysts.

Although dentigerous cysts generally involve permanent teeth, deciduous teeth are also involved (56). In an evaluation of over 2,000 dentigerous cysts, most occurred in young males (57). About 2.5 percent of these cases represented multiple cysts in the same patient, and 0.5 percent occurred with other odontogenic cysts or tumors at the same site or the opposite side of the jaw. Although most dentigerous cysts are clearly developmental, Benn et al. (58) reported on 15 examples that developed around the crown of an unerupted tooth as a result of an adjacent inflammatory condition such as a nonvital tooth.

Clinical Features. There is usually enlargement of the buccal cortical plate of the maxilla or mandible. The cysts are asymptomatic, unless they become secondarily inflamed. They are often identified on radiographs made for other reasons such as orthodontic treatment or when a tooth fails to erupt.

Radiographic Features. Radiographically, dentigerous cysts usually appear as a well-circumscribed radiolucency associated with the crown of an unerupted or impacted tooth (figs. 3-10, 3-11). The radiolucency has a well-defined and corticated border, and may be unilocular or multilocular depending on the size of the lesion. Anatomic structures such as the inferior alveolar nerve and adjacent teeth are usually displaced rather than resorbed by the slow rate of cystic expansion. Even large cysts that have displaced the associated tooth several centimeters appear to originate from the cementoenamel junction.

Radiographic findings alone are not diagnostic because many odontogenic cysts and tumors developing in tooth follicles have identical features. The normal radiographic follicular space around third molars is generally regarded as 2.0 to 2.5 mm. Spaces larger than this suggest cyst or tumor formation. In impacted canines, the follicular space is not considered abnormal until it reaches a diameter greater than 3.0 mm. There is considerable overlap in the appearance of small dentigerous cysts and enlarged or hyperplastic tooth follicles (56,59).

Microscopic Findings. The dentigerous cyst has a nonkeratinized, stratified squamous epithelial lining with a surrounding fibrovascular connective tissue wall (figs. 3-12–3-14). Occasionally, cuboidal, columnar, mucous goblet, or even sebaceous epithelial cell metaplasia is a component of the cyst lining. Cholesterol slits and their associated multinucleated giant cells may be present in inflamed cysts (fig. 3-15). Rushton body formation can be seen. Rushton bodies are hyalinized, eosinophilic, angulated, linear, or curved amorphous foci within the epithelium (fig. 3-16). Rushton bodies are not specific to dentigerous cysts, and are found in a variety of other developmental and inflammatory cysts. They are of unknown origin (60). The fibrous wall, which is, at least in part, formed by a residual dental follicle, may contain odontogenic rests.

One study reported that 17 percent of ameloblastomas were associated with an existing dentigerous cyst (61); this figure varies by study, however (62,63). Both squamous cell carcinomas and mucoepidermoid carcinomas have been reported arising from dentigerous cysts (64–68).

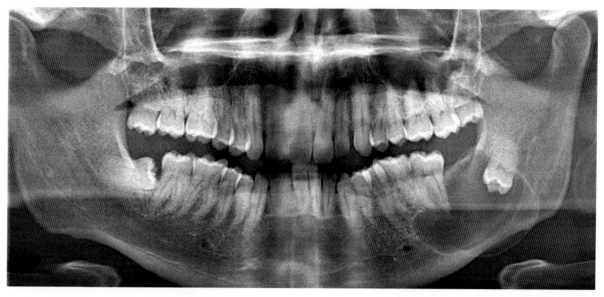

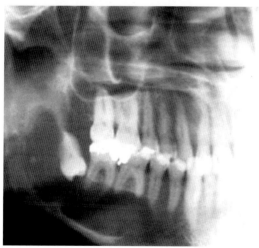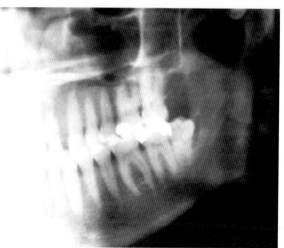

Figure 3-10

DENTIGEROUS CYST

Top: A well-corticated radiolucency of the left posterior mandible is displacing the impacted third molar.

Bottom: A corticated radiolucency involving the crown of the right mandibular third molar is resorbing the roots of the first and second molars.

Immunohistochemical Findings. In a recent evaluation of p63 immunoreactivity within the follicles of impacted mandibular third molars, more reactivity was identified in the follicles of complete impactions (64 percent) than partial bony impactions (40 percent) (69). This activity may contribute to the formation of dentigerous cysts and odontogenic neoplasms, and is considered to be further justification for prophylactic removal of impacted teeth with normal radiographic follicles.

Treatment and Prognosis. Dentigerous cysts are best treated by removal of the impacted/unerupted tooth and curettage of the cystic lining (70). For large lesions, marsupialization with subsequent enucleation may be appropriate. Iatrou et al. (71) reported on the management of 47 central bony cystic lesions, including 20 dentigerous cysts, in children aged 2 to 14 years. All were treated successfully with simple enucleation or marsupialization, preserving the adjacent teeth whenever possible.

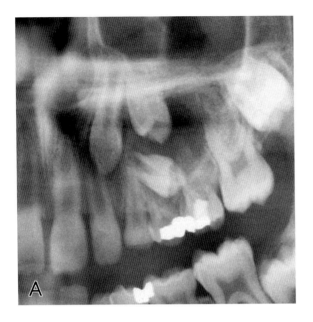

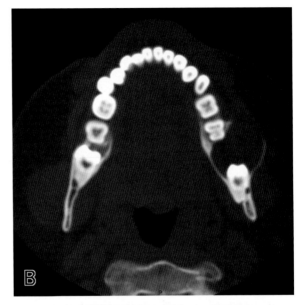

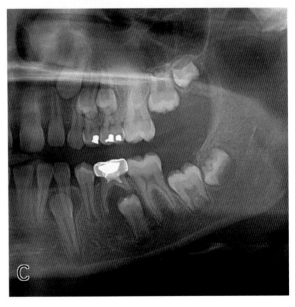

Figure 3-11

DENTIGEROUS CYST

A: A well-demarcated radiolucency involving the crown of a maxillary second premolar is displacing the unerupted first premolar and canine.

B: Axial computerized tomography (CT) shows a well-demarcated radiolucency in the body of the mandible displacing the third molar into the ramus.

C: A radiolucency involves the crown of an unerupted premolar and the roots of a nonvital primary molar.

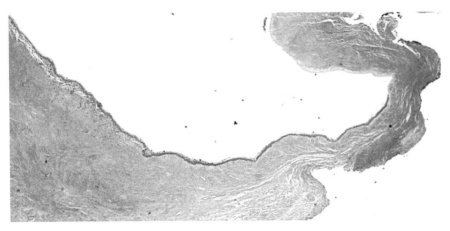

Figure 3-12

DENTIGEROUS CYST

Walls of fibrovascular connective tissue surround a central lumen lined by epithelium.

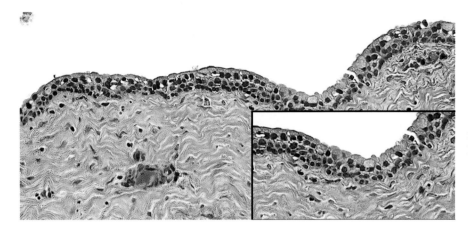

Figure 3-13

DENTIGEROUS CYST

Foci of mucous goblet cell metaplasia are noted. Higher power is shown in inset.

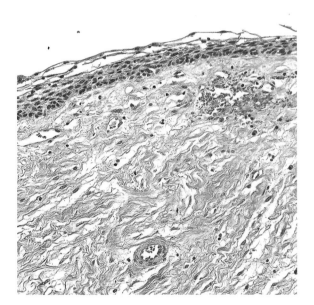
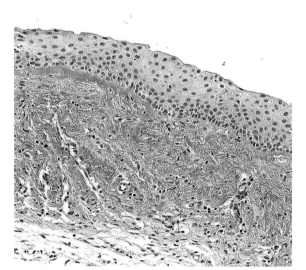

Figure 3-14

DENTIGEROUS CYST

Left: The luminal lining is nonkeratinized stratified squamous epithelium.

Right: The cyst lining shows no evidence of a uniform basal cell layer, parakeratin, or corrugation at the luminal surface.

Eruption Cyst

Definition. An *eruption cyst* is a variant of a dentigerous cyst and occurs when an erupting tooth attempts to push through a dentigerous cyst near the crest of the alveolus. It is most often identified in children and can involve either primary or permanent teeth (72–75). The cyst often involves only the gingival soft tissues (76,77).

Clinical Features. In a series of 24 cases, the most common location for eruption cysts was the central incisor and primary first molar region (78). Patients ranged from 1 month to 12 years in age. Two cysts were associated with natal teeth, 10 with primary teeth, and 12 with permanent teeth. The female to male ratio was 2 to 1. According to some studies, eruption cysts occur in the maxilla more often than the mandible (79). Eruption cysts that are inflamed may be difficult to distinguish from paradental cysts (80). The cyst is a smooth-surfaced swelling with a bluish hue (fig. 3-17). They are asymptomatic unless secondarily inflamed due to trauma or communication with the oral cavity.

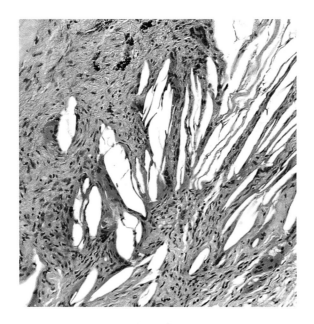

Figure 3-15

DENTIGEROUS CYST AND CHOLESTEROL CLEFTS

Chronic inflammation and tissue degeneration often lead to the formation of cholesterol clefts, surfaced focally by multinucleated giant cells.

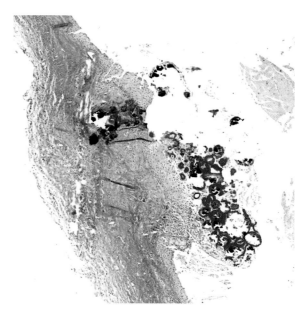

Figure 3-16

DENTIGEROUS CYST WITH RUSHTON BODIES

Eosinophilic, angular hyalinized entities (Rushton bodies) are seen focally within the stratified squamous epithelium.

Figure 3-17

ERUPTION CYST

A blue soft tissue enlargement involves the gingiva overlying an unerupted maxillary canine.

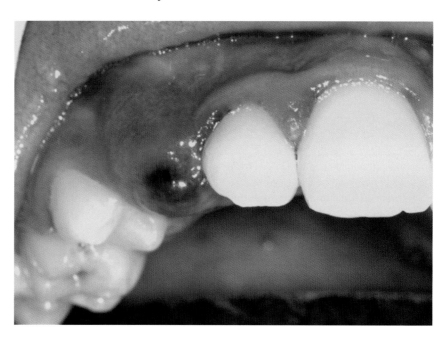

Radiographic Features. The cysts usually present as a well-demarcated radiolucency associated with the crown of an erupting tooth. As with dentigerous cysts, the radiolucency can usually be traced to the cementoenamel junction of the involved tooth.

Microscopic Findings. Microscopically, these cysts are identical to intrabony dentigerous cysts. Nonkeratinizing atrophic or hyperplastic epithelium surfaces fibrovascular connective tissue with varying numbers of epithelial rests characteristic of a dental follicle. Cuboidal or

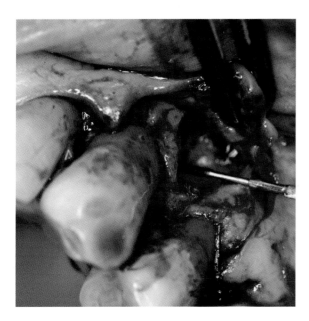

Figure 3-18

LATERAL PERIODONTAL CYST

At surgery, a smooth, bony cavity lined by thin soft tissue was uncovered.

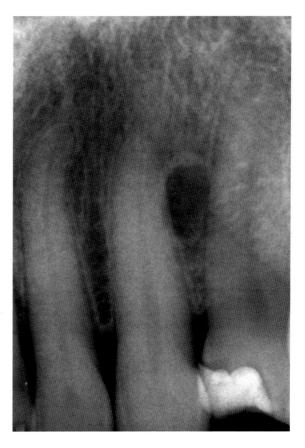

Figure 3-19

LATERAL PERIODONTAL CYST

A well-corticated radiolucency is between the maxillary canine and premolar roots.

mucous cell metaplasia may be seen. Some eruption cysts have infiltrates of acute and chronic inflammatory cells in the surrounding fibrous connective tissue.

Treatment and Prognosis. Many eruption cysts do not require treatment because they rupture and resolve on their own. For lesions that persist, simple incision or marsupialization of the cyst allowing the underlying tooth to continue to erupt is indicated (78,81). Prophylactic management of these cysts in immunocompromised children is indicated to avoid the possible spread of a localized infection (82).

Lateral Periodontal Cyst

Definition. *Lateral periodontal cysts* develop in association with the lateral root surface of erupted teeth. The cysts arise from the epithelial rests of Malassez in the periodontal ligament. The vitality of the tooth is irrelevant. In the past, some radicular cysts identified on the lateral aspect of the tooth root were termed lateral periodontal cysts; however, current classification schemes identify lateral periodontal cysts as developmental with characteristic microscopic features identical to the multilocular botryoid odontogenic cyst and some gingival cysts.

Clinical Features. Lateral periodontal cysts most often occur in the mandibular premolar/canine area and the maxillary lateral incisor region (fig. 3-18); however, any tooth may be involved (83,84). The cyst can form in the interproximal area between tooth roots and is usually an incidental radiographic finding (85,86). Males are more often affected, with a 2 to 1 ratio. The peak incidence is in the fifth and sixth decades (87).

Radiographic Features. The cyst presents as a unilocular radiolucency associated with the lateral periodontal ligament space of an erupted tooth. The radiolucency has a well-corticated periphery (fig. 3-19). Larger lesions may displace adjacent tooth roots. Multilocular lesions are a special subset and are classified as botryoid odontogenic cysts (see following section on botryoid odontogenic cysts) (88).

23

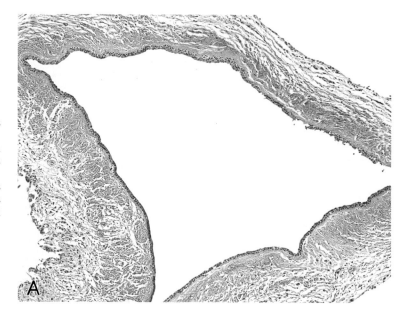

Figure 3-20

LATERAL PERIODONTAL CYST

A: Fibrovascular connective tissue has a luminal surface of epithelium.

B: Nonkeratinized, uniformly thin stratified squamous epithelium surfaces fibrovascular connective tissue.

C: The fibrovascular connective tissue is lined by a thin layer of stratified squamous and cuboidal epithelium, with occasional tufts of clear cells.

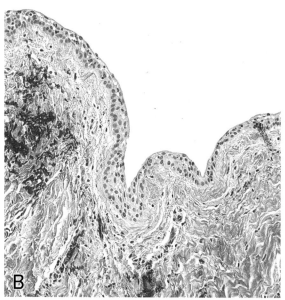

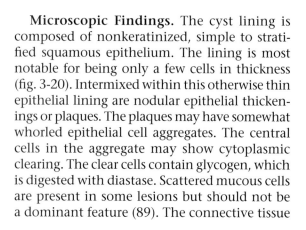

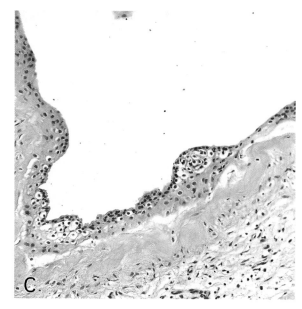

Microscopic Findings. The cyst lining is composed of nonkeratinized, simple to stratified squamous epithelium. The lining is most notable for being only a few cells in thickness (fig. 3-20). Intermixed within this otherwise thin epithelial lining are nodular epithelial thickenings or plaques. The plaques may have somewhat whorled epithelial cell aggregates. The central cells in the aggregate may show cytoplasmic clearing. The clear cells contain glycogen, which is digested with diastase. Scattered mucous cells are present in some lesions but should not be a dominant feature (89). The connective tissue wall may contain epithelial rests but these are not required for diagnosis.

Treatment and Prognosis. These cysts are treated with simple enucleation and recurrent lesions are infrequent (90). If multilocularity is noted radiographically or at the time of surgery, a botryoid variant should be suspected and more aggressive curettage of the bony walls performed.

Botryoid Odontogenic Cyst

Definition. The *botryoid odontogenic cyst* is a multilocular variant of the lateral periodontal cyst. Botryoid refers to the grape-like clusters that

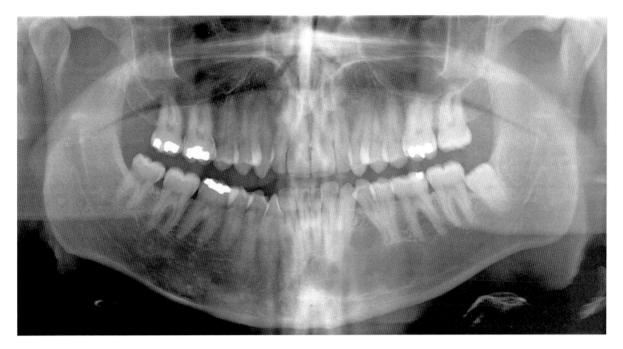

Figure 3-21

BOTRYOID ODONTOGENIC CYST

A well-circumscribed, multiloculated radiolucency in the left body of the mandible displaces the roots of the premolar and canine teeth.

describes these cysts radiographically, grossly, and microscopically. It has been suggested that the multilocular nature of this cyst may be due to the neoplastic growth potential (91,92).

Clinical Features. Most cysts are diagnosed in the fifth or sixth decade, and many are found in the mandibular premolar region (93–95). In a retrospective analysis of 67 cases published between 1973 and 2005, 85 percent were located in the mandible, 55 percent occurred in females, and most were diagnosed in the fifth decade of the life (96).

Radiographic Features. The cysts characteristically present adjacent to the lateral root surfaces of erupted teeth. The multiple lobules may envelop the tooth root and significantly displace adjacent teeth (fig. 3-21). The classic lesions are radiographically multilocular, although unilocular lesions are possible (97). The borders are well defined and usually well corticated. Root resorption is uncommon.

Microscopic Findings. At low power, multiple cystic lumens, or small "daughter" cysts, are often seen (fig. 3-22). At higher power, the cyst has the same microscopic features as lateral periodontal cysts, which includes a thin nonkeratinizing stratified squamous epithelium with areas of cuboidal and ovoid clear cell metaplasia and focal epithelial tufts (fig. 3-23). Clusters of glycogen-rich epithelial cells may be noted in nodular thickenings of the cyst lining.

Immunohistochemical Findings. Although the microscopic features alone should be adequate for diagnosis, expression of cytokeratin (CK) 19 and the lack of expression of p53, as well as the higher proliferation rate of the basal epithelial cell layer, are useful for differentiating botryoid odontogenic cysts from keratocystic odontogenic tumors (98). The presence of CK13 confirms that salivary gland epithelium plays no role in the origin of these multilocular cysts (98).

Treatment and Prognosis. Like the lateral periodontal cyst, the treatment for smaller lesions usually consists of enucleation with bony curettage. Recurrence, especially for larger multiloculated lesions, has been reported up to 9 years following initial surgery (93,99), indicating a need for more aggressive treatment, especially for larger, multicystic lesions (96)

Glandular Odontogenic Cyst

Definition. *Glandular odontogenic cysts* are nonkeratinizing cysts that have features of ductal and secretory cell differentiation (100–102). The terms *sialo-odontogenic cyst* and *mucoepidermoid cyst* have also been used (103,104).

Clinical Features. Although few cases have been reported, the anterior mandible is the most frequently reported site. The lesion occurs in the second to the ninth decade but the most cases occur in the fifth and sixth decades. Males are most often affected. The cyst is noticed initially because of cortical plate enlargement or secondary inflammation that causes pain. Tooth displacement, root resorption, and an association with unerupted teeth occur with some frequency (105). Perforation and thinning of cortical plates has been reported and may be an indicator of aggressive behavior (106).

In a series of 46 cases by Fowler et al. (106a), the mean age at diagnosis was 51 years, with 71 percent of cases in the fifth to seventh decades. No gender predilection was noted. Thirty-seven cases occurred in the mandible, and 28 of the lesions involved the anterior regions of the jaws. Swelling/expansion was the most common presenting complaint. The canine area was a common location for maxillary cases.

Radiographic Features. These lesions present as unilocular or multilocular radiolucencies with well-defined sclerotic borders, identical to other cysts and benign tumors of the jaws (fig. 3-24). In the series by Fowler et al. (106a), most presented as well-defined unilocular or multilocular radiolucencies involving the periapical area of multiple teeth. Some had a dentigerous or lateral periodontal presentation.

Microscopic Findings. Microscopically, glandular odontogenic cysts show a nonkeratinizing squamous-lined lumen (fig. 3-25). The most superficial layer of lining epithelium is sometimes cuboidal, with mucous goblet cell metaplasia (102,107,108). Cilia may be present focally. The

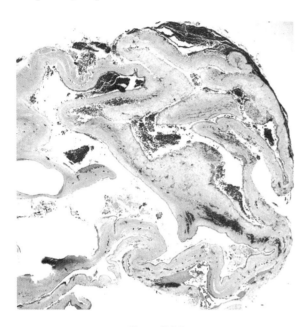

Figure 3-22

BOTRYOID ODONTOGENIC CYST

Multiple cystic spaces are surrounded by fibrovascular connective tissue septa.

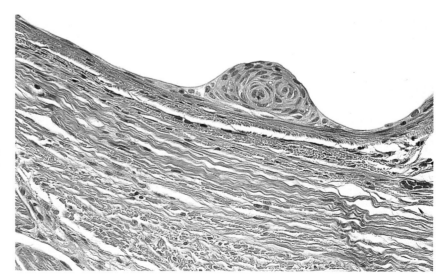

Figure 3-23

BOTRYOID ODONTOGENIC CYST

The cystic spaces are lined by squamous and cuboidal epithelium of variable thickness, with occasional epithelial tufts.

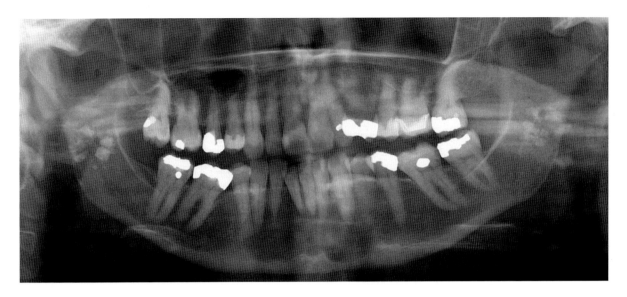

Figure 3-24

GLANDULAR ODONTOGENIC CYST

A panoramic radiograph shows a multilocular radiolucency of the anterior mandible.

epithelium also shows multiple cyst-like spaces lined by cuboidal cells (fig. 3-26). Spherical squamous tufts within the epithelial lining can be seen. Foci of hyaline may be present (109). Daughter cysts in the walls have been reported (110). No keratinization is present nor is there evidence of stellate reticulum or a uniform basal cell layer.

In the Fowler et al. series (106a), the focal presence of seven or more microscopic parameters described below was highly predictive of a diagnosis of glandular odontogenic cyst while the focal presence of five or fewer microscopic parameters was highly predictive of a nonglandular odontogenic cyst . These parameters included: 1) microcysts (duct-like structures) within the epithelial lining; 2) epithelial spheres or plaques; 3) clear cells; 4) variable thickness of the epithelial cyst lining; and 5) multiple epithelial-lined compartments similar to botryoid odontogenic cysts.

The most important entity in the differential diagnosis is intraosseous mucoepidermoid carcinoma (figs. 3-27, 3-28). Glandular odontogenic cysts have a thin squamous lining with little tendency to form the larger thickenings of squamous, intermediate, and mucous cells seen in mucoepidermoid carcinoma (111).

Immunohistochemical Findings. Expression of cytokeratins, Ki-67, and p53 helps differ-

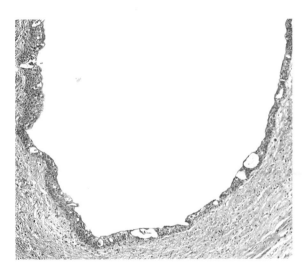

Figure 3-25

GLANDULAR ODONTOGENIC CYST

A cystic lumen lined by epithelium is surrounded by fibrovascular connective tissue.

entiate glandular odontogenic cysts from cysts with foci of mucous metaplasia, botryoid cysts, surgical ciliated cysts, and low-grade mucoepidermoid carcinomas (95,106,112,113). High levels of maspin in the cytoplasm and nuclei of epithelial mucous cells in mucoepidermoid carcinoma also distinguishes this tumor from glandular odontogenic cyst (114).

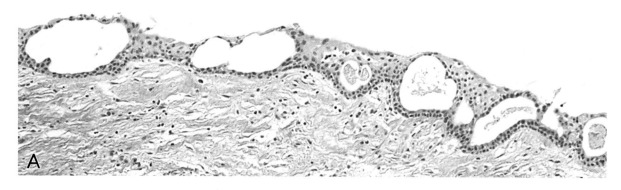

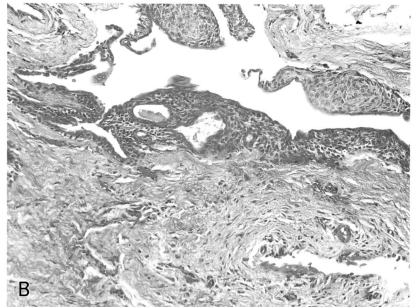

Figure 3-26

**GLANDULAR
ODONTOGENIC CYST**

A: The squamous epithelial
lining shows numerous duct-like
structures and evidence of mucous
cell metaplasia.

B: Ductal structures are seen in
areas of epithelial tufting.

C: Ductal structures are focally
rimmed by cuboidal epithelium in
areas of epithelial tufting.

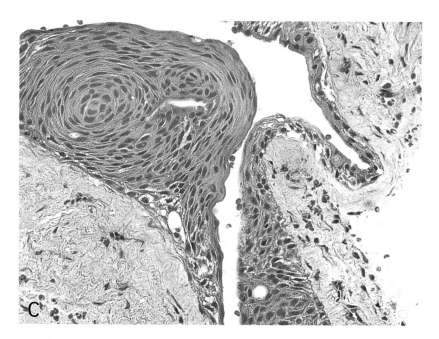

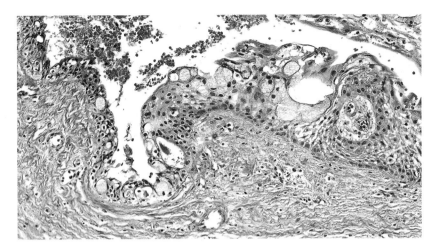

Figure 3-27

GLANDULAR ODONTOGENIC CYST

In some areas, mucous metaplasia and ducts closely mimic the features of low-grade mucoepidermoid carcinoma.

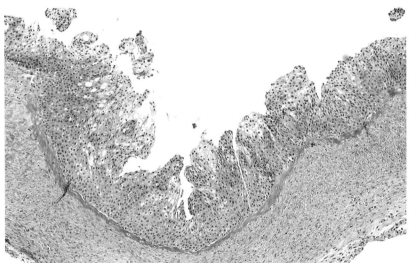

Figure 3-28

INTRAOSSEOUS LOW-GRADE MUCOEPIDERMOID CARCINOMA

Top: Compared to glandular odontogenic cysts, rare intraosseous mucoepidermoid carcinomas show a greater proliferation of squamous, intermediate, and mucous cells.

Bottom: Squamous, intermediate, and mucous cells predominate in this low-grade variant.

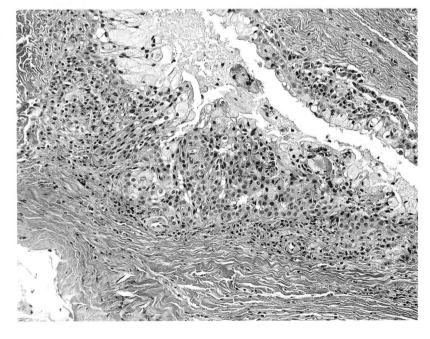

Treatment and Prognosis. The recurrence rate of glandular odontogenic cysts as described in the literature varies from 20 to 30 percent based on different initial treatments (104–106,115,116). In the series by Fowler et al. (106a), all cases were treated conservatively (enucleation, curettage, cystectomy, excision). Follow-up on 18 cases revealed a recurrence rate of 50 percent, with 6 cases recurring more than once (range of follow-up: 2 months to 20 years; average length of follow-up: 8.75 years). The mean interval from initial treatment to first recurrence was 8 years, and from first recurrence to second recurrence was 5.8 years. Two cases recurred three times and the interval from second to third recurrence was 7 years. Islands resembling mucoepidermoid carcinoma were identified in the cyst wall of three cases, only one of which had follow-up (no evidence of disease at 74 months). There were no statistically significant differences microscopically between lesions that recurred and those that did not.

Treatment by enucleation or curettage carries the highest risk for recurrence, especially for large and multilocular lesions (117,118). Peripheral ostectomy with Carnoy solution or marginal resection have both been suggested as treatment of choice (106,115,116,119–122). Long-term follow-up is necessary because of the multiple recurrences (123).

Primordial Cyst (Odontogenic Cyst of Undetermined Origin)

Definition. A *primordial cyst* is a nonkeratinized cyst that forms in place of a developing tooth. In practice, this diagnosis describes any developmental cyst that cannot be further defined based on clinical, radiographic, and microscopic findings. The identification of a missing tooth is not necessary because the definition technically includes supernumerary teeth.

Clinical Features. Most previously diagnosed primordial cysts, when examined microscopically, are odontogenic keratocysts now classified by the WHO as keratocystic odontogenic tumors (72,124–128). Because this term can no longer be used to describe keratocystic odontogenic tumors very few true primordial cysts are now diagnosed. In an early analysis of 312 keratocystic odontogenic tumors, 44 percent fit the radiographic and clinical criteria for primordial cysts (129). In 1982, Altini et al. (130) described a series of primordial cysts that appeared radiographically as follicular (dentigerous) cysts, but were microscopically extrafollicular.

Radiographic Features. This cyst occurs wherever odontogenesis occurs. A unilocular or multilocular radiolucency is seen, with well-demarcated, corticated borders. Slow growth usually results in displacement of the adjacent anatomy, including teeth, but resorption of tooth roots also occurs.

Microscopic Findings. The microscopic features alone are nondiagnostic. Primordial cysts show a lining of nonkeratinizing stratified squamous epithelium, with or without cuboidal or focal mucous goblet cell metaplasia. The underlying connective tissue is nonspecific and may contain epithelial rests similar to other developmental cysts.

Treatment and Prognosis. Treatment usually involves simple enucleation although larger lesions may be better managed with marsupialization or curettage.

Orthokeratinizing Odontogenic Cyst

Definition. When the *odontogenic keratocyst* was first defined, it was not separated into parakeratinized and orthokeratinized types (131–133). Wright (134) was the first to formally separate these two groups of cysts and proposed the name *odontogenic keratocyst, orthokeratinizing variant* (134). He noted different histopathologic features and the lack of recurrences associated with orthokeratinizing cysts following simple enucleation. Orthokeratinizing odontogenic cysts are rare, comprising only 10 to 12 percent of keratinizing cystic lesions (135,136).

Following the reclassification of parakeratinizing odontogenic keratocysts as keratocystic odontogenic tumors by the WHO in 2005, the confusion regarding the diagnosis of cystic keratinizing lesions has decreased. It is important, however, to recognize that there remain some overlapping features, including focal areas of orthokeratosis in keratocystic odontogenic tumors. The original series of 60 orthokeratinizing odontogenic keratocysts described by Wright (134) included 7 with focal areas of parakeratin. Thus classification based solely on the type of keratin alone is unwise. The separation of

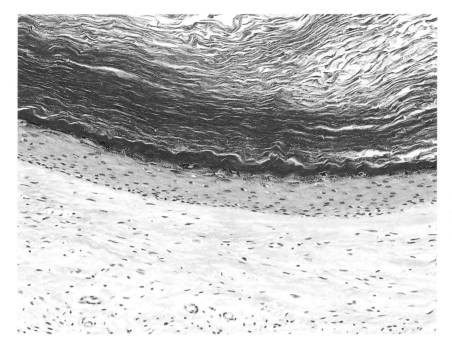

Figure 3-29

ORTHOKERATINIZING ODONTOGENIC CYST

The stratified squamous epithelium is of uniform thickness. A prominent granular cell layer and layers of orthokeratin are at the luminal surface. No prominent basal cell layer is seen.

orthokeratinizing odontogenic cysts from keratocystic odontogenic tumors is vitally important because of significant differences in recurrence rates following simple enucleation.

Clinical Features. According to Brannon (129), the peak incidence of orthokeratinizing odontogenic cyst is in the third through fifth decades. About 75 percent form in the follicles of unerupted or impacted teeth, appearing radiographically indistinguishable from dentigerous cysts. Most are asymptomatic, although pain and swelling are reported in 22 and 13 percent of cases, respectively. Most occur in males and are most often identified in the mandibular third molar region (136). Orthokeratinizing odontogenic cysts are not associated with basal cell nevus syndrome.

Radiographic Features. Orthokeratinizing odontogenic cysts show well-defined radiolucencies with a corticated border. If associated with an unerupted tooth, the cyst is indistinguishable from a dentigerous cyst. Because of their slow growth rate, these cysts have a tendency to displace normal anatomic structures, such as the mandibular canal or teeth roots, but some can cause resorption.

Microscopic Findings. The epithelial lining is most often a uniformly thin, stratified squamous epithelium with a prominent granular cell layer and a surface showing layers of orthokeratin (fig. 3-29). Keratin production varies and may only occur in focal areas of the epithelial lining. In areas of nonkeratinization, mucous cell metaplasia may be seen. Some cases mimic epidermal cysts, with sebaceous or even dermal appendage formation (137). Most important is the absence of a prominent basal layer with hyperchromatic palisaded nuclei characteristic of keratocystic odontogenic tumors.

Immunohistochemical Findings. Staining of the epithelial lining for cytokeratins, epithelial membrane antigen (EMA), carcinoembryonic antigen (CEA), and involucrin has shown significant differences between orthokeratinizing odontogenic cysts and keratocystic odontogenic tumors (137). Orthokeratinizing odontogenic cysts express lower levels of Ki-67 and p63 than keratocystic odontogenic tumors (136).

Treatment and Prognosis. The importance in distinguishing orthokeratinizing odontogenic cysts from keratocystic odontogenic tumors involves primarily their recurrence rates following conservative treatment. Orthokeratinizing cysts have a recurrence rate of only about 2 percent following simple enucleation. In Wright's original description, follow-up for 24 cases revealed only 1 recurrence (134). In an analysis of 54 cases, a recurrence rate of only 2.2 percent following initial treatment was reported (135). In another series, follow-up of nine cases treated by simple enucleation revealed no recurrences over a period of 3.5 to 12.0 years (138). In an evaluation of 42 cases followed for an average of more than 6 years after conservative treatment, there were no recurrences (136).

REFERENCES

1. Kramer IR, Pindborg JJ, Shear M. The WHO histological typing of odontogenic tumours. A commentary on the second edition. Cancer 1992;70:2988-2994.
2. Shear M. The aggressive nature of the odontogenic keratocyst: is it a benign cystic neoplasm? Part 2. Proliferation and genetic studies. Oral Oncol 2002;38:323-331.
3. Shear M. The aggressive nature of the odontogenic keratocyst: is it a benign cystic neoplasm? Part 3. Immunocytochemistry of cytokeratin and other epithelial cell markers. Oral Oncol 2002;38:407-415.
4. Shear M. The aggressive nature of the odontogenic keratocyst: is it a benign cystic neoplasm? Part 1. Clinical and early experimental evidence of aggressive behaviour. Oral Oncol 2002;38:219-226.
5. Barnes L, Eveson JW, Reichart P, Sidransky D, eds. World Health Organization classification of tumours. Pathology and genetics of head and neck tumours. Lyon: IARC Press; 2005.
6. Browne RM. Some observations on the fluids of odontogenic cysts. J Oral Pathol 1976;5:74-87.
7. Toller P. Permeability of cyst walls in vivo: investigations with radioactive tracers. Proc R Soc Med 1966;59:724-729.
8. Toller PA. Newer concepts of odontogenic cysts. Int J Oral Surg 1972;1:3-16.
9. Toller PA. Immunological factors in cysts of the jaws. Proc R Soc Med 1971;64:555-559.
10. Toller PA. Protein substances in odontogenic cyst fluids. Br Dent J 1970;128:317-322.
11. Stoelinga PJ. Studies on the dental lamina as related to its role in the etiology of cysts and tumors. J Oral Pathol 1976;5:65-73.
12. Morgenroth K. [Odontogenic cysts.] Pathologe 2008;29:214-220. [German]
13. Li T, Browne RM, Matthews JB. Immunocytochemical expression of growth factors by odontogenic jaw cysts. Mol Pathol 1997;50:21-27.
14. Mason GI, Matthews JB. In situ determination of different dehydrogenase activity profiles in the linings of odontogenic keratocysts and radicular cysts. Histochem J 1996;28:187-193.
15. Ricucci D, Mannocci F, Ford TR. A study of periapical lesions correlating the presence of a radiopaque lamina with histological findings. Oral Surg Oral Med Oral Pathol Oral Radiol Endod 2006;101:389-394.
16. Slabbert H, Shear M, Altini M. Vacuolated cells and mucous metaplasia in the epithelial linings of radicular and residual cysts. J Oral Pathol Med 1995;24:309-312.
17. Bhaskar SN. Periapical lesions—types, incidence, and clinical features. Oral Surg Oral Med Oral Pathol 1966;21:657-671.
18. Shear M. Cholesterol in dental cysts. Oral Surg Oral Med Oral Pathol 1963;16:1465-1473.
19. Shear M. Inflammation in dental cysts. Oral Surg Oral Med Oral Pathol 1964;17:756-767.
20. Garcia CC, Diago MP, Mira BG, Sebastian JV, Sempere FV. Expression of cytokeratins in epithelialized periapical lesions. Oral Surg Oral Med Oral Pathol Oral Radiol Endod 2009;107:e43-6.
21. Carrillo C, Penarrocha M, Penarrocha M, Vera F, Penarrocha D. Immunohistochemical study of Langerhans cells in periapical lesions: correlation with inflammatory cell infiltration and epithelial cell proliferation. Med Oral Patol Oral Cir Bucal 2010;15:e335-9.
22. Teixeira-Salum TB, Rodrigues DB, Gervasio AM, Souza CJ, Rodrigues V Jr, Loyola AM. Distinct Th1, Th2 and Treg cytokines balance in chronic periapical granulomas and radicular cysts. J Oral Pathol Med 2010;39:250-256.
23. Lee FM. Ameloblastoma of the maxilla with probable origin in a residual cyst. Oral Surg Oral Med Oral Pathol 1970;29:799-805.
24. Ahlstrom U, Johansen CC, Lantz B. Radicular and residual cysts of the jaws. A long term roentgenographic study following cystectomies. Odontol Revy 1969;20:111-117.
25. High AS, Hirschmann PN. Symptomatic residual radicular cysts. J Oral Pathol 1988;17:70-72.
26. Weine FS, Silverglade LB. Residual cysts masquerading as periapical lesions: three case reports. J Am Dent Assoc 1983;106:833-835.

27. Boffano P, Gallesio C. Exposed inferior alveolar neurovascular bundle during surgical removal of a residual cyst. J Craniofac Surg 2010;21:270-273.

28. Galzignato PF, Sivolella S, Cavallin G, Ferronato G. Dental implant failure associated with a residual maxillary cyst. Br Dent J 2010;208:153-154.

29. Muglali M, Sumer AP. Squamous cell carcinoma arising in a residual cyst: a case report. J Contemp Dent Pract 2008;9:115-121.

30. Craig GT. The paradental cyst. A specific inflammatory odontogenic cyst. Br Dent J 1976;141:9-14.

31. Main DM. Epithelial jaw cysts: a clinicopathological reappraisal. Br J Oral Surg 1970;8:114-125.

32. Bsoul SA, Flint DJ, Terezhalmy GT, Moore WS. Paradental cyst (inflammatory collateral, mandibular infected buccal cyst). Quintessence Int 2002;33:782-783.

33. Ackermann G, Cohen MA, Altini M. The paradental cyst: a clinicopathologic study of 50 cases. Oral Surg Oral Med Oral Pathol 1987;64:308-312.

34. Philipsen HP, Reichart PA, Ogawa I, Suei Y, Takata T. The inflammatory paradental cyst: a critical review of 342 cases from a literature survey, including 17 new cases from the author's files. J Oral Pathol Med 2004;33:147-155.

35. Colgan CM, Henry J, Napier SS, Cowan CG. Paradental cysts: a role for food impaction in the pathogenesis? A review of cases from Northern Ireland. Br J Oral Maxillofac Surg 2002;40:163-168.

36. Morimoto Y, Tanaka T, Nishida I, et al. Inflammatory paradental cyst (IPC) in the mandibular premolar region in children. Oral Surg Oral Med Oral Pathol Oral Radiol Endod 2004;97:286-293.

37. de Sousa SO, Correa L, Deboni MC, de Araujo VC. Clinicopathologic features of 54 cases of paradental cyst. Quintessence Int 2001;32:737-741.

38. Reichart PA, Philipsen HP. [Inflammatory paradental cyst. Report of 6 cases.] Mund Kiefer Gesichtschir 2003;7:171-174. [German]

39. Fowler CB, Brannon RB. The paradental cyst: a clinicopathologic study of six new cases and review of the literature. J Oral Maxillofac Surg 1989;47:243-248.

40. Bohay RN, Weinberg S, Thorner PS. The paradental cyst of the mandibular permanent first molar: report of a bilateral case. ASDC J Dent Child 1992;59:361-365.

41. da Graca Naclerio-Homem M, Deboni MC, Simoes AW, Traina AA, Chin V. Paradental cyst: case report and review of the literature. J Clin Pediatr Dent 2004;29:83-86.

42. Baughman R. Diagnostic quiz. Case No. 2: mandibular buccal cyst (buccal bifurcation cyst.) Today's FDA 2007;19:20-23.

43. Santos SE, Sato FR, Sawazaki R, Asprino L, de Moraes M, Moreira RW. Mandibular buccal bifur-

44. Magnusson B, Borrman H. The paradental cyst a clinicopathologic study of 26 cases. Swed Dent J 1995;19:1-7.

45. Lacaita MG, Capodiferro S, Favia G, Santarelli A, Lo Muzio L. Infected paradental cysts in children: a clinicopathological study of 15 cases. Br J Oral Maxillofac Surg 2006;44:112-115.

46. Stoneman DW, Worth HM. The mandibular infected buccal cyst—molar area. Dent Radiogr Photogr 1983;56:1-14.

47. Zadik Y, Yitschaky O, Neuman T, Nitzan DW. On the self-resolution nature of the buccal bifurcation cyst. J Oral Maxillofac Surg 2011;69: e282-284.

48. Corona-Rodriguez J, Torres-Labardini R, Velasco-Tizcareno M, Mora-Rincones O. Bilateral buccal bifurcation cyst: case report and literature review. J Oral Maxillofac Surg 2011;69:1694-1696.

49. Vedtofte P, Holmstrup P. Inflammatory paradental cysts in the globulomaxillary region. J Oral Pathol Med 1989;18:125-127.

50. Vedtofte P, Praetorius F. The inflammatory paradental cyst. Oral Surg Oral Med Oral Pathol 1989;68:182-188.

51. David LA, Sandor GK, Stoneman DW. The buccal bifurcation cyst: in non-surgical treatment an option? J Can Dent Assoc 1998;64:712-716.

52. Shohat I, Buchner A, Taicher S. Mandibular buccal bifurcation cyst: enucleation without extraction. Int J Oral Maxillofac Surg 2003;32:610-613.

53. Thikkurissy S, Glazer KM, McNamara KK, Tatakis DN. Buccal bifurcation cyst in a 7-year-old: surgical management and 14-month follow-up. J Periodontol 2010;81:442-446.

54. Pompura JR, Sandor GK, Stoneman DW. The buccal bifurcation cyst: a prospective study of treatment outcomes in 44 sites. Oral Surg Oral Med Oral Pathol Oral Radiol Endod 1997;83:215-221.

55. Toller PA. Epithelial discontinuities in cysts of the jaws. Br Dent J 1966;120:74-78.

56. Daley TD, Wysocki GP. The small dentigerous cyst. A diagnostic dilemma. Oral Surg Oral Med Oral Pathol Oral Radiol Endod 1995;79:77-81.

57. Zhang LL, Yang R, Zhang L, Li W, Macdonald-Jankowski D, Poh CF. Dentigerous cyst: a retrospective clinicopathological analysis of 2082 dentigerous cysts in British Columbia, Canada. Int J Oral Maxillofac Surg 2010;39:878-882.

58. Benn A, Altini M. Dentigerous cysts of inflammatory origin. A clinicopathologic study. Oral Surg Oral Med Oral Pathol Oral Radiol Endod 1996;81:203-209.

59. Fukuta Y, Totsuka M, Takeda Y, Yamamoto H. Pathological study of the hyperplastic dental follicle. J Nihon Univ Sch Dent 1991;33:166-173.

60. Barsky SH, Hannah JB. Extracellular hyaline bodies are basement membrane accumulations. Am J Clin Pathol 1987;87:455-460.

61. McMillan MD, Smillie AC. Ameloblastomas associated with dentigerous cysts. Oral Surg Oral Med Oral Pathol 1981;51:489-496.

62. Paul JK, Fay JT, Stamps P. Recurrent dentigerous cyst evidencing ameloblastic proliferation: report of case. J Oral Surg 1969;27:211-214.

63. Taylor RN, Callins JF, Menell HB, Williams AC. Dentigerous cyst with ameloblastomatous proliferation: report of a case. J Oral Surg 1971;29:136-140.

64. Chretien PB, Carpenter DF, White NS, Harrah JD, Lightbody PM. Squamous carcinoma arising in a dentigerous cyst. Presentation of a fatal case and review of four previously reported cases. Oral Surg Oral Med Oral Pathol 1970;30:809-816.

65. Copete MA, Cleveland DB, Orban RE Jr, Chen SY. Squamous carcinoma arising from a dentigerous cyst: report of a case. Compend Contin Educ Dent 1996;17:202-204.

66. Johnson LM, Sapp JP, McIntire DN. Squamous cell carcinoma arising in a dentigerous cyst. J Oral Maxillofac Surg 1994;52:987-990.

67. Maxymiw WG, Wood RE. Carcinoma arising in a dentigerous cyst: a case report and review of the literature. J Oral Maxillofac Surg 1991;49:639-643.

68. Waldron CA, Koh ML. Central mucoepidermoid carcinoma of the jaws: report of four cases with analysis of the literature and discussion of the relationship to mucoepidermoid, sialodontogenic, and glandular odontogenic cysts. J Oral Maxillofac Surg 1990;48:871-877.

69. Brkic A, Mutlu S, Kocak-Berberoglu H, Olgac V. Pathological changes and immunoexpression of p63 gene in dental follicles of asymptomatic impacted lower third molars: an immunohistochemical study. J Craniofac Surg 2010;21:854-857.

70. Clauser C, Zuccati G, Barone R, Villano A. Simplified surgical-orthodontic treatment of a dentigerous cyst. J Clin Orthod 1994;28:103-106.

71. Iatrou I, Theologie-Lygidakis N, Leventis M. Intraosseous cystic lesions of the jaws in children: a retrospective analysis of 47 consecutive cases. Oral Surg Oral Med Oral Pathol Oral Radiol Endod 2009;107:485-492.

72. Robinson HB. Classification of cysts of the jaws. Am J Orthod Oral Surt 1945;31:370-375.

73. Clark CA. A survey of eruption cysts in the newborn. Oral Surg Oral Med Oral Pathol 1962;15:917.

74. Ramon Boj J, Garcia-Godoy F. Multiple eruption cysts: report of a case. ASDC J Dent Child 2000;67:282-284, 232.

75. Puranik RS, Vanaki SS. Dentigerous cyst vs. eruption cyst. Aust Dent J 2007;52:345.

76. Aguilo L, Cibrian R, Bagan JV, Gandia JL. Eruption cysts: retrospective clinical study of 36 cases. ASDC J Dent Child 1998;65:102-106.

77. Nortje CJ. General practitioner's radiology. Case 49. Eruption cyst. SADJ 2007;62:82.

78. Bodner L, Goldstein J, Sarnat H. Eruption cysts: a clinical report of 24 new cases. J Clin Pediatr Dent 2004;28:183-186.

79. Anderson RA. Eruption cysts: a retrograde study. ASDC J Dent Child 1990;57:124-127.

80. Slater LJ. Dentigerous cyst versus paradental cyst versus eruption pocket cyst. J Oral Maxillofac Surg 2003;61:149.

81. Ricci HA, Parisotto TM, Giro EM, de Souza Costa CA, Hebling J. Eruption cysts in the neonate. J Clin Pediatr Dent 2008;32:243-246.

82. Karp JM, Milner LA. Oral eruption cysts in a child with hepatoblastoma. J Pediatr Hematol Oncol 2009;31:509-511.

83. Angelopoulou E, Angelopoulos AP. Lateral periodontal cyst. Review of the literature and report of a case. J Periodontol 1990;61:126-131.

84. Altini M, Shear M. The lateral periodontal cyst: an update. J Oral Pathol Med 1992;21:245-250.

85. Cohen DA, Neville BW, Damm DD, White DK. The lateral periodontal cyst. A report of 37 cases. J Periodontol 1984;55:230-234.

86. Carter LC, Carney YL, Perez-Pudlewski D. Lateral periodontal cyst. Multifactorial analysis of a previously unreported series. Oral Surg Oral Med Oral Pathol Oral Radiol Endod 1996;81:210-216.

87. Eliasson S, Isacsson G, Kondell PA. Lateral periodontal cysts. Clinical, radiographical and histopathological findings. Int J Oral Maxillofac Surg 1989;18:191-193.

88. Phelan JA, Kritchman D, Fusco-Ramer M, Freedman PD, Lumerman H. Recurrent botryoid odontogenic cyst (lateral periodontal cyst). Oral Surg Oral Med Oral Pathol 1988;66:345-348.

89. Shear M, Pindborg JJ. Microscopic features of the lateral periodontal cyst. Scand J Dent Res 1975;83:103-110.

90. Formoso Senande MF, Figueiredo R, Berini Aytes L, Gay Escoda C. Lateral periodontal cysts: a retrospective study of 11 cases. Med Oral Patol Oral Cir Bucal 2008;13:E313-7.

91. Weathers DR, Waldron CA. Unusual multilocular cysts of the jaws (botryoid odontogenic cysts). Oral Surg Oral Med Oral Pathol 1973;36:235-241.

92. Phelan JA, Kritchman D, Fusco-Ramer M, Freedman PD, Lumerman H. Recurrent botryoid odontogenic cyst (lateral periodontal cyst). Oral Surg Oral Med Oral Pathol 1988;66:345-348.

93. Gurol M, Burkes EJ Jr, Jacoway J. Botryoid odontogenic cyst: analysis of 33 cases. J Periodontol 1995;66:1069-1073.

94. Ucok O, Yaman Z, Gunhan O, Ucok C, Dogan N, Baykul T. Botryoid odontogenic cyst: report of a case with extensive epithelial proliferation. Int J Oral Maxillofac Surg 2005;34:693-695.

95. de Sousa SO, Cabezas NT, de Oliveira PT, de Araujo VC. Glandular odontogenic cyst: report of a case with cytokeratin expression. Oral Surg Oral Med Oral Pathol Oral Radiol Endod 1997;83:478-483.

96. Mendez P, Junquera L, Gallego L, Baladron J. Botryoid odontogenic cyst: clinical and pathological analysis in relation to recurrence. Med Oral Patol Oral Cir Bucal 2007;12:E594-8.

97. Redman RS, Whitestone BW, Winne CE, Hudec MW, Patterson RH. Botryoid odontogenic cyst. Report of a case with histologic evidence of multicentric origin. Int J Oral Maxillofac Surg 1990;19:144-146.

98. Weibrich G, Kleis WK, Otto M, et al. [Cytokeratin expression in botryoid odontogenic cyst. A rare differential keratocyst and ameloblastoma diagnosis.] Mund Kiefer Gesichtschir 2000;4:309-314. [German]

99. Chbicheb S, Bennani A, Taleb B, Wady WE. [Botryoid odontogenic cyst.] Rev Stomatol Chir Maxillofac 2008;109:114-116. [French]

100. Gardner DG, Kessler HP, Morency R, Schaffner DL. The glandular odontogenic cyst: an apparent entity. J Oral Pathol 1988;17:359-366.

101. Patron M, Colmenero C, Larrauri J. Glandular odontogenic cyst: clinicopathologic analysis of three cases. Oral Surg Oral Med Oral Pathol 1991;72:71-74.

102. Gardner DG, Morency R. The glandular odontogenic cyst, a rare lesion that tends to recur. J Can Dent Assoc 1993;59:929-930.

103. Babburi S, Krishnan PA, Sundharam BS. Sialo-odontogenic cyst—a case report. Indian J Dent Res 2003;14:298-300.

104. Koppang HS, Johannessen S, Haugen LK, Haanaes HR, Solheim T, Donath K. Glandular odontogenic cyst (sialo-odontogenic cyst): report of two cases and literature review of 45 previously reported cases. J Oral Pathol Med 1998;27:455-462.

105. Macdonald-Jankowski DS. Glandular odontogenic cyst: systematic review. Dentomaxillofac Radiol 2010;39:127-139.

106. Kaplan I, Anavi Y, Hirshberg A. Glandular odontogenic cyst: a challenge in diagnosis and treatment. Oral Dis 2008;14:575-581.

106a. Fowler CB, Brannon RB, Kessler HP, Castle JT, Kahn MA. Glandular odontogenic cyst: analysis of 46 cases with special emphasis on microscopic criteria for diagnosis. Head Neck Pathol 2011;5:364-375.

107. Savage NW, Joseph BK, Monsour PA, Young WG. The glandular odontogenic jaw cyst: report of a case. Pathology 1996;28:370-372.

108. de Sousa SO, Cabezas NT, de Oliveira PT, de Araujo VC. Glandular odontogenic cyst: report of a case with cytokeratin expression. Oral Surg Oral Med Oral Pathol Oral Radiol Endod 1997;83:478-483.

109. Ide F, Shimoyama T, Horie N. Glandular odontogenic cyst with hyaline bodies: an unusual dentigerous presentation. J Oral Pathol Med 1996;25:401-404.

110. Magnusson B, Goransson L, Odesjo B, Grondahl K, Hirsch JM. Glandular odontogenic cyst. Report of seven cases. Dentomaxillofac Radiol 1997;26:26-31.

111. Waldron CA, Koh ML. Central mucoepidermoid carcinoma of the jaws: report of four cases with analysis of the literature and discussion of the relationship to mucoepidermoid, sialo-dontogenic, and glandular odontogenic cysts. J Oral Maxillofac Surg 1990;48:871-877.

112. Pires FR, Chen SY, da Cruz Perez DE, de Almeida OP, Kowalski LP. Cytokeratin expression in central mucoepidermoid carcinoma and glandular odontogenic cyst. Oral Oncol 2004;40:545-551.

113. Tosios KI, Kakarantza-Angelopoulou E, Kapranos N. Immunohistochemical study of bcl-2 protein, Ki-67 antigen and p53 protein in epithelium of glandular odontogenic cysts and dentigerous cysts. J Oral Pathol Med 2000;29:139-144.

114. Vered M, Allon I, Buchner A, Dayan D. Is maspin immunolocalization a tool to differentiate central low-grade mucoepidermoid carcinoma from glandular odontogenic cyst? Acta Histochem 2010;112:161-168.

115. Kaplan I, Gal G, Anavi Y, Manor R, Calderon S. Glandular odontogenic cyst: treatment and recurrence. J Oral Maxillofac Surg 2005;63:435-441.

116. Boffano P, Cassarino E, Zavattero E, Campisi P, Garzino-Demo P. Surgical treatment of glandular odontogenic cysts. J Craniofac Surg 2010;21:776-780.

117. Gardner DG, Kessler HP, Morency R, Schaffner DL. The glandular odontogenic cyst: an apparent entity. J Oral Pathol 1988;17:359-366.

118. Gardner DG, Morency R. The glandular odontogenic cyst, a rare lesion that tends to recur. J Can Dent Assoc 1993;59:929-930.

119. Hussain K, Edmondson HD, Browne RM. Glandular odontogenic cysts. Diagnosis and treatment. Oral Surg Oral Med Oral Pathol Oral Radiol Endod 1995;79:593-602.

120. Qin XN, Li JR, Chen XM, Long X. The glandular odontogenic cyst: clinicopathologic features and treatment of 14 cases. J Oral Maxillofac Surg 2005;63:694-699.

121. Abu-Id MH, Kreusch T, Bruschke C. [Glandular odontogenic cyst of the mandible. Case report.] Mund Kiefer Gesichtschir 2005;9:188-192. [German]

122. Thor A, Warfvinge G, Fernandes R. The course of a long-standing glandular odontogenic cyst: marginal resection and reconstruction with particulated bone graft, platelet-rich plasma, and additional vertical alveolar distraction. J Oral Maxillofac Surg 2006;64:1121-1128.

123. Osny FJ, Azevedo LR, Sant'Ana E, Lara VS. Glandular odontogenic cyst: case report and review of the literature. Quintessence Int 2004;35:385-389.

124. Cohen MA, Shear M. Histological comparison of parakeratinised and orthokeratinised primordial cysts (keratocysts). J Dent Assoc S Afr 1980;35:161-165.

125. De Veer I, Lobos N. [Tumors of the jaw: general, neoplastic, odontogenic and primordial cysts]. Odontol Chil 1982;30:55-65. [Spanish]

126. Femiano F, Serpico R, Laino G. [Keratocysts: primordial cysts? Nosological problems and clinical aspects]. Arch Stomatol (Napoli) 1986;27:157-167. [Italian]

127. Partridge M, Towers JF. The primordial cyst (odontogenic keratocyst): its tumour-like characteristics and behaviour. Br J Oral Maxillofac Surg 1987;25:271-279.

128. Gordeeff M, Clergeau-Guerithault S. Expression of certain cytokeratins in the epithelium of dentigerous and primordial cysts. J Biol Buccale 1990;18:59-67.

129. Brannon RB. The odontogenic keratocyst. A clinicopathologic study of 312 cases. Part I. Clinical features. Oral Surg Oral Med Oral Pathol 1976;42:54-72.

130. Altini M, Cohen M. The follicular primordial cyst—odontogenic keratocyst. Int J Oral Surg 1982;11:175-182.

131. Gorlin RJ. Potentialities of oral epithelium namifest by mandibular dentigerous cysts. Oral Surg Oral Med Oral Pathol 1957;10:271-284.

132. Onuki M, Saito A, Hosokawa S, et al. A case of orthokeratinized odontogenic cyst suspected to be a radicular cyst. Bull Tokoyo Dent Coll 2009;50:31-35.

133. Vuhahula E, Nikai H, Ijuhin N, et al. Jaw cysts with orthokeratinization: analysis of 12 cases. J Oral Pathol Med 1993;22:35-40.

134. Wright JM. The odontogenic keratocyst: orthokeratinized variant. Oral Surg Oral Med Oral Pathol 1981;51:609-618.

135. Crowley TE, Kaugars GE, Gunsolley JC. Odontogenic keratocysts: a clinical and histologic comparison of the parakeratin and orthokeratin variants. J Oral Maxillofac Surg 1992;50:22-26.

136. Dong Q, Pan S, Sun LS, Li TJ. Orthokeratinized odontogenic cyst: a clinicopathologic study of 61 cases. Arch Pathol Lab Med 2010;134:271-275.

137. Vuhahula E, Nikai H, Ijuhin N, et al. Jaw cysts with orthokeratinization: analysis of 12 cases. J Oral Pathol Med 1993;22:35-40.

138. Li TJ, Kitano M, Chen XM, et al. Orthokeratinized odontogenic cyst: a clinicopathological and immunocytochemical study of 15 cases. Histopathology 1998;32:242-251.

4   NONODONTOGENIC CYSTS OF THE JAWS

NASOPALATINE DUCT CYST (MEDIAN ANTERIOR MAXILLARY CYST, INCISIVE CANAL CYST)

Definition. The *nasopalatine duct cyst* is a nonodontogenic cyst arising in the midline of the anterior maxilla posterior to the central incisors. Alternative terms include *median anterior maxillary cyst* and *incisive canal cyst*.

Clinical Features. Nasopalatine duct cysts are usually asymptomatic and often identified as a result of dental radiographs (1). Occasionally patients complain of a "bitter taste" as a result of periodic cyst drainage. They are common cysts and in one study accounted for 72 percent of nonodontogenic jaw cysts (2). Most are less than 1 cm in diameter but some exceed 2 cm (3,4). The majority occur within bone, but they also occur in the midline soft tissues of the anterior hard palate.

Radiographic Features. Radiographs reveal a well-demarcated, corticated enlargement involving the midline of the anterior maxilla (fig. 4-1). Larger radiolucencies may cause divergence or resorption of the central incisor roots. Nasopalatine duct cysts have been reported in association with mesiodens (5).

Microscopic Findings. Microscopic examination reveals a cystic cavity lined by stratified squamous, cuboidal, mucous goblet, or pseudostratified ciliated columnar epithelium (figs. 4-2–4-5). Dendritic cells containing melanin pigment have been demonstrated in the epithelial lining (6). The fibrous connective tissue wall often contains the contents of the nasopalatine ducts including hyaline cartilage, adipose tissue, and minor mucous salivary gland acini.

Treatment and Prognosis. Therapeutic management involves simple enucleation and recurrence rates are low. There are isolated reports of aggressive lesions and even squamous cell carcinomas arising from these cysts (7–9).

NASOLABIAL CYST

Definition and Clinical Features. The *nasolabial cyst* is a lesion of soft tissue adjacent to the ala of the nose. Clinically, the cyst presents as an asymptomatic fluctuant enlargement involving the maxillary vestibule in the canine region (fig. 4-6). Secondary inflammation can cause pain, erythema, and swelling (10). Radiographs seldom reveal any evidence of underlying bony involvement (11). Although benign and slowly growing, these soft tissue cysts can enlarge to more than 1 cm in diameter (12–14). One such cyst has been reported in association with a unilateral cleft lip and palate (15).

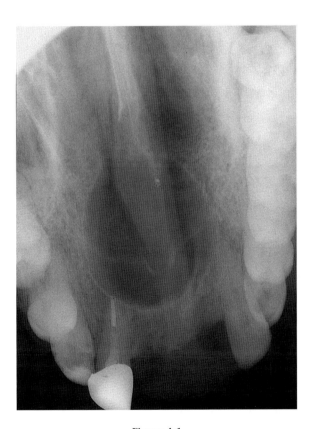

Figure 4-1

NASOPALATINE DUCT CYST

An anterior maxillary occlusal radiograph shows a well-demarcated radiolucency in the midline.

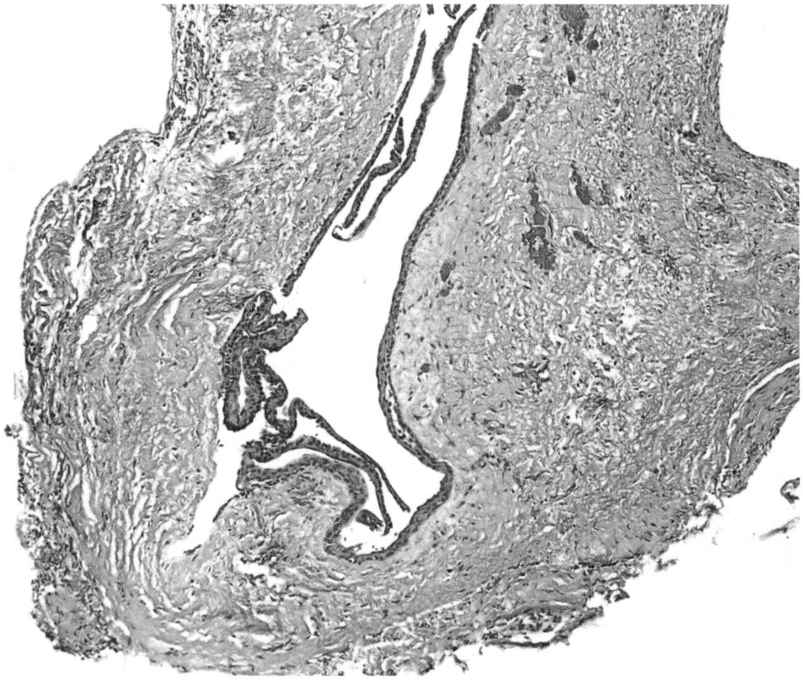

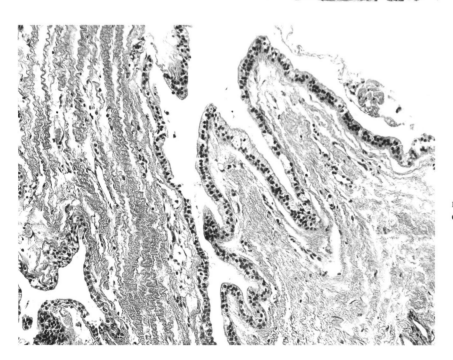

Figure 4-2

NASOPALATINE DUCT CYST

At low power, the cystic space has a thin epithelial lining.

Figure 4-3

NASOPALATINE DUCT CYST

Cuboidal, low columnar, and mucous goblet cells are in the cyst lining.

Microscopic Findings. The cysts are most often lined by pseudostratified ciliated columnar, stratified squamous, or simple cuboidal epithelium (fig. 4-7). Foci of mucous goblet cell or apocrine metaplasia have been reported, but these are not common findings (16). Inflammation of the connective tissue wall is not characteristic but can be identified if the cyst lining has been disrupted.

Treatment and Prognosis. Intraoral conservative excision is the recommended treatment of choice and recurrence rates are low. Recently, Chao et al. (17) advocated transnasal marsupialization as an alternative treatment.

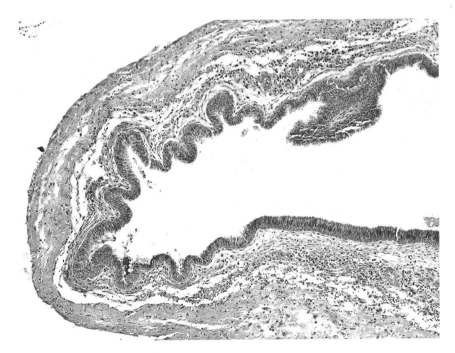

Figure 4-4

NASOPALATINE DUCT CYST

Most of this cyst shows a lining of pseudostratified ciliated columnar epithelium.

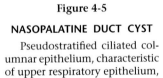

Figure 4-5

NASOPALATINE DUCT CYST

Pseudostratified ciliated columnar epithelium, characteristic of upper respiratory epithelium, focally lines this cyst.

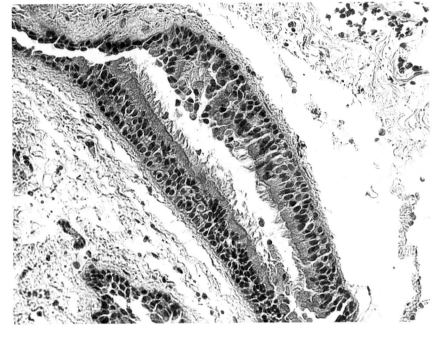

SURGICAL CILIATED CYST

Definition. *Surgical ciliated cysts* occur in the maxilla at a site of previous trauma or surgery including extraction of teeth. Surgical ciliated cysts have been identified following Caldwell-Luc surgery, orthognathic surgery, and surgery for chronic sinus inflammatory disease (18,19). The antral lining directly adjacent to molar and premolar roots becomes detached and persists, forming a cyst in the healing surgical site. In a series of 60 cases, most of the patients were in their 20s and 30s at the time of diagnosis (20,21).

Radiographic Features. The lesions are characteristically asymptomatic and usually identified incidentally on dental radiographs made for other reasons (22). These cysts are slow growing

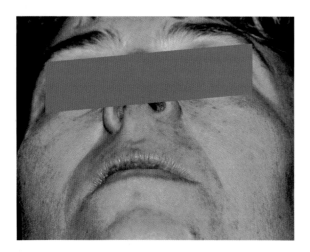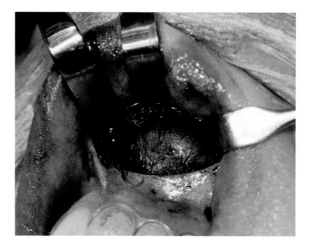

Figure 4-6

NASOLABIAL CYST

Left: Facial vew shows filling-out of the nasolabial fold and slight displacement of the left ala of the nose.
Right: Intraoperative view of the cyst shown on the left. (Fig. 4-7 from Fascicle 29, Third Series.)

Figure 4-7

NASOLABIAL CYST

Photomicrograph demonstrates metaplastic cyst epithelium with mucous cells.

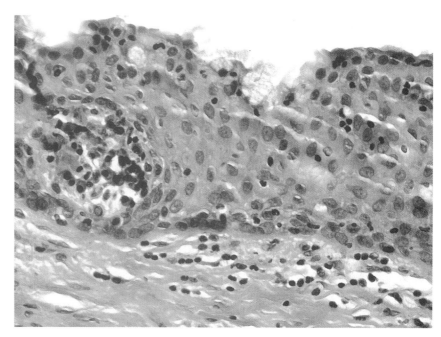

or static lesions presenting as a radiolucency with a well-corticated border.

Microscopic Findings. The cystic lumen is lined by pseudostratified ciliated columnar epithelium and mucous goblet cells characteristic of maxillary sinus lining (fig. 4-8). Occasional areas of squamous metaplasia and secondary inflammation are identified. Dysplastic epithelium has also been reported (21). Although seldom necessary for diagnosis, a characteristic electrophoretic pattern of glycosaminoglycans from fluid aspirates has been reported (23).

Treatment and Prognosis. Surgical enucleation is the treatment of choice and recurrent lesions are not expected. Marsupialization is also an effective treatment (24).

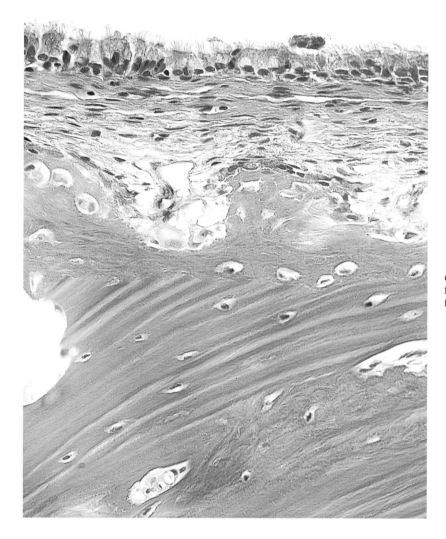

Figure 4-8

SURGICAL CILIATED CYST

A cyst wall lined by ciliated columnar epithelium is separated from the maxillary alveolar bone by fibrovascular connective tissue.

REFERENCES

1. Allard RH. Naso-palatine duct cyst. Int J Oral Surg 1981;10(Suppl 1):131-133.
2. Daley TD, Wysocki GP, Pringle GA. Relative incidence of odontogenic tumors and oral and jaw cysts in a Canadian population. Oral Surg Oral Med Oral Pathol 1994;77:276-280.
3. Anneroth G, Hall G, Stuge U. Nasopalatine duct cyst. Int J Oral Maxillofac Surg 1986;15:572-580.
4. Swanson KS, Kaugars GE, Gunsolley JC. Nasopalatine duct cyst: an analysis of 334 cases. J Oral Maxillofac Surg 1991;49:268-271.
5. Damm DD, Lu RJ, Rhoton RC. Concurrent nasopalatine duct cyst and bilateral mesiodens. Oral Surg Oral Med Oral Pathol 1988;65:264-265.
6. el-Bardaie A, Nikai H, Takata T. Pigmented nasopalatine duct cyst. Report of 2 cases. Int J Oral Maxillofac Surg 1989;18:138-139.
7. Takeda Y. Intra-osseous squamous cell carcinoma of the maxilla: probably arisen from non-odontogenic epithelium. Br J Oral Maxillofac Surg 1991;29:392-394.
8. Takagi R, Ohashi Y, Suzuki M. Squamous cell carcinoma in the maxilla probably originating from a nasopalatine duct cyst: report of case. J Oral Maxillofac Surg 1996;54:112-115.

9. Tanaka S, Iida S, Murakami S, Kishino M, Yamada C, Okura M. Extensive nasopalatine duct cyst causing nasolabial protrusion. Oral Surg Oral Med Oral Pathol Oral Radiol Endod 2008;106:e46-50.

10. Barzilai M. Case report: bilateral nasoalveolar cysts. Clin Radiol 1994;49:140-141.

11. Adams A, Lovelock DJ. Nasolabial cyst. Oral Surg Oral Med Oral Pathol 1985;60:118-119.

12. Camerlinck M, Vanhoenacker FM, Demuynck K. Nasolabial cyst. JBR-BTR 2008;91:268.

13. Aquilino RN, Bazzo VJ, Faria RJ, Eid NL, Boscolo FN. Nasolabial cyst: presentation of a clinical case with CT and MR images. Braz J Otorhinolaryngol 2008;74:467-471.

14. Sumer AP, Celenk P, Sumer M, Telcioglu NT, Gunhan O. Nasolabial cyst: case report with CT and MRI findings. Oral Surg Oral Med Oral Pathol Oral Radiol Endod 2010;109:e92-4.

15. Aikawa T, Iida S, Fukuda Y, et al. Nasolabial cyst in a patient with cleft lip and palate. Int J Oral Maxillofac Surg 2008;37:874-876.

16. Lopez-Rios F, Lassaletta-Atienza L, Domingo-Carrasco C, Martinez-Tello FJ. Nasolabial cyst: report of a case with extensive apocrine change. Oral Surg Oral Med Oral Pathol Oral Radiol Endod 1997;84:404-406.

17. Chao WC, Huang CC, Chang PH, Chen YL, Chen CW, Lee TJ. Management of nasolabial cysts by transnasal endoscopic marsupialization. Arch Otolaryngol Head Neck Surg 2009;135:932-935.

18. Hayhurst DL, Moenning JE, Summerlin DJ, Bussard DA. Surgical ciliated cyst: a delayed complication in a case of maxillary orthognathic surgery. J Oral Maxillofac Surg 1993;51:705-8; discussion 708-9.

19. Cano J, Campo J, Alobera MA, Baca R. Surgical ciliated cyst of the maxilla. Clinical case. Med Oral Patol Oral Cir Bucal 2009;14:E361-4.

20. Kaneshiro S, Nakajima T, Yoshikawa Y, Iwasaki H, Tokiwa N. The postoperative maxillary cyst: report of 71 cases. J Oral Surg 1981;39:191-198.

21. Yamamoto H, Takagi M. Clinicopathologic study of the postoperative maxillary cyst. Oral Surg Oral Med Oral Pathol 1986;62:544-548.

22. Miller R, Longo J, Houston G. Surgical ciliated cyst of the maxilla. J Oral Maxillofac Surg 1988;46:310-312.

23. Smith G, Smith AJ, Basu MK, Rippin JW. The analysis of fluid aspirate glycosaminoglycans in diagnosis of the postoperative maxillary cyst (surgical ciliated cyst). Oral Surg Oral Med Oral Pathol 1988;65:222-224.

24. Yoshikawa Y, Nakajima T, Kaneshiro S, Sakaguchi M. Effective treatment of the postoperative maxillary cyst by marsupialization. J Oral Maxillofac Surg 1982;40:487-491.

5 IDIOPATHIC AND DEVELOPMENTAL ABNORMALITIES

IDIOPATHIC BONE CAVITY (SIMPLE BONE CYST, TRAUMATIC BONE CYST, HEMORRHAGIC BONE CYST, SOLITARY BONE CYST)

Definition. *Idiopathic bone cavities* are common lesions involving the mandible. As the names imply, they are of unknown cause.

Clinical Features. These lesions characteristically involve individuals under 20 years of age and are reported more often in males. The mandibular molar and premolar regions are the most common sites. A recent study suggested these cavities may be causally related to orthodontic treatment, but since these asymptomatic lesions are often noted on dental panoramic radiographs made for young people undergoing orthodontics, this suggestion may be the result of sampling error (1).

Radiographic Features. Radiographs reveal a unilocular, well-demarcated radiolucency, often with scalloped margins, between the roots of molar and premolar teeth (figs. 5-1, 5-2). The vitality of the teeth are irrelevant since there is no evidence of an inflammatory origin. Even with large lesions greater than 2 cm in radiographic diameter, clinical expansion of the buccal or lingual cortical plates is seldom identified. This is an important factor and can often be used to help clinically differentiate these lesions from true central bony cysts or tumors (2,3).

Microscopic Findings. At the time of surgery, an empty bony cavity lined by fibrous connective tissue and containing inspissated fluid and hemosiderin is found (fig. 5-3). Most surgeons include a portion of the surrounding cortical bone in a biopsy specimen, which should exhibit no microscopic abnormalities (fig. 5-4).

Treatment and Prognosis. The biopsy procedure is all that is necessary for treatment because these lesions characteristically resolve spontaneously. Larger lesions treated with graft material have been reported (4).

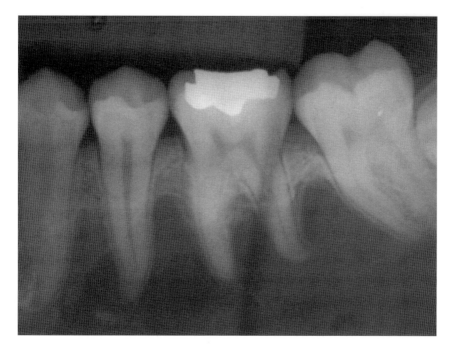

Figure 5-1

IDIOPATHIC BONE CAVITY

An intraoral radiograph shows a well-defined radiolucency that appears to scallop between the roots of multiple teeth.

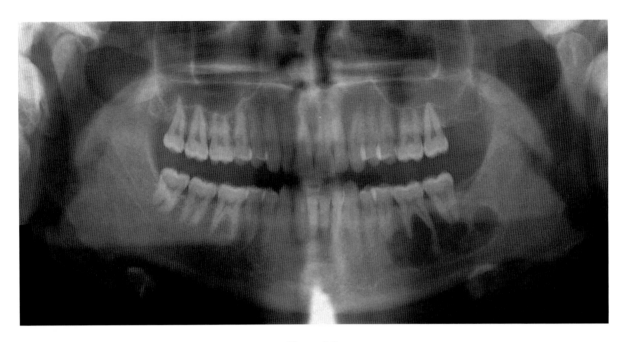

Figure 5-2

IDIOPATHIC BONE CAVITY

A panoramic radiograph shows a well-demarcated radiolucency of the left posterior mandibular body.

Figure 5-3

IDIOPATHIC BONE CAVITY

At surgery, the buccal cortex of the mandible reveals no cyst lining and no tumor.

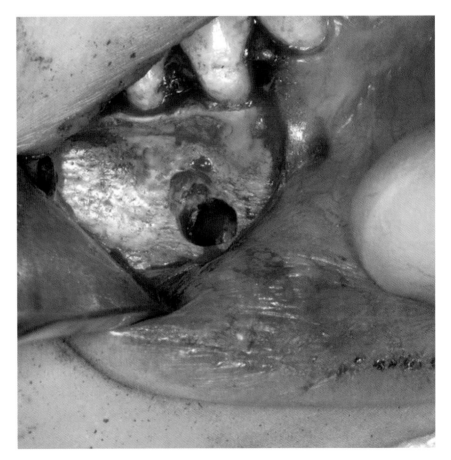

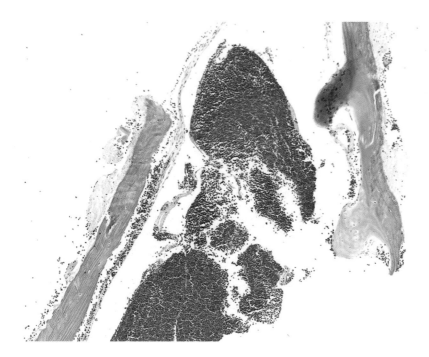

Figure 5-4

IDIOPATHIC BONE CAVITY

Biopsy of the tissue lining the cavity reveals only fibrous connective tissue, hemorrhage, and vital lamellar bone.

LINGUAL SALIVARY GLAND DEFECT (STAFNE BONE DEFECT, LATENT BONE CYST)

Definition. While the *lingual salivary gland defect* appears as a central osseous radiolucency, it is in fact the result of a developmental concavity on the lingual aspect of the mandible. The concavity forms around a portion of the submandibular gland in the posterior mandible or sublingual gland in the anterior mandible. Synonymous terms include *Stafne bone defect, salivary gland depression,* and *latent bone cyst.* These defects have been identified in the jaws of ancient humans (5).

Clinical Features. This entity was first described in 1942 by Stafne (6). It usually presents inferior to the mandibular canal in the molar or premolar region. Fewer examples are identified in the mandibular incisor region (7–9). Multiple concurrent lesions are rare but have been reported (10). Some cases may result in an extraosseous course for the mandibular neurovascular bundle (11).

Radiographic Features. These lesions are well-demarcated radiolucencies with a dense sclerotic corticated border, an indication of their static, developmental nature (figs. 5-5, 5-6). They range in size from 1 to 3 cm in diameter. In most cases, the radiographic features are sufficient for a diagnosis, but advanced imaging

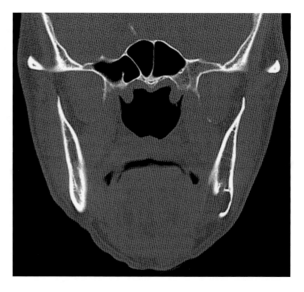

Figure 5-5

LINGUAL SALIVARY GLAND DEFECT

A coronal computerized tomography (CT) image shows an invagination of the lingual cortical plate in the left posterior mandible.

modalities, especially computerized tomography (CT) and magnetic resonance imaging (MRI) scans are useful to access unusual lesions in an effort to avoid unnecessary surgery (fig. 5-7) (12–14). Sialograms also help provide a nonsurgical diagnosis (15,16).

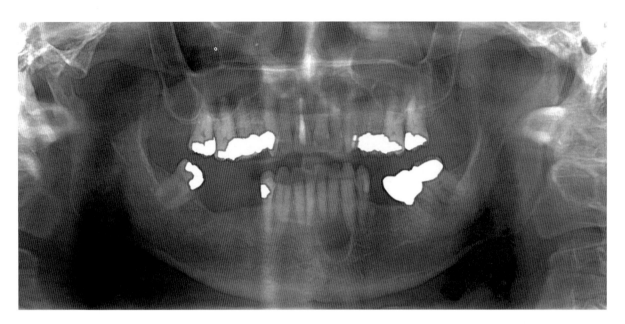

Figure 5-6

LINGUAL SALIVARY GLAND DEFECT

A corticated radiolucency is seen in the anterior mandible near the roots of the teeth.

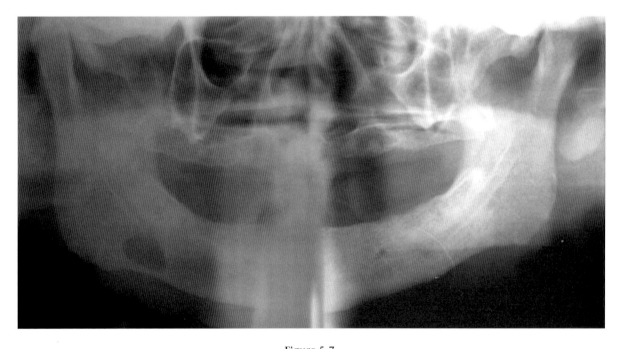

Figure 5-7

LINGUAL SALIVARY GLAND DEFECT

A thickly corticated radiolucency is noted in the right posterior mandible near the inferior border.

Microscopic Findings. While the majority of these lesions are identified by their radiographic features, in some instances, lesions are evaluated microscopically. Soft tissues submitted for microscopic examination include loose fibrous connective tissue, fat, skeletal

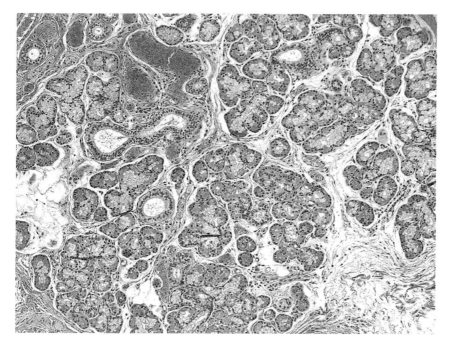

Figure 5-8

LINGUAL SALIVARY GLAND DEFECT

The soft tissue removed from a defect consists of normal salivary gland.

muscle, and normal salivary gland acini (fig. 5-8) (17).

Treatment and Prognosis. Therapeutic management is unnecessary since these lesions are not a true pathologic condition. In the posterior mandible, however, their presence may increase the likelihood of fracture during surgical removal of impacted third molars (18).

REFERENCES

1. Velez I, Siegel MA, Mintz SM, Rolle R. The relationship between idiopathic bone cavity and orthodontic tooth movement: analysis of 44 cases. Dentomaxillofac Radiol 2010;39:162-166.
2. Harris SJ, O Carroll MK, Gordy FM. Idiopathic bone cavity (traumatic bone cyst) with the radiographic appearance of a fibro-osseous lesion. Oral Surg Oral Med Oral Pathol 1992;74:118-123.
3. Manganaro AM. Review of the idiopathic bone cavity of the jaws. Mil Med 1997;162:734-736.
4. Kraut R, Robin C. Idiopathic bone cavity. A report of recurrent lesions and their management. N Y State Dent J 2003;69:30-33.
5. Jordana X, Garcia Sivoli C, Galtes I, Palacios M, Cos M, Malgosa A. Report on a Stafne defect in a man from medieval age. J Oral Maxillofac Surg 2007;65:556-559.
6. Stafne EC. Cavities situated near the angle of the mandible. J Am Dent Assoc 1942;29:1969-72.
7. Apruzzese D, Longoni S. Stafne cyst in an anterior location. J Oral Maxillofac Surg 1999;57:333-338.
8. Katz J, Chaushu G, Rotstein I. Stafne's bone cavity in the anterior mandible: a possible diagnostic challenge. J Endod 2001;27:304-307.
9. de Courten A, Kuffer R, Samson J, Lombardi T. Anterior lingual mandibular salivary gland defect (Stafne defect) presenting as a residual cyst. Oral Surg Oral Med Oral Pathol Oral Radiol Endod 2002;94:460-464.
10. Boyle CA, Horner K, Coulthard P, Fleming GJ. Multiple Stafne bone cavities: a diagnostic dilemma. Dent Update 2000;27:494-497.
11. Reuter I. An unusual case of Stafne bone cavity with extra-osseous course of the mandibular neurovascular bundle. Dentomaxillofac Radiol 1998;27:189-191.

12. Branstetter BF, Weissman JL, Kaplan SB. Imaging of a Stafne bone cavity: what MR adds and why a new name is needed. AJNR Am J Neuroradiol 1999;20:587-589.

13. Ogunsalu C, Pillai K, Barclay S. Radiological assessment of type II Stafne idiopathic bone cyst in a patient undergoing implant therapy: a case report. West Indian Med J 2006;55:447-450.

14. Sisman Y, Etoz OA, Mavili E, Sahman H, Tarim Ertas E. Anterior Stafne bone defect mimicking a residual cyst: a case report. Dentomaxillofac Radiol 2010;39:124-126.

15. Quesada-Gómez C, Valmaseda-Castellón E, Berini-Aytés L, Gay-Escoda C. Stafne bone cavity: a retrospective study of 11 cases. Med Oral Patol Oral Cir Bucal 2006;11:E277-80.

16. Segev Y, Puterman M, Bodner L. Stafne bone cavity—magnetic resonance imaging. Med Oral Patol Oral Cir Bucal 2006;11:E345-7.

17. Krafft T, Eggert J, Karl M. A Stafne bone defect in the anterior mandible—a diagnostic dilemma. Quintessence Int 2010;41:391-393

18. Kao YH, Huang IY, Chen CM, Wu CW, Hsu KJ, Chen CM. Late mandibular fracture after lower third molar extraction in a patient with Stafne bone cavity: a case report. J Oral Maxillofac Surg 2010;68:1698-1700.

EPITHELIAL ODONTOGENIC NEOPLASMS

AMELOBLASTOMA

Intraosseous Ameloblastoma

Definition. *Ameloblastoma* is a neoplasm that recapitulates enamel organ development during tooth crown formation. Phenotyping and in situ hybridization analysis of messenger RNA have shown that amelogenin, a gene transcribed solely by differentiated ameloblasts, is expressed by the tumor cells of ameloblastomas (1). These neoplasms are entirely epithelial, originating from reduced enamel epithelium of the follicle, epithelial rests, the lining of an odontogenic cyst, or possibly, the basal cells of the overlying alveolar mucosa.

Since its early description, the similarity of ameloblastoma with other tumors of neural crest origin, including craniopharyngioma, has been reported (2,3). Three main clinical types exist: *intraosseous*, sometimes referred to as *solid* or *multicystic*; *unicystic*; and *peripheral*. Features of the intraosseous neoplasm are discussed here. The unicystic and peripheral variants, because of behavioral and prognostic differences, are discussed separately.

General Features. Ameloblastomas comprised 11.7 percent of 1,088 odontogenic neoplasms in one evaluation (4). If odontomas are considered to be hamartomas, ameloblastomas became the most common odontogenic neoplasm in the survey, accounting for 48.5 percent.

Intraosseous ameloblastomas occur in all tooth-forming locations of the jaws, although most (80 percent) occur in the mandible. The desmoplastic variant of ameloblastoma is more common in the maxilla and anterior portions of the jaws. The overall ratio of ameloblastoma in the mandible versus the maxilla is about 5 to 1. Patient age ranges from 2 to 92 years, with a median age of 35. The distribution among males and females is approximately equal. Tumors of the mandible occur in younger patients than tumors of the maxilla (5,6).

Clinical Features. A painless swelling or expansion of the buccal cortical plate is the most common clinical presentation. As with other odontogenic tumors and cysts, ameloblastomas are usually asymptomatic unless secondarily inflamed. Perforation of the cortex, although reported, is not a common finding. Although infiltrative at the margins, there is seldom any paresthesia. The tumor is more aggressive than most other odontogenic tumors, however, its growth rate is slow. Tumors are often first identified on radiographs made for other reasons such as caries or third molar assessment. Due to the lack of symptoms and slow growth, patients seldom self-identify these neoplasms.

Radiographic Features. Small ameloblastomas appear as unilocular radiolucencies with well-demarcated, corticated borders, indistinguishable from other benign tumors or cysts of the jaws. Larger lesions may show a "soap bubble" or honeycomb, multilocular appearance (fig. 6-1). The roots of adjacent teeth may be pushed aside by the expanding tumor, or may show evidence of resorption. Impacted or unerupted teeth developing adjacent to an ameloblastoma are often displaced as the tumor expands. Ameloblastomas forming in the dental follicle prevent the eruption of the tooth. Recurrent lesions show similar radiographic findings (fig. 6-2).

These radiographic features are characteristic of all histolopathologic variants except for some desmoplastic ameloblastomas. Desmoplastic ameloblastomas that are more than 2 cm in diameter often have a mixed radiolucent-radiopaque appearance, probably due primarily to the density of collagen. This feature can often lead to an initial impression that the lesion is an alternative odontogenic neoplasm capable of mineralization, such as an adenomatoid odontogenic tumor, ameloblastic fibro-odontoma, or even a benign fibro-osseous lesion such as a cemento-ossifying fibroma.

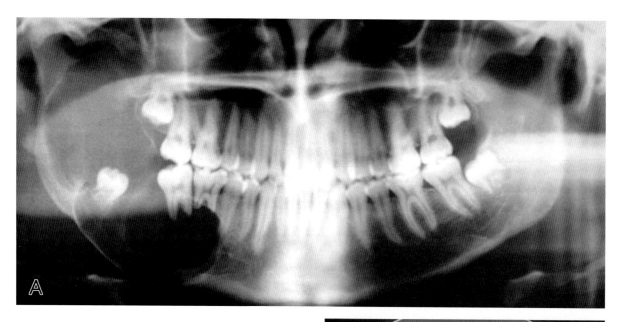

Figure 6-1

AMELOBLASTOMA

A: A large well-circumscribed radiolucency involves the right ramus and body of the mandible. It displaces the third molar and resorbs the roots of the first and second molars.

B: An axial computerized tomography (CT) scan shows a well-circumscribed radiolucency of the right posterior mandible with buccal and lingual expansion surrounding a molar tooth.

C: A well-demarcated radiolucency of the left third molar region with pathologic fracture of the mandible is seen.

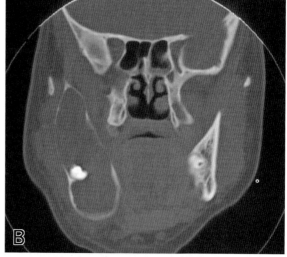

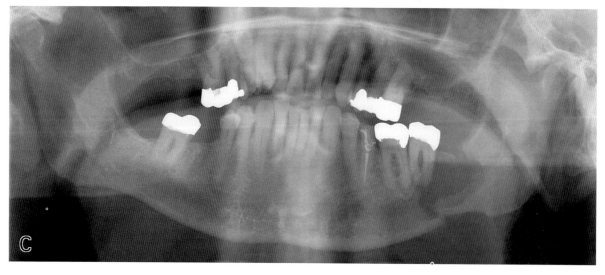

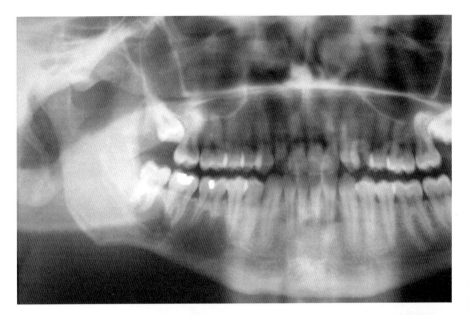

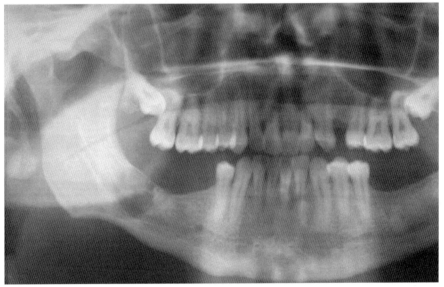

Figure 6-2

**AMELOBLASTOMA
AND RECURRENCE**

Top: A well-demarcated radiolucency of the right posterior mandible involves the roots of the molar teeth. The tumor was excised, the tooth removed, and the bony defect curetted.

Bottom: One year later, a progressive radiolucency was identified. The biopsy revealed recurrent ameloblastoma.

Gross Findings. Incisional biopsies fixed in formalin appear as solid, gray-tan soft tissues. Some tumors have large or small cystic spaces. In resected specimens, the tumors appear well demarcated from the surrounding bone, even though marginal infiltration into bone or soft tissue is often encountered during microscopic examination (fig. 6-3).

Microscopic Findings. The classic features of ameloblastoma were described by Vickers and Gorlin (3). These features include columnar palisading basal cells, hyperchromatic nuclei polarized away from the basement membrane, and focal vacuolization of the cytoplasm. The columnar cells often surround epithelium that can appear identical to the stellate reticulum of the enamel organ, with squamous cells with keratinization, basal cells, or granular cells.

Although there are multiple microscopic subtypes of intraosseous ameloblastoma, the subtype has no bearing on the prognosis. Many tumors show a combination of histopathologic patterns. The subtypes of intraosseous ameloblastoma include: *follicular, acanthomatous, plexiform, granular cell, basal cell,* and *desmoplastic.*

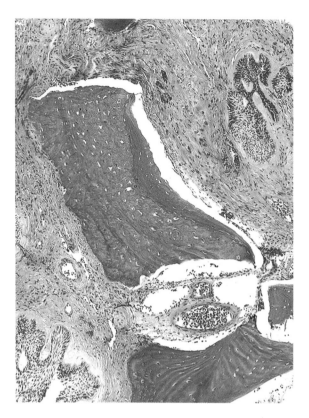 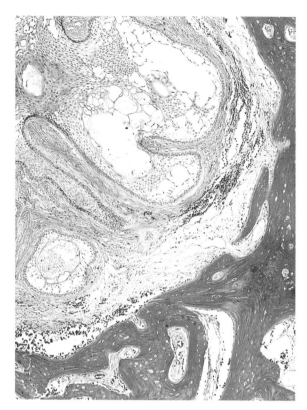

Figure 6-3

AMELOBLASTOMA INFILTRATION

Left: Islands of desmoplastic ameloblastoma infiltrate trabecular bone at the margin of the tumor.
Right: Follicular ameloblastoma islands at the tumor margin are in close proximity to medullary bone trabeculae.

Follicular. Follicular ameloblastoma is the most common variant and most closely resembles embryonic tooth-forming structures. Large and small epithelial islands, in a background of loose and dense fibrocollagenous connective tissue, show a peripheral layer of columnar palisaded cells which resemble ameloblasts (fig. 6-4). The nuclei of these columnar cells are polarized centrally, oriented away from the peripheral basement membrane. This feature gives rise to the term "reverse polarity" in reference to secretory cells in exocrine glands which have nuclei polarized away from the central lumen. These columnar cells also show cytoplasmic clearing and vacuolization. While the nucleus may appear hyperchromatic, there should be little, if any, mitotic activity. The central portions of the epithelial islands show a loose arrangement of stellate epithelial cells reminiscent of embryonic stellate reticulum. Microcyst formation is common in this subtype. Other cell types, including mucous cells, are rarely seen (7).

Acanthomatous. This microscopic subtype is identical to the follicular variant, but includes extensive areas of squamous metaplasia in areas normally occupied by stellate reticulum–like cells (figs. 6-5, 6-6). Keratin pearls are often noted. These features can be extensive in some tumors, giving the impression of a squamous malignancy at low power. The lack of marked nuclear atypia or mitotic activity and the presence of the peripheral columnar cell arrangement should clearly differentiate these two neoplasms. *Keratoameloblastoma* describes ameloblastomas with extensive keratinization of the islands central to the peripheral ameloblasts (fig. 6-7)

Plexiform. This histologic variant is the second most common after the follicular pattern. The plexiform variant shows long anastomosing double columns and sheets of cuboidal or

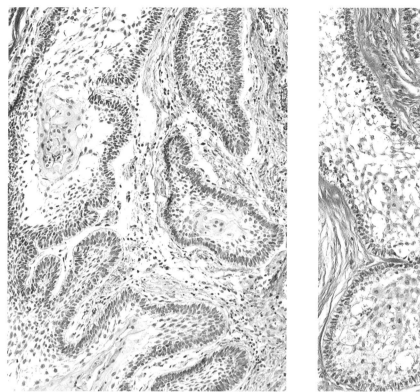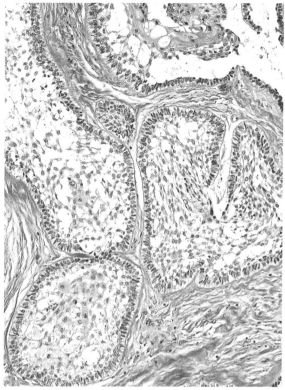

Figure 6-4

FOLLICULAR AMELOBLASTOMA

Left: Large and small epithelial islands made up predominantly of stellate cells are rimmed focally by tall columnar cells with centrally polarized, hyperchromatic nuclei.

Right: The peripheral ameloblasts show centrally polarized nuclei and vacuolated cytoplasm.

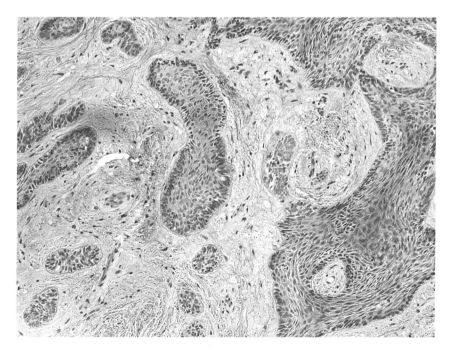

Figure 6-5

ACANTHOMATOUS AMELOBLASTOMA

Islands of primarily squamous epithelium are rimmed focally by columnar ameloblasts.

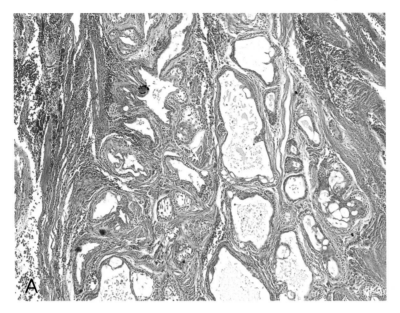

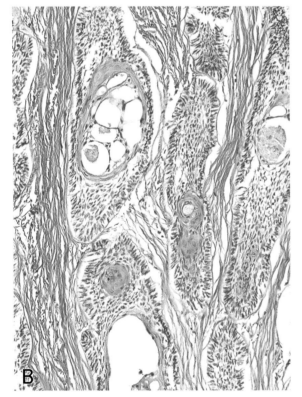

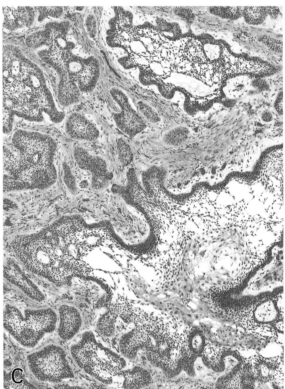

Figure 6-6

ACANTHOMATOUS AMELOBLASTOMA

A: Islands rimmed focally by columnar cells with centrally polarized nuclei show keratinocyte metaplasia and cystic degeneration.

B: Islands of stellate reticulum-like or squamous epithelial cells are rimmed by columnar ameloblasts with hyperchromatic nuclei.

C: Epithelial islands with peripheral rims of columnar cells border central stellate and squamous epithelium with keratinization.

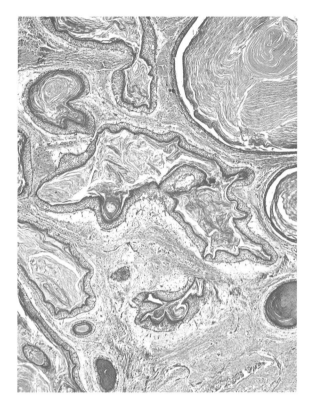

Figure 6-7

KERATOAMELOBLASTOMA

Islands rimed by columnar and cuboidal epithelial cells show central parakeratin formation.

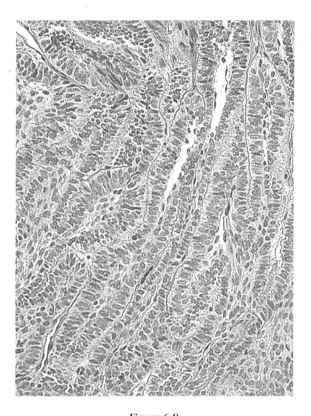

Figure 6-8

PLEXIFORM AMELOBLASTOMA

Double strands of tall columnar epithelial cells with centrally polarized nuclei surround foci of stellate epithelial cells with squamous metaplasia.

columnar epithelial cells with centrally polarized hyperchromatic nuclei and little or no evidence of stellate reticulum differentiation (fig. 6-8). In areas, the double columns separate to surround a variety of epithelial cell types (fig. 6-9).

Granular Cell. The granular cell pattern has varying numbers of eosinophilic, cytoplasmic granules (lysosomes) centrally within the follicular epithelial islands, or within the columnar and cuboidal cells of the follicular or plexiform variants (fig. 6-10). Peripheral columnar and cuboidal cells retain their reverse polarity and focal cytoplasmic vacuolization.

Basal Cell. The basal cell pattern is the least common variant. Small, ovoid, basal-like cells are in areas of the follicular epithelial islands normally occupied by stellate reticulum–like cells (fig. 6-11).The resemblance to some forms of basal cell carcinoma of skin can be striking. Basal cell ameloblastomas are more common as a peripheral ameloblastoma variant.

Desmoplastic. Small nests of tumor cells are present within a very sclerotic and dense collagen background (fig. 6-12). Islands of ameloblastic epithelium show less frequent peripheral palisading, and may appear cuboidal, ovoid, or even squamous, often making evaluation of additional sections necessary to confirm the diagnosis (8). Extensive crush artifact of these islands is often a feature further complicating microscopic analysis. The desmoplasia seen in these ameloblastomas is caused by active de novo synthesis of extracellular matrix proteins (9).

The desmoplastic variant accounts for 4 to 13 percent of all ameloblastomas and has differing epidemiologic and clinical features compared to the other intraosseous variants. The average age at initial diagnosis is slightly higher, at 42.9 years, than for patients with other intraosseous ameloblastomas. The male to female ratio is equal and they occur with equal frequency in the maxilla and mandible (10).

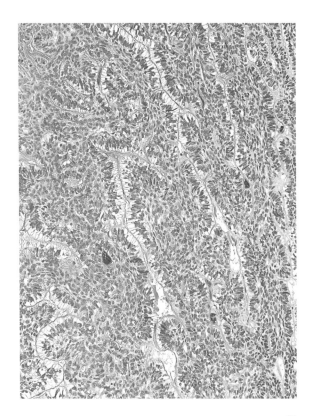 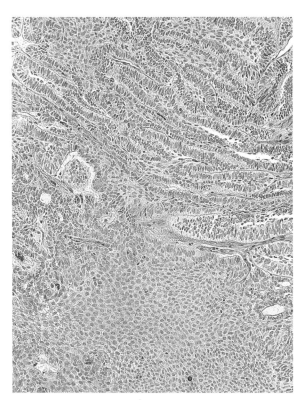

Figure 6-9

PLEXIFORM/ACANTHOMATOUS AMELOBLASTOMA

Left: Trabeculae of columnar cells with vesicular cytoplasm border sheets of squamous epithelium.
Right: Double-stranded trabeculae of columnar cells border sheets of squamous epithelium.

The term *mural ameloblastoma* describes islands of ameloblastoma in the fibrous wall of an odontogenic cyst, or a unicystic ameloblastoma (see fig. 6-18, Unicystic Ameloblastoma). Most evidence suggests that these lesions are best treated as solid ameloblastomas, and the modifier is seldom utilized (11).

The subtypes described above seldom, if ever, dominate an entire tumor. Many tumors show features of two or three subtypes (fig. 6-13) (12). Fortunately, no subtype or combination of subtypes has been shown to have clinically significant differences in behavior or prognosis.

Schafer et al. (13) have reported extragnathic ameloblastomas originating in the sinonasal tract. There were 5 females and 19 males with an age range of 43 to 81 years, and a mean age at presentation of 59.7 years. Unilateral opacification of the maxillary sinus (n = 12) was the most common radiographic finding. Fifteen ameloblastomas seemed to be derived from surface epithelium.

Immunohistochemical and Ultrastructural Findings. Many studies have shed light on the nature and aggressive local behavior of ameloblastomas. CD34, used to evaluate angiogenesis, has shown microvessel density to be significantly higher in ameloblastomas when compared to keratocystic odontogenic tumors and dentigerous cysts (14). Studies involving proliferating cell nuclear antigen (PCNA) and *p53* gene status and expression in ameloblastomas, malignant ameloblastomas, and tooth germs have suggested that *p53* mutation plays a role in neoplastic changes of odontogenic epithelium (15,16). Murine double minute 2 (MDM2), which is able to physically associate with p53 tumor suppressor gene and block growth suppressive functions, has increased expression in ameloblastoma, especially in the basal cell variants (17). Expression of Ki-67 as a measure of proliferation is higher in follicular variants compared to plexiform or unicystic variants (18). The proliferation index of ameloblastomas, as measured using proliferating cell

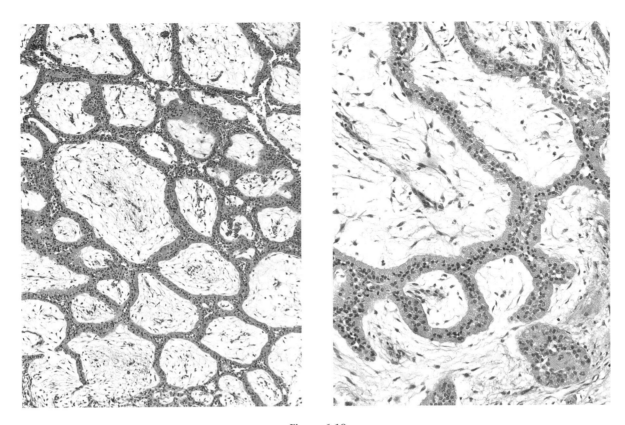

Figure 6-10

GRANULAR CELL AMELOBLASTOMA

Left: Epithelial cells are arranged in anastomosing, double-stranded trabeculae.

Right: Columnar and cuboidal epithelial cells arranged in double-stranded trabeculae show eosinophilic granular cytoplasm.

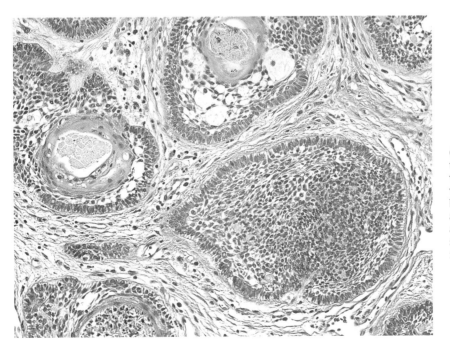

Figure 6-11

BASAL CELL AMELOBLASTOMA

An island of ameloblastoma (lower right) has a periphery of typical columnar ameloblasts with central polarized nuclei and vesicular cytoplasm surrounding basaloid cells with ovoid nuclei and scant cytoplasm. Adjacent are three islands with classic stellate reticulum and squamous metaplasia.

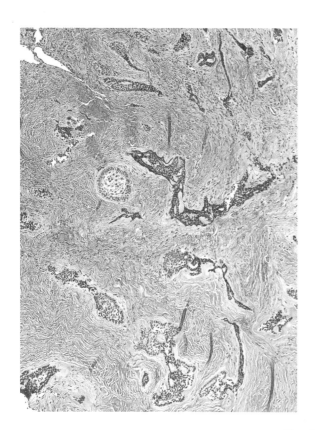
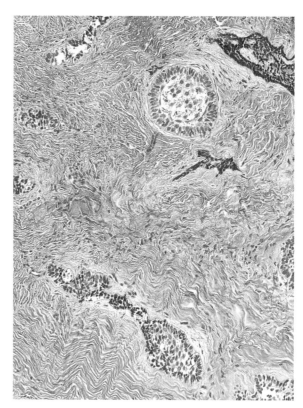

Figure 6-12

DESMOPLASTIC AMELOBLASTOMA

Left: Nests, strands, and islands of epithelial cells are scattered throughout dense collagenous connective tissue.

Right: At higher power, some islands and strands show evidence of columnar ameloblastic differentiation and surround stellate reticulum–like cells.

Figure 6-13

BIPHASIC AMELOBLASTOMA

Foci of plexiform and follicular ameloblastoma are seen.

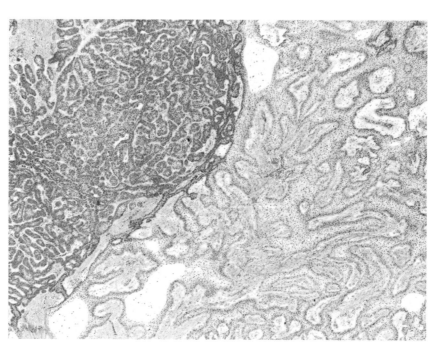

nuclear antigen monoclonal antibody (clone IPO 38), is similar to keratocystic odontogenic tumors, with increased activity in the peripheral columnar cells (19).

Studies involving metalloproteinases 1, 2, and 9 in ameloblastomas suggest these may play a part in tumor growth and progression (20). Expression of E-cadherin and beta-catenin is similar in tooth germs, and unicystic and solid ameloblastomas (21). A study of alpha5 beta1 integrin suggests that it may be a contributor to the local invasiveness of ameloblastomas (22). Acanthomatous, follicular, and unicystic ameloblastomas have shown integrin staining patterns similar to the adult oral mucosa while plexiform ameloblastomas staining was similar to the dental lamina (23). Calponin stains are positive in most ameloblastomas (24).

Calretinin, a calcium-binding protein that is expressed in cells of the central and peripheral nervous systems as well as in many other normal and pathologic human tissues, is present in over 90 percent of ameloblastomas (25,26). The protein is almost always restricted to the stellate reticulum–like epithelium. Since keratocystic odontogenic tumors show no calretinin staining this has been suggested as a useful marker to differentiate these tumors from cystic ameloblastomas.

The *Notch* gene family, already identified in plexiform and follicular ameloblastomas, may play a role in the tissue-specific cellular characteristics of desmoplastic ameloblastomas (27). Desmoplastic variants have been shown to have a lower Ki-67 proliferation index and higher levels of syndecan-1 expression compared to other ameloblastomas (28).

New research involving the inhibition of neoplastic signaling pathways such as the sonic hedgehog and PI3K/Akt/mTOR could eventually lead to methods of nonsurgical management for ameloblastomas (29).

Treatment and Prognosis. Gardner (30,31) pointed out two important issues to consider for the proper surgical management of ameloblastomas. First is the tumor's ability to infiltrate medullary bone and inability to infiltrate compact bone. The second is the location of the tumor. Dense compact bone, such as that of the inferior border of the mandible or ramus, acts as a first-line barrier to prevent tumor spread. The periosteum is a secondary barrier (44). In the maxilla, only a thin cortical plate exists between contiguous bones and is generally thought of as a poor barrier to prevent the spread of ameloblastomas (32,33).

Many reports regarding the treatment of ameloblastoma indicate significant recurrence rates following simple curettage, ranging from 30 to 90 percent (34–39). Despite some reports of successful treatment with enucleation and curettage (40,41), the standard treatment for intraosseous ameloblastomas in most centers is to include 1 cm of normal tissue beyond the radiographic margin (42,43). Unfortunately, there are no well-controlled studies comparing the resected specimen dimensions with presurgical radiographs or correlating the actual microscopic tumor margin with the radiographic margin (32). Whether ameloblastoma invades nerve bundles, including the mandibular nerve, is controversial (44), but Nakamura et al. (40,45) suggest that a conservative approach in preserving the inferior alveolar nerve is recommended when possible.

Hong et al. (39) reported on the surgical management outcomes of 305 cases of ameloblastoma (239 patients: males,139; females, 100). Segmental resection or maxillectomy was performed in 22 patients, resection with bone margin was performed in 43 patients, and more conservative treatment was carried out in 174 patients. Recurrences were observed in 57 patients. These included 1 patient who underwent segmental resection, 5 patients who were treated by resection with bone margin, and 51 patients who had more conservative treatment.

More than 10 cases of recurrent ameloblastoma in bone grafts have been published. A single recurrence 16 years after initial surgery was published by Martins and Favaro (46). They concluded that the recurrence most likely arose from the soft tissues peripheral to the tumor, including the adjacent periosteum. In his published evaluation of the Reichart retrospective analysis of 3,677 cases of ameloblastoma in 1995 (5), Gardner (47) suggested that additional knowledge regarding the biologic profile of ameloblastomas would necessitate large, long-term prospective studies.

Unicystic Ameloblastoma

Definition. *Unicystic ameloblastomas* are unilocular cystic lesions lined by ameloblastomatous epithelium (48). To qualify as a unicystic ameloblastoma, the lesion must be unilocular

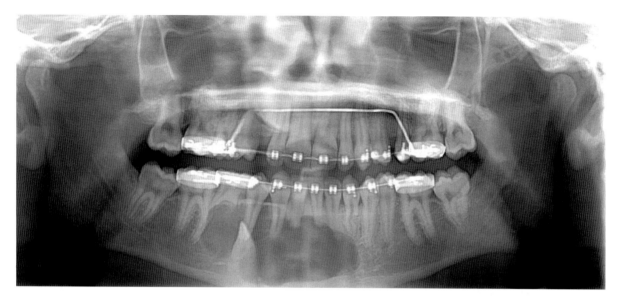

Figure 6-14

UNICYSTIC AMELOBLASTOMA

A well-demarcated radiolucency of the right anterior mandible suggestive of a dentigerous cyst is associated with the crown of an impacted tooth.

radiographically and have a single cystic lining microscopically. Because the treatment and clinical course of solid intraosseous ameloblastoma and unicystic ameloblastoma are different, distinction is vitally important.

Clinical Features. Unicystic ameloblastomas account for approximately 5 to 15 percent of all ameloblastomas and generally occur in younger patients when compared to solid or multicystic intraosseous ameloblastomas (5,49–52). In an evaluation of 193 published cases, Philipsen et al. (53) found the average age at diagnosis was 16.5 years. Most tumors occurred in the mandible and over 50 percent occurred in association with an impacted or unerupted tooth. As with other odontogenic cysts and tumors, unicystic ameloblastomas are usually asymptomatic unless secondarily inflamed.

Prior to 1981, cases of dentigerous cyst showing a plexiform epithelial pattern resembling some cases of intraosseous ameloblastoma were difficult to classify and were often felt to be the result of simple hyperplasia. However, in an evaluation of 19 cases, Gardner et al. (54) coined the term *plexiform unicystic ameloblastoma* to describe these lesions as a variant of unicystic ameloblastoma. An additional 10 cases were published in 1983 and 28 examples in 1984

(55–57). Most were diagnosed in the second or third decade and were located in the posterior mandible. Initially, some felt this entity represented mural and luminal ameloblastomatous change in a preexisting cyst.

In an evaluation of 57 unicystic ameloblastomas by Ackermann et al. (58), 30 occurred in males and 23 in females of a mean age at diagnosis of 24 years. The lesions were classified histologically into three groups: group 1 (42 percent), a cyst lined by ameloblastomatous epithelium; group 2 (9 percent), a cyst showing intraluminal plexiform proliferation of epithelium; and group 3 (49 percent), a cyst with mural invasion of epithelium into the cyst wall in either a follicular or plexiform pattern.

Radiographic Features. Unicystic ameloblastomas present as radiolucent, unilocular lesions, with well-demarcated, corticated borders, indistinguishable from most other odontogenic cysts or tumors (fig. 6-14). As with other slow-growing odontogenic neoplasms and cysts, unicystic ameloblastomas usually displace normal anatomy, such as tooth roots, although resorption is also seen. When the tumors develop in association with a tooth follicle they appear identical to dentigerous cysts. The nonspecific radiographic appearance clearly justifies submission of

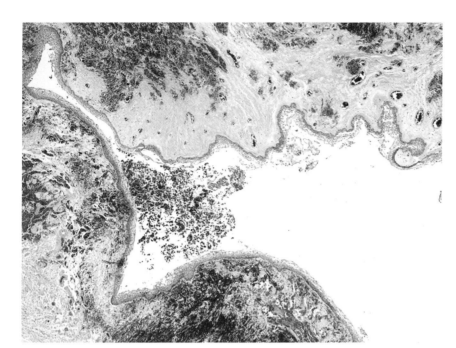

Figure 6-15

UNICYSTIC AMELOBLASTOMA

At low power, a cystic lumen is surrounded by dense fibrovascular connective tissue.

periapical and pericoronal soft tissues for microscopic examination (59,60).

In an evaluation of unicystic ameloblastomas versus keratocystic odontogenic tumors using contrast-enhanced magnetic resonance imaging (MRI), unicystic ameloblastomas showed low signal intensity on T1-weighted images and high signal intensity on T2-weighted images, with thick rim-enhancement sometimes including small intraluminal nodules (61). These features suggest a unicystic ameloblastoma prior to surgical biopsy.

Gross Findings. Most unicystic ameloblastomas are indistinguishable grossly from other cysts of the jaws. Intraluminal outgrowths may be present but are not pathognomonic.

Microscopic Findings. The microscopic features summarized by Vickers and Gorlin (3) for follicular variants of solid tumors are found focally in unicystic ameloblastomas. These features include palisading of basal cells and polarization of the nuclei away from the basement membrane zone, hyperchromasia of the nuclei of the basal cells, vacuolization of the cytoplasm of the basal cells, and a stratum spinosum showing cells with a loose, sometimes fusiform configuration similar to the stratum intermedium or stellate reticulum of a developing tooth (figs. 6-15, 6-16). In many unicystic ameloblastomas, much of the cystic lining is

not diagnostic, but a careful search, sometimes including additional sections, reveals the microscopic features necessary for diagnosis (62).

The plexiform unicystic variant shows luminal tufts of anastomosing double columns and sheets of cuboidal or columnar epithelium, central polarization of hyperchromatic nuclei, and little or no evidence of stellate reticulum differentiation. These features are identical to those of the multicystic plexiform variant of intraosseous ameloblastoma (fig. 6-17).

A report of hard tissue, identified as dentin in the connective tissue wall of a plexiform variant, has been published (63). Another published case showed the presence of mucous goblet cells in an otherwise typical unicystic lining epithelium (64).

Secondary inflammation, seen focally in many odontogenic tumors and cysts, alters the diagnostic features of unicystic ameloblastoma in a manner similar to keratocystic odontogenic tumors. Additionally, the identification of islands of ameloblastoma in the fibrous connective tissue wall, so-called *mural ameloblastoma*, is of prognostic significance (fig. 6-18). Many practitioners believe mural growth should be an indication for more aggressive treatment, similar to the intraosseous tumor variants (53,58).

Immunohistochemical Findings. While most of these lesions are identified based on

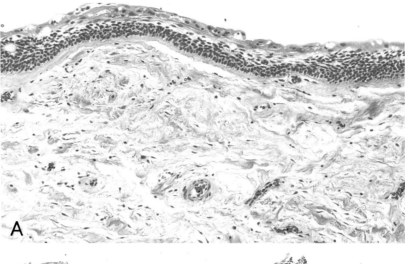

Figure 6-16

UNICYSTIC AMELOBLASTOMA

A: The cyst lumen is lined by epithelium with a prominent basal cell layer, which focally appears columnar with polarized nuclei.

B: The basal cell layer is prominent and the superficial layers are stellate, with evidence of keratin formation.

C: The cystic lining consists of a basal cell layer of columnar cells with nuclei polarized away from the basement membrane. The more superficial epithelial cells resemble stellate reticulum and have focal keratinization.

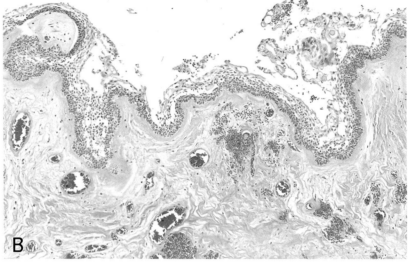

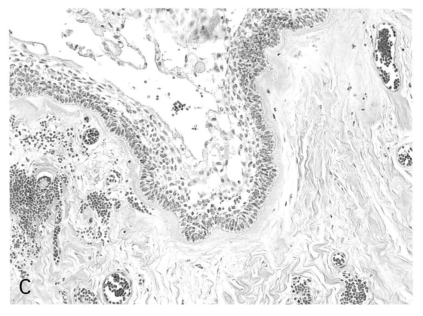

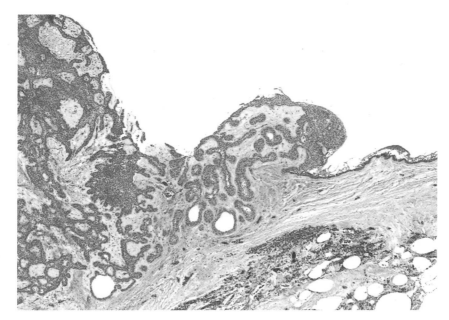

Figure 6-17

PLEXIFORM UNICYSTIC AMELOBLASTOMA

A luminal proliferation consists of double strands of columnar epithelial cells.

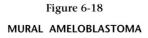

Figure 6-18

MURAL AMELOBLASTOMA

During serial sectioning, a cystic lumen (left) with mural islands of follicular ameloblastoma in the fibrous connective tissue wall (right) is seen.

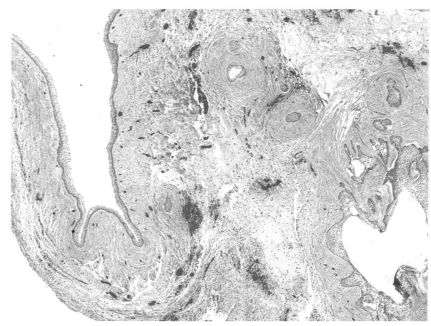

their hematoxylin and eosin (H&E) features, calretinin, a 29-kDa calcium-binding protein expressed in normal human tissues and tumors helps distinguish unicystic ameloblastomas from other cystic lesions. Altini et al. (25) evaluated the lining epithelium in unicystic ameloblastomas, keratocystic odontogenic tumors, residual cysts, and dentigerous cysts for expression of calretinin (65). No positive epithelial staining was observed in any of the cysts, but 81 percent of the unicystic ameloblastomas and 93 percent

of intraosseous or multicystic ameloblastomas showed retention of stain.

Treatment and Prognosis. Unicystic ameloblastoma was separated from the "standard" ameloblastoma by Robinson and Martinez in 1977 (48). The subtitle of that publication included "a prognostically distinct entity," indicating that this type of ameloblastoma deserved separation from intraosseous ameloblastomas. The authors suggested a recurrence rate following conservative enucleation of about 20 percent compared with the published recurrence rates for intraosseous ameloblastomas treated in a similar manner of 55 to 90 percent. The original paper allowed for mural tumor cell islands and radiographic multilocularity, which are now exclusion factors. Two of their three lesions described as "large dentigerous cysts" recurred. Eversole and Leider (66) later used 2-cm size as a cutoff point and found that "cystogenic" ameloblastomas over that size have a propensity to recur with simple enucleation.

In an evaluation of 28 cases treated with enucleation and curettage, 3 recurred (10.7 percent) (56). Connective tissue involvement (mural invasion) is an important predictor of recurrence (5,53,67,68). Unicystic tumors with mural growth should be treated as intraosseous ameloblastomas (58). Philipsen and Reichart (53) arrived at a similar conclusion following a review of 193 cases.

In an evaluation of 100 cases with a minimum of 5 years follow-up, Lau et al. (69) found recurrence rates for all unicystic ameloblastoma variants of 3.6 percent following resection, 30.5 percent following enucleation alone, 16 percent after enucleation followed by application of Carnoy solution, and 18 percent following marsupialization. Covani (70) described an intraluminal unicystic ameloblastoma in a 22-year-old treated with surgical enucleation and osteotomy with use of a piezoelectric knife. Five-year follow-up showed no sign of recurrent tumor.

ADENOMATOID ODONTOGENIC TUMOR

Definition. *Adenomatoid odontogenic tumors* are infrequent odontogenic neoplasms. In past classifications, they have been referred to as *adenoameloblastomas* (71) or *ameloblastic adenomatoid tumors* because of their similarity to ameloblastomas. The microscopic similarity is limited and the behavior of this neoplasm is more like hamartomatous odontomas.

General Features. In a study by Buchner et al. (4) involving 1,088 odontogenic tumors, adenomatoid odontogenic tumors were the third most common tumor following ameloblastomas and myxomas. Depending on the study, the tumors comprise a small portion of all odontogenic tumors, ranging from 2.2 to 7.3 percent (72). The neoplasms are sometimes referred to as the "two-thirds tumor" because about two thirds

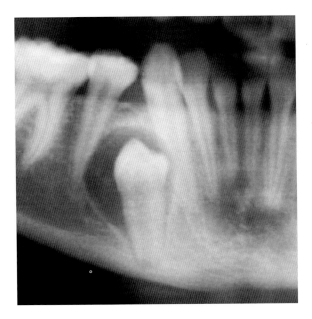

Figure 6-19

ADENOMATOID ODONTOGENIC TUMOR

A well-demarcated, corticated radiolucency is associated with the crown of the impacted mandibular right canine. Faint "snowflake" radiopacities are adjacent to the tooth crown.

occur in females, two thirds are in the maxilla, two thirds are associated with impacted teeth especially the maxillary canines, and two thirds are found in teenagers.

Clinical Features. The neoplasm may occur in any tooth-forming region, but there is a preference for the anterior maxilla (64 percent). The patients are younger than those with ameloblastomas (73,74). Adenomatoid odontogenic tumors have been further classified in terms of their development location, whether follicular or extrafollicular, and whether extraosseous although this has little or no bearing on histopathologic appearance or clinical behavior (72,74).

Radiographic Features. Adenomatoid odontogenic tumors most often appear as unilocular radiolucencies with well-circumscribed, corticated borders indicative of their very slow growth rates. They are often associated with the crowns of unerupted or impacted teeth, especially maxillary canines, leading to the impression that they represent dentigerous cysts (75). Depending on the amount of mineralized tissue within the tumor, small radiopacities often described as "snowflake" in appearance may be seen (fig. 6-19). Similar to other benign tumors

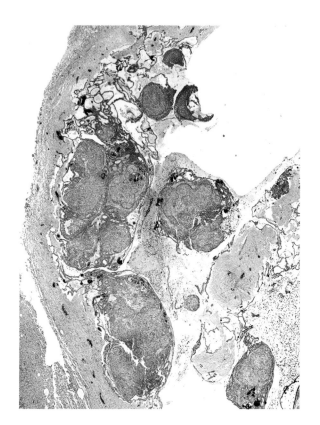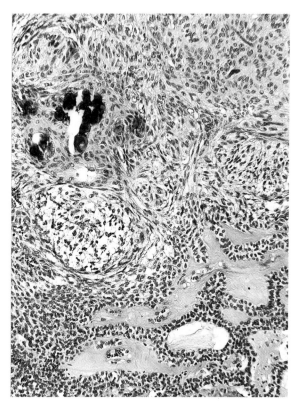

Figure 6-20

ADENOMATOID ODONTOGENIC TUMOR

Left: At low power, the tumors often have a cystic appearance, with islands and nests of epithelial cells surfacing thick, fibrovascular connective tissue.

Right: Trabecular nests and cords of columnar, cuboidal, and spindle cells have hyaline and mineralizations.

and cysts, these slow-growing neoplasms are more likely to displace rather than resorb adjacent anatomy including teeth.

Gross Findings. Adenomatoid odontogenic tumors often appear as cystic cavities, with walls that vary dramatically in thickness. The varying amounts of mineralization may require demineralization prior to final processing and sectioning.

Microscopic Findings. Most adenomatoid odontogenic tumors consist predominantly of spindle-shaped epithelial cells arranged in haphazard whorled masses, sometimes forming small rosettes in a loose fibrovascular stroma (figs. 6-20, 6-21). Duct-like structures lined by cuboidal or columnar epithelial cells are found in varying numbers (fig. 6-22). Foci of amyloid, varying amounts of eosinophilic amorphous material, and dystrophic mineralizations or lamellar psammoma-like bodies are seen (fig. 6-23) (76). Circular arrangements of tall columnar

cells producing enamel-like material are identified (77). Much of the laminated eosinophilic material most likely represents mineralized amyloid (76) or a form of enamel matrix (fig. 6-23) (74,78). Some show focal positive Congo red staining (fig. 6-24). Areas of calcifying epithelial odontogenic tumor–like tissue are commonly identified (79).

Immunohistochemical and Ultrastructural Findings. Adenomatoid odontogenic tumors stain focally for a variety of cytokeratins including 5, 8, 14, 17, and 19 as well as vimentin, and bcl-2 (77). Multiple matrix components, including proteoglycans biglycan and decorin and glycoproteins osteonectin, osteopontin, bone sialoprotein, and osteocalcin have been identified in the eosinophilic amorphous areas and connective tissue foci of adenomatoid odontogenic tumors (80). A low proliferation index observed using Ki-67 could account for the low

Figure 6-21

**ADENOMATOID
ODONTOGENIC TUMOR**

Large and small duct-like
structures are in a background of
spindle cells forming nests and
occasional rosettes.

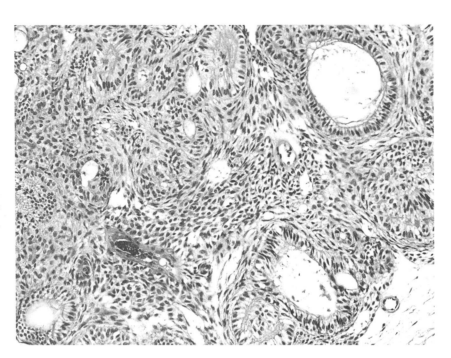

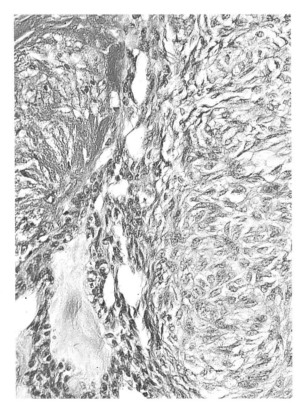
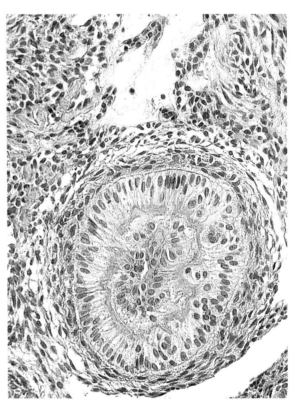

Figure 6-22

ADENOMATOID ODONTOGENIC TUMOR

Left: Sheets of spindle cells and trabeculae of cuboidal cells border eosinophilic mineralized material.

Right: Ovoid and spindle cells surround a duct-like structure that has peripheral palisading of the nuclei and vesicular
cytoplasm.

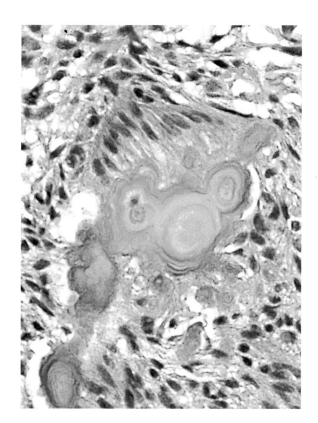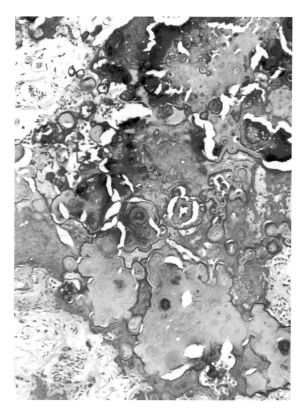

Figure 6-23

ADENOMATOID ODONTOGENIC TUMOR

Left: Annular calcification juxtaposes spindle and columnar epithelial cells.
Right: Calcification is dystrophic in nature and uneven in its distribution.

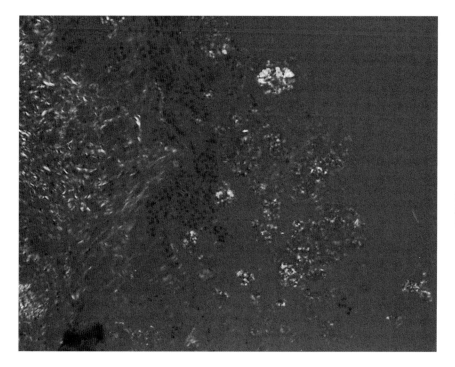

Figure 6-24

ADENOMATOID ODONTOGENIC TUMOR

Under polarized light, Congo red staining shows the apple-green birefringence typical of amyloid.

recurrence rate following conservative treatment (79,81). The absence of hormonal receptor reactivity in adenomatoid odontogenic tumors would seem to exclude hormones as a reason for the observed female predominance (81).

Treatment and Prognosis. Adenomatoid odontogenic tumor is best treated with conservative surgical curettage. These tumors often have a thick, fibrous capsule separating tumor cells from the surrounding bone and making simple curettage easy. Recurrence rates following conservative enucleation are about 2 percent (82).

CALCIFYING EPITHELIAL ODONTOGENIC TUMOR (CALCIFYING ODONTOGENIC TUMOR, PINDBORG TUMOR)

Definition. *Calcifying epithelial odontogenic tumor* is an unusual odontogenic neoplasm characterized by sheets of hyperchromatic, pleomorphic cells with foci of mineralization. The cytologic and morphologic resemblance to any structures identified in embryologic tooth development is minimal.

Clinical Features. The tumor occurs more often in the mandible than the maxilla (ratio of about 2 to 1) usually in the molar-premolar region (83). The tumor most often occurs in the third through fifth decades and can sometimes be seen peripherally as a gingival or alveolar ridge mass (84–86).

In an evaluation of 1,088 odontogenic neoplasms excluding odontomas as hamartomas, calcifying epithelial odontogenic tumors comprised less than 4 percent of the total (4). In an evaluation of 181 cases, Philipsen et al. (87) found that 94 percent of calcifying epithelial odontogenic tumors occurred within bone in patients with a mean age at initial diagnosis of 39 years. About 60 percent were associated with unerupted teeth.

Gross Findings. Most calcifying epithelial odontogenic tumors consist of nondescript tan soft tissue containing small foci to large nodules of bony hard tissue. Although most appear as fragmented tumor masses, some have a prominent cystic lumen (88). Most calcifying epithelial odontogenic tumors are diagnosed based on incisional or excisional biopsy although the characteristic features are also identified by fine needle aspiration cytology (89).

Radiographic Features. As with other odontogenic neoplasms, calcifying epithelial odontogenic tumors present most often as a well-circumscribed, corticated, unilocular or multilocular radiolucency (fig. 6-25). Some tumors produce enough mineralization that small radiopacities are detected within the radiolucent area. Tumors with little or no evidence of mineralization have been reported and may have a distinct predilection for occurrence in the anterior and premolar regions of the maxilla (90).

Microscopic Findings. The tumor is characterized by islands and sheets of polygonal epithelial cells dispersed throughout a nonspecific fibrous stroma. In many instances the polygonal epithelial cells show remarkable pleomorphism and nuclear hyperchromasia (figs. 6-26, 6-27). The borders of the epithelial cells are well defined and have prominent intercellular bridges (fig. 6-28). Some tumors have areas dominated by cells with clear cytoplasm (87). Foci of homogenous eosinophilic material, shown to be amyloid based on Congo red stains, are found within the tumor (fig. 6-29). Also noted are small round globules of mineralized material exhibiting a Leisegang ring phenomenon (83,85).

Malignant features, including more prominent nuclear pleomorphism, vascular invasion, frequent mitotic figures, and increased proliferative activity as assessed by Ki-67, are present in the rare *malignant calcifying odontogenic tumor* (91,92).

Immunohistochemical Findings. Some calcifying epithelial odontogenic tumors show immunologic features similar to those of myoepithelial-derived salivary gland neoplasms (93). Staining reveals focal positivity for calponin, glial fibrillary acidic protein, and low molecular weight cytokeratin in some calcifying odontogenic tumors (24). The tumor cells express laminins 1 and 5, fibronectin, and vimentin (94). Dendritic Langerhans cells with strong staining for S-100 protein and CD1a have been identified (90).

The green birefringent congophilic amyloid in calcifying odontogenic tumors, which has also been detected in unerupted tooth follicles, is composed of N-terminal fragments of a putative 153-residue protein specified by a gene designated *FLJ20513* and now known to represent exons 5 through 10 of the odontogenic ameloblast-associated protein (ODAM) locus that en-

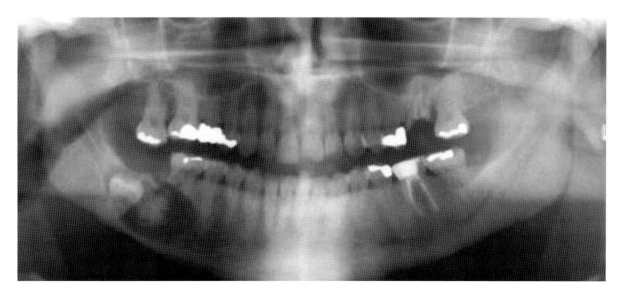

Figure 6-25

CALCIFYING EPITHELIAL ODONTOGENIC TUMOR

A well-demarcated combination radiolucency/radiopacity is associated with the crown of the impacted mandibular right second molar. There is resorption of the first molar roots.

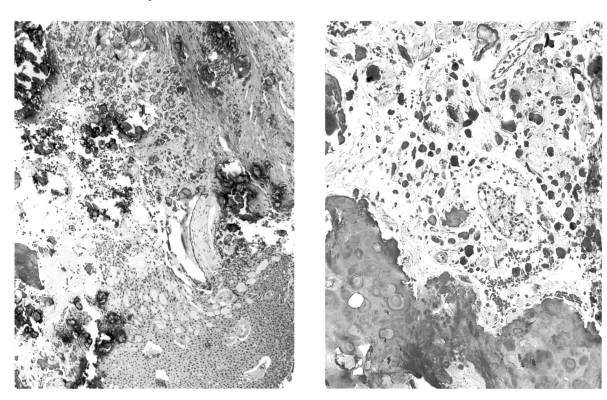

Figure 6-26

CALCIFYING EPITHELIAL ODONTOGENIC TUMOR

Left: Mineralizations and sheets of squamous epithelium are seen.

Right: Much of this tumor consists of islands and sheets of mineralized material, some of which show a concentric appositional pattern often referred to as Liesegang rings.

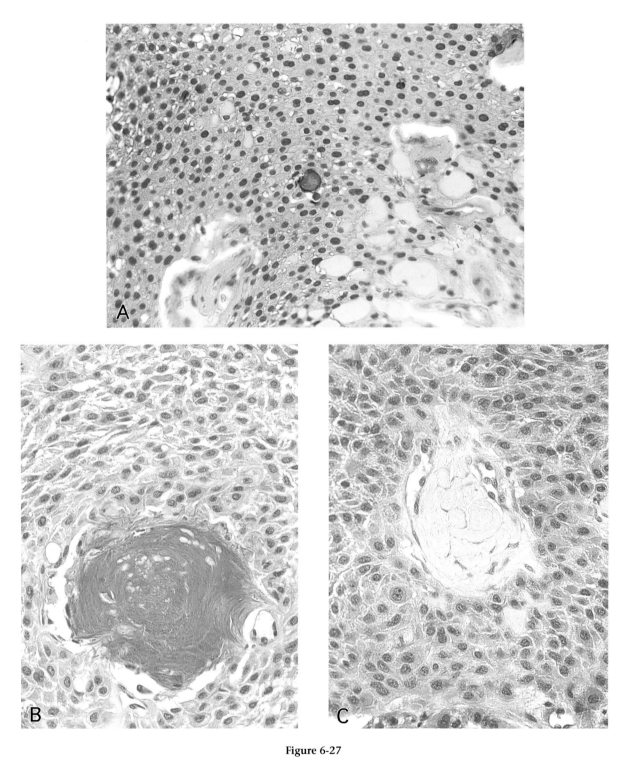

Figure 6-27

CALCIFYING EPITHELIAL ODONTOGENIC TUMOR

A: Hyalinized nodules, mineralizations, and sheets of squamous epithelial cells with prominent intercellular bridges and hyperchromatic nuclei are seen.

B: Sheets of squamous epithelial cells with prominent intercellular bridges and hyperchromatic nuclei surround an area of eosinophilic mineralized material.

C: Squamous epithelial cells with prominent intercellular bridges and ovoid nuclei surround amyloid.

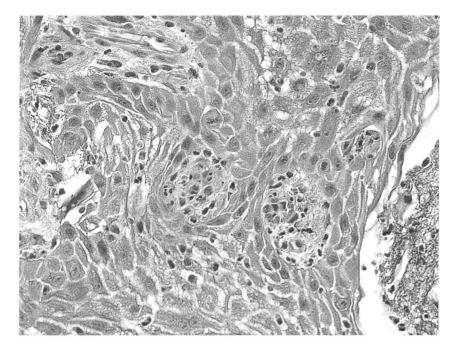

Figure 6-28

CALCIFYING EPITHELIAL ODONTOGENIC TUMOR

The squamous epithelial cells have prominent intercellular bridges, cellular pleomorphism, and mitotic activity.

Figure 6-29

CALCIFYING EPITHELIAL ODONTOGENIC TUMOR

Congo red staining under polarized light shows the apple-green birefringence typical of amyloid.

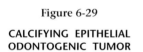
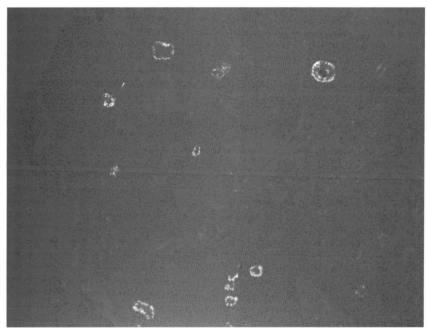

codes a 279-residue polypeptide (95). Solomon et al. (96) used microanalytic techniques to characterize the associated amyloid and found some fibrils to be composed of a polypeptide of approximately 46 repeat polypeptides.

Perdigao et al. (97) have identified alterations in the *ameloblastin* (*AMBN*) gene, which regulates an important protein that acts as a cell adhesion molecule in calcifying epithelial odontogenic tumors. Similar to other odontogenic neoplasms, gene mutations in *PTCH1* are present in the calcifying epithelial odontogenic tumor (98). Expression of *HOXC13* mRNA has recently been identified in 43 percent of seven normal oral mucosal samples and 100 percent of calcifying epithelial odontogenic tumors (99).

Treatment and Prognosis. As with most other odontogenic tumors, therapeutic management consists of conservative surgical removal. Recurrence rates are 10 to 14 percent following enucleation combined with curettage/peripheral ostectomy. Long-term follow-up is necessary since occasional recurrences occur more than 10 years following initial treatment (82,83,85,87).

KERATOCYSTIC ODONTOGENIC TUMOR (KERATINIZING CYSTIC ODONTOGENIC TUMOR, PARAKERATINIZING ODONTOGENIC KERATOCYST)

Definition. *Keratocystic odontogenic tumor* has undergone the most noticeable change in classification of odontogenic lesions in recent years. What was previously classified an odontogenic cyst that behaved in a more aggressive manor than many benign odontogenic neoplasms is now classified by the World Health Organization (WHO) as a benign neoplasm that is grossly and microscopically a cyst (100,101).

Keratocystic odontogenic tumors were first described by Philipsen in 1956 but even five decades later the debate continues as to the pathogenesis, behavior, treatment, and classification of this cystic neoplasm (102–105).

Clinical Features. The mandible is the site of most keratocystic odontogenic tumors, with approximately 75 percent of reported cases occurring in the posterior body. As with other odontogenic neoplasms and cysts, they arise in any tooth-bearing site including in the maxilla. They expand superiorly to involve the maxillary sinuses, nasal antrum, and even the floor of the orbit. Most patients are male and most tumors are first diagnosed in the second through fourth decades of life.

Keratocystic odontogenic tumors are usually asymptomatic unless secondarily inflamed. Usually, the buccal cortical plate is expanded and sometimes exhibits crepitus when palpated. Cortical plate perforation by these tumors is uncommon, but can be an important prognostic factor because keratocystic odontogenic tumors proliferate within muscle tissue (106). If multiple odontogenic cysts are present, the consideration of basal cell nevus (Gorlin) syndrome should be considered.

Radiographic Features. Keratocystic odontogenic tumors appear radiographically as well-demarcated radiolucencies with thin, well-defined, corticated borders (fig. 6-30). The tumor usually displaces normal anatomy, including teeth, but resorption can also occur with greater frequency compared to other odontogenic tumors. The radiolucency may appear multilocular depending primarily on the size of the lesion. Computerized tomography (CT) scans are valuable for assessing these lesions in three dimensions prior to surgical management (fig. 6-31).

Gross Findings. At the time of surgery and at gross inspection, keratocystic odontogenic tumors present as tissue paper–thin strips and sheets of soft tissue. Care should be taken to inspect the formalin transport container because the lining epithelium often separates from the connective tissue and appears as a translucent membrane in the fixative. The entire specimen should be processed for microscopic examination not only to ensure that diagnostic areas are identified, but also to check for budding or other tumors, including ameloblastoma. The formalin also often contains varying amounts of amorphous "cheese-like" material, which if processed, is identified as keratin. This material is often described by surgeons in the biopsy submission information.

Microscopic Findings. The epithelial lining is composed of a uniform layer of stratified squamous epithelium 6 to 10 cells in thickness (fig. 6-32). There is no rete ridge formation. The surface of the parakeratinized epithelium is often corrugated or wavy. Important findings are a palisaded basal epithelial layer and hyperchromatic nuclei. The underlying fibrovascular connective tissue can contain varying numbers of epithelial rests or small microcysts (fig. 6-33). In the past, the presence of microcysts was postulated as a reason for the high recurrence rate (107), but this has not been supported by follow-up reports.

The secondary inflammation seen focally in many keratocystic odontogenic tumors will substantially alter the microscopic features, sometimes causing large areas to become nondiagnostic (fig. 6-34). Following marsupialization, a technique sometimes used prior to definitive surgery for larger lesions, the microscopic features of the tumor are altered (fig. 6-35).

Immunohistochemical Findings. Several studies have described the immunohistochemical nature of keratocystic odontogenic tumor

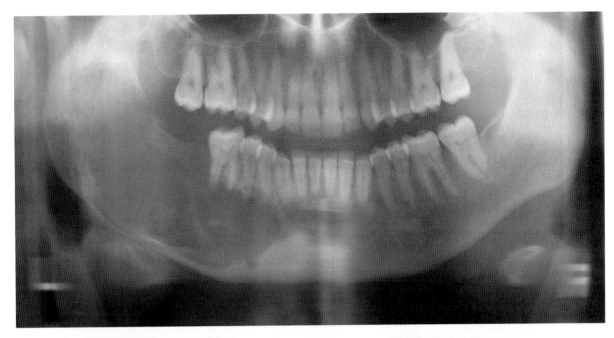

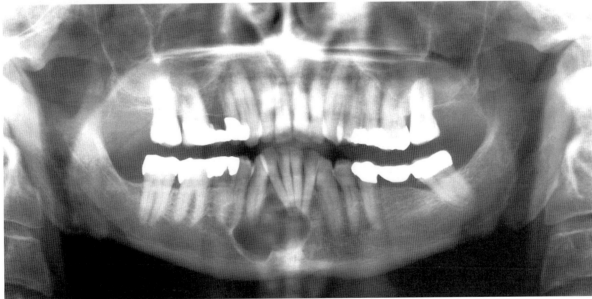

Figure 6-30

KERATOCYSTIC ODONTOGENIC TUMOR

Top: A panoramic radiograph shows a well-circumscribed radiolucency of the right body and ramus of the mandible. Bottom: A well-demarcated, corticated radiolucency displaces the roots of the canine and incisor teeth.

and supported its reclassification as a neoplasm (108,109). As early as 1989, Scharffetter et al. (110) documented increased mitotic activity within the epithelial lining of the tumors.

Proliferating cell nuclear antigen (PCNA), COX-2, cell proliferation markers (Ki-67), and tumor suppressor protein (p53) positivity occur more frequently and more intensely in keratocystic odontogenic tumors than in other odontogenic lesions (111–116). High expression of Ki-67 and expression of p53 are often identified in recurrent tumors (117).

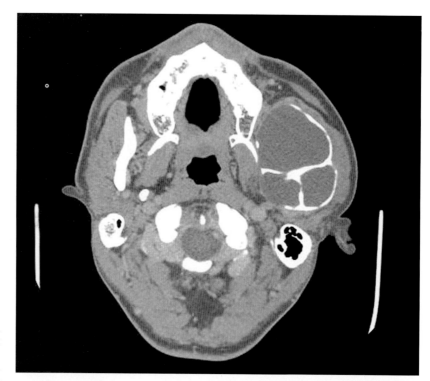

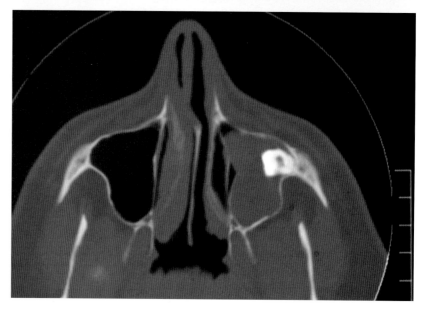

Figure 6-31

KERATOCYSTIC ODONTOGENIC TUMOR

Top: An axial CT image shows a multilocular radiolucency of the left mandibular body and ramus.

Bottom: A cystic lesion associated with an impacted tooth expands into the left maxillary sinus, as seen on axial CT.

The presence of aberrant sonic hedgehog signaling proteins SHH, PTCH1, SMO, GLI1, and NMYC in keratocystic odontogenic tumors also supports the view that the tumors are neoplastic (108,118,119). Epithelial expression of sonic hedgehog transcriptional effector GlI2 has been identified in keratocystic odontogenic tumors induced from rests of Malassez in transgenic mice (120).

Vascular endothelial growth factor (VEGF) is more prominent in keratocystic odontogenic tumors than in dentigerous cysts (114). The use of CD34 to evaluate angiogenesis has shown microvessel density to be higher in keratocystic odontogenic tumors compared to dentigerous cysts, although the density of both was lower than ameloblastoma (14). Podoplanin, a

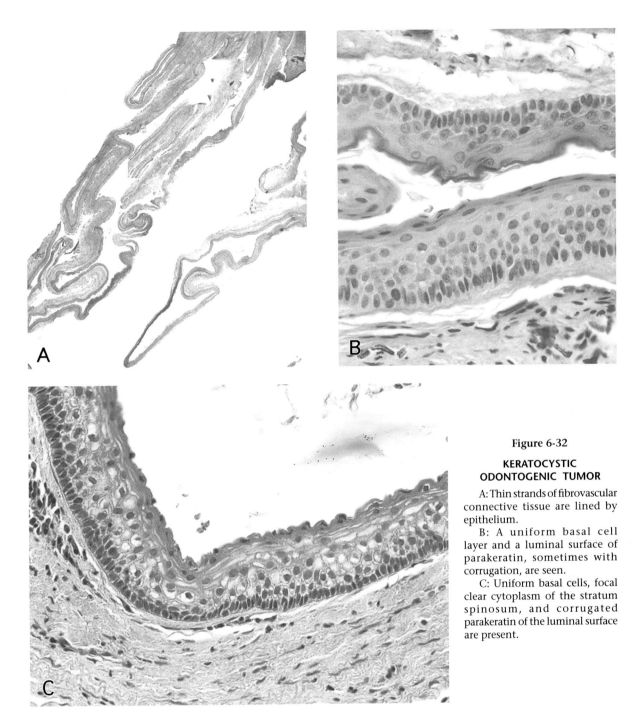

Figure 6-32

KERATOCYSTIC ODONTOGENIC TUMOR

A: Thin strands of fibrovascular connective tissue are lined by epithelium.

B: A uniform basal cell layer and a luminal surface of parakeratin, sometimes with corrugation, are seen.

C: Uniform basal cells, focal clear cytoplasm of the stratum spinosum, and corrugated parakeratin of the luminal surface are present.

lymphatic endothelial marker highly expressed in ameloblastomas, is also identified in the cytoplasm of most basal and suprabasal cells in keratocystic odontogenic tumors (121).

The epithelial proliferation and apoptotic indices of both sporadic keratocystic odontogenic tumors and tumors associated with basal cell nevus syndrome have been shown to be similar to ameloblastomas and higher than dentigerous cyst epithelium (19,122). Survivin, an inhibitor of apoptosis, is present in keratocystic odontogenic tumors but not in nonkeratinizing periapical cysts (123).

An evaluation of common tumor suppressor genes has concluded that clonal deletion mutations of genomic DNA indicate a neoplastic rather

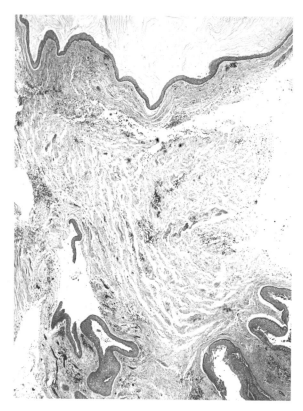

Figure 6-33

KERATOCYSTIC ODONTOGENIC TUMOR

Satellite tumors are seen in the fibrovascular connective tissue wall.

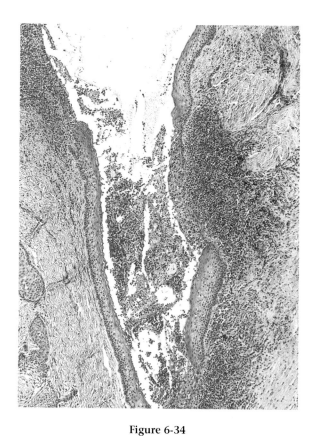

Figure 6-34

KERATOCYSTIC ODONTOGENIC TUMOR

Foci of inflammation cause the epithelium to lose its diagnostic features.

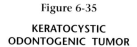

Figure 6-35

KERATOCYSTIC ODONTOGENIC TUMOR

Three months following marsupialization, the epithelial lining shows evidence of hyperplasia in the stratum spinosum and the formation of rete.

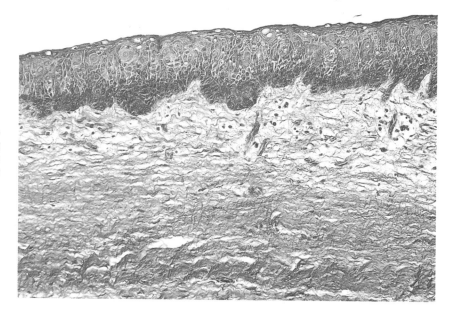

than cystic origin (101). Immunoreactivity for bcl-2 was detected in the basal layer of keratocystic odontogenic tumors while orthokeratinizing odontogenic cysts were negative (124).

Keratocystic odontogenic tumors, gingival mucosa, odontogenic rests, and dentigerous cysts all show evidence of a p63-positive, high molecular weight cytokeratin (CK5/6)-positive immunophenotype (24). Keratinocyte growth factor and receptor have been identified in the epithelium of more keratocystic odontogenic tumors than dentigerous cyst epithelium, and the intensity of growth factor staining is significantly reduced following marsupialization of the tumors (125).

There is significant downregulation in the expression of cell adhesion proteins beta-catenin and E-cadherin along with alteration of Wnt-1 and Wnt-10A signaling pathways when compared to dentigerous cysts (126). Cytoplasmic osteopontin, often found in malignant epithelial tumors and important in bone metastasis through a process of osteoclast activation, has been identified in the epithelium of 8 of 20 keratocystic odontogenic tumors, but in no dentigerous or radicular cysts (90).

Treatment and Prognosis. Early attempts to explain the high recurrence rates (sometimes as high as 60 percent) included the presence of epithelial rests or satellite cyst formation in the fibrous connective tissue walls (107), incomplete removal of the paper-thin epithelial lining, collagenase activity (127), or prostaglandin-induced bone resorption (128).

In a recent series of 120 keratocystic odontogenic tumors treated with simple enucleation, 28 (26 percent) recurred (129). Average follow-up was 86 months, with a range of 18 to 151 months. There was no correlation between tumor site, cortical perforation, or radiographic features. In another series of 32 keratocystic odontogenic tumors treated by enucleation, 4 recurred during follow-up ranging from 1 to 114 months (117).

Marsupialization of large lesions, which results in a decrease in tumor size of up to 47 percent making follow-up enucleation much simpler, has been advocated (130). Some investigators have claimed success with decompression and subsequent enucleation while others advocate enucleation and excision of overlying mucosa, peripheral ostectomy, and chemical curettage (131–136).

Regardless of the initial treatment provided, patients need to be followed with periodic radiography for a minimum of 10 years so recurrent lesions can be identified and treated when they are small. Intracranial extension of keratocystic odontogenic tumors has been reported (137). Clinical work-up to assess for basal cell nevus syndrome is always prudent when multiple concurrent or sequential keratocystic odontogenic tumors are diagnosed. All tumors should still be examined histopathologically to confirm the diagnosis.

BASAL CELL NEVUS SYNDROME (NEVOID BASAL CELL CARCINOMA SYNDROME, GORLIN SYNDROME)

Definition. *Basal cell nevus syndrome* is called by many names, and the nomenclature often depends on what portions of the syndrome, such as bifid ribs and keratocystic odontogenic tumors, are present. Gorlin et al. described no less than 37 anomalies associated with this syndrome (138–142).

Mutations in the *PTCH1* gene are responsible for basal cell nevus syndrome. Li et al. (143) detected 26 *PTCH1* mutations in 10 of 34 (29.4 percent) sporadic and 14 of 16 (87.5 percent) syndromic keratocystic odontogenic tumors. The results indicate that defects of *PTCH1* are involved in the pathogenesis of syndromic as well as sporadic keratocystic odontogenic tumors.

Clinical Features. Features that are seen in over 50 percent of patients are shown in Table 6-1 (144). Medulloblastomas are a less frequent finding. Bilateral hyperplasia of the mandibular coronoid processes has also been described (145).

Keratocystic odontogenic tumors sometimes present in childhood and often aid in establishing a diagnosis. This is especially true in those cases in which there are new mutations with no prior familial history (146,147). In an analysis of 312 cases of keratocystic odontogenic tumor, 5.1 percent were from patients with basal cell nevus syndrome and 5.8 percent were from patients with multiple keratocysts but with no other features of the syndrome (148). There was a wide age range, with a peak incidence in the second and third decades of life. The cysts usually occur about a decade earlier in patients with the syndrome than in those without the syndrome. The mandible to maxilla ratio was 2 to 1, with the mandibular third molar area and ramus being the most common sites.

Up to 40 percent of cases may be new mutations. Although genetic testing is advancing, there may be large variations in expression in this autosomal dominant disease (149). In contrast to expression, penetrance is considered complete. The defect is located on chromosome 9, q22.3 (150,151). This syndrome group served as the basis for finding the chromosomal dam-

age responsible for actinically induced basal cell carcinomas.

Evaluation PCNA, Ki-67, and p53 suggests that there are no differences in the growth potential or aggressive behavior of syndromic and nonsyndromic keratocystic odontogenic tumors (152). The epithelial proliferation index in both sporadic and syndrome-associated tumors is higher than in dentigerous cysts (122). The apoptotic index is the same in the basal and suprabasal cell layers for all three lesions, and is higher in the superficial epithelial layers of both types of keratocystic odontogenic tumor compared to dentigerous cysts.

Radiographic Features. The radiographic features of syndromic keratocystic odontogenic tumors are identical to those described for the nonsyndromic tumors. Well-demarcated, expansile radiolucencies, unilocular or multilocular depending primarily on size, are identified in the tooth-bearing areas of the mandible and maxilla (fig. 6-37). Lam et al. (153) evaluated the radiographic features of 43 keratocystic odontogenic tumors identified in 11 syndromic patients on plain film radiographs and CT: 25 developed in the mandible and 18 in the maxillae. Five developing keratocystic odontogenic tumors were only evident on CT images, indicating that early CT analysis of the jaws for patients with basal cell nevus syndrome is of value for identifying tumor development and minimizing surgical complications associated with the treatment of larger tumors.

Table 6-1

COMMON FEATURES OF
BASAL CELL NEVUS SYNDROME[a]

Frontal and/or occipital bossing

Hypertelorism

Multiple basal cell carcinomas, especially at a young age (fig. 6-36)

Odontogenic keratocysts of the jaws, especially at a young age

Epidermal cysts of skin

Palmar and/or plantar pits

Calcified ovarian fibromas

Calcified falx cerebri

Rib anomalies (especially bifid)

Spina bifida occulta

Bridged sella or fused clinoids

[a]Data from reference 144.

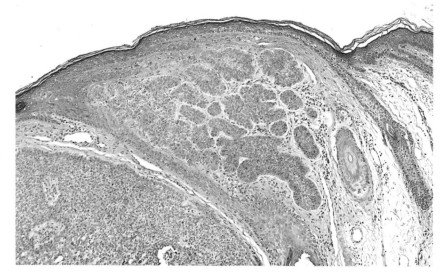

Figure 6-36

**BASAL CELL
NEVUS SYNDROME**

Typical basal cell carcinoma of the skin.

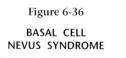

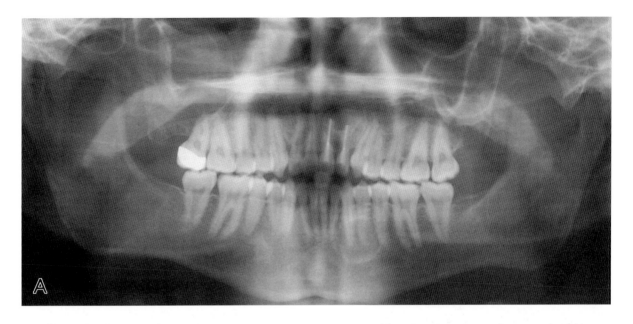

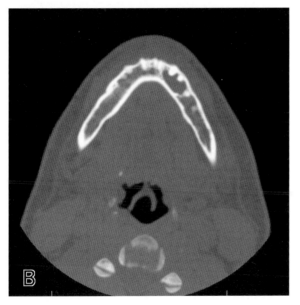
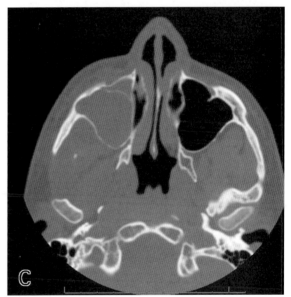

Figure 6-37

BASAL CELL NEVUS SYNDROME

A: Panoramic radiograph shows well-defined radiolucencies in the left premolar region of the mandible and right posterior maxilla, extending into the maxillary sinus.

B: The mandibular lesion is visualized on an axial CT image.

C: The right maxillary lesion displaces most of the sinus antrum. Incisional biopsies showed both to be keratocystic odontogenic tumors.

Microscopic Findings. The microscopic features of syndromic and nonsyndromic keratocystic odontogenic tumors are identical (see fig. 6-32). The cyst-like lumen is lined by stratified squamous epithelium with a uniform basal cell layer of cuboidal cells showing palisaded hyperchromatic nuclei. The epithelium is usually 7 to 10 cell layers thick, with a layer of corrugated parakeratin at the surface. Similar to nonsyndromic keratocystic odontogenic

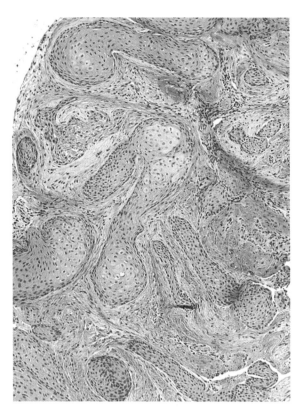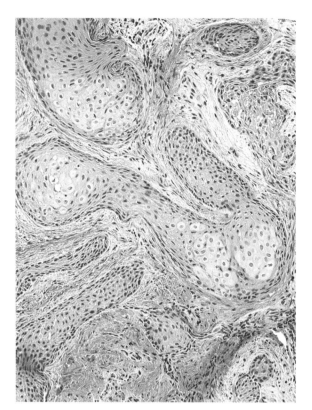

Figure 6-38

SQUAMOUS ODONTOGENIC TUMOR

Left: Large and small islands of squamous epithelial cells are seen.
Right: The squamous islands show no periphery of columnar ameloblasts and no evidence of cellular atypia.

tumors, these features can be rendered nondiagnostic by secondary inflammation.

Treatment and Prognosis. Therapeutic management of syndrome-associated keratocystic odontogenic tumors is identical to that of nonsyndromic tumors. Once the syndrome has been diagnosed, the patient should undergo clinical and radiographic screening on a regular basis. Tumors that seem to recur are most likely new tumors and each patient has an extremely variable overall prognosis.

SQUAMOUS ODONTOGENIC TUMOR

Definition. *Squamous odontogenic tumor* is a rare, benign epithelial neoplasm first characterized by Pullon et al. in 1975 (154). These tumors occur most often in the anterior maxilla or posterior mandible, or rarely, from rests in the periodontal soft tissues, accounting for reports of lesions peripheral to bone (155–158).

The importance of the tumor is that the squamous epithelial islands seen microscopically may be misinterpreted as invasion of a primary carcinoma or metastasis. The appearance may also lead to misdiagnosis of acanthomatous ameloblastoma.

Radiographic Features. Radiographically, squamous odontogenic tumors have the same general appearance as other benign tumors of the jaws, which includes a well-demarcated radiolucency with a sclerotic, osseous border, an indication of its slow growth rate.

Microscopic Findings. The microscopic features include islands of bland squamous epithelium, and no cellular pleomorphism, nuclear hyperchromasia, dyskeratosis, keratin pearl formation, or noticeable mitotic activity (fig. 6-38). The tumors should have no peripheral palisading columnar cells suggestive of an acanthomatous ameloblastoma. The diagnosis is based entirely on the H&E appearance and special stains are of no value.

Squamous odontogenic tumor-like epithelial islands are present in other neoplasms, as well as developmental or inflammatory cysts. They most likely represent hyperplastic odontogenic rests, and do not have therapeutic significance (159–161).

Treatment and Prognosis. Most tumors are easily treated with enucleation and simple conservative curettage (155,162). Rarely, reports describe unusually aggressive behavior requiring additional surgical management (158).

REFERENCES

1. Snead ML, Luo W, Hsu DD, Melrose RJ, Lau EC, Stenman G. Human ameloblastoma tumors express the amelogenin gene. Oral Surg Oral Med Oral Pathol 1992;74:64-72.

2. Gorlin RJ, Chaudhry AP. The ameloblastoma and the craniopharyngioma; their similarities and differences. Oral Surg Oral Med Oral Pathol 1959;12:199-205.

3. Vickers RA, Gorlin RJ. Ameloblastoma: delineation of early histopathologic features of neoplasia. Cancer 1970;26:699-710.

4. Buchner A, Merrell PW, Carpenter WM. Relative frequency of central odontogenic tumors: a study of 1,088 cases from Northern California and comparison to studies from other parts of the world. J Oral Maxillofac Surg 2006;64:1343-1352.

5. Reichart PA, Philipsen HP, Sonner S. Ameloblastoma: biological profile of 3677 cases. Eur J Cancer B Oral Oncol 1995;31B:86-99.

6. Fregnani ER, da Cruz Perez DE, de Almeida OP, Kowalski LP, Soares FA, de Abreu Alves F. Clinicopathological study and treatment outcomes of 121 cases of ameloblastomas. Int J Oral Maxillofac Surg 2010;39:145-149.

7. Punnya AV, Rekha K. "Ameloblastoma with mucous cells": review of literature and presentation of 2 cases. Oral Surg Oral Med Oral Pathol Oral Radiol Endod 2008;106:e20-26.

8. Eversole LR, Leider AS, Hansen LS. Ameloblastomas with pronounced desmoplasia. J Oral Maxillofac Surg 1984;42:735-740.

9. Philipsen HP, Ormiston IW, Reichart PA. The desmo- and osteoplastic ameloblastoma. Histologic variant or clinicopathologic entity? Case reports. Int J Oral Maxillofac Surg 1992;21:352-357.

10. Philipsen HP, Reichart PA, Takata T. Desmoplastic ameloblastoma (including "hybrid" lesion of ameloblastoma). Biological profile based on 100 cases from the literature and own files. Oral Oncol 2001;37:455-460.

11. Shteyer A, Lustmann J, Lewin-Epstein J. The mural ameloblastoma: a review of the literature. J Oral Surg 1978;36:866-872.

12. dos Santos JN, De Souza VF, Azevedo RA, Sarmento VA, Souza LB. "Hybrid' lesion of desmoplastic and conventional ameloblastoma: immunohistochemical aspects. Braz J Otorhinolaryngol 2006;72:709-713.

13. Schafer DR, Thompson LD, Smith BC, Wenig BM. Primary ameloblastoma of the sinonasal tract: a clinicopathologic study of 24 cases. Cancer 1998;82:667-674.

14. Alaeddini M, Salah S, Dehghan F, Eshghyar N, Etemad-Moghadam S. Comparison of angiogenesis in keratocystic odontogenic tumours, dentigerous cysts and ameloblastomas. Oral Dis 2009;15:422-427.

15. Kumamoto H, Izutsu T, Ohki K, Takahashi N, Ooya K. p53 gene status and expression of p53, MDM2, and p14 proteins in ameloblastomas. J Oral Pathol Med 2004;33:292-299.

16. Barboza CA, Pereira Pinto L, Freitas Rde A, Costa Ade L, Souza LB. Proliferating cell nuclear antigen (PCNA) and p53 protein expression in ameloblastoma and adenomatoid odontogenic tumor. Braz Dent J 2005;16:56-61.

17. Sandra F, Mitsuyasu T, Nakamura N, Shiratsuchi Y, Ohishi M. Immunohistochemical evaluation of PCNA and Ki-67 in ameloblastoma. Oral Oncol 2001;37:193-198.

18. Han B, Li L, Wang H. [Expression of Ki-67 antigen in ameloblastoma and its clinical significance.] Hua Xi Kou Qiang Yi Xue Za Zhi 2003;21:153-154. [Chinese]

19. Thosaporn W, Iamaroon A, Pongsiriwet S, Ng KH. A comparative study of epithelial cell proliferation between the odontogenic keratocyst, orthokeratinized odontogenic cyst, dentigerous cyst, and ameloblastoma. Oral Dis 2004;10:22-26.

20. Ribeiro BF, Iglesias DP, Nascimento GJ, Galvao HC, Medeiros AM, Freitas RA. Immunoexpression of MMPs-1, -2, and -9 in ameloblastoma and odontogenic adenomatoid tumor. Oral Dis 2009;15:472-477.

21. Alves Pereira KM, do Amaral BA, dos Santos BR, Galvao HC, Freitas Rde A, de Souza LB. Immunohistochemical expression of E-cadherin and beta-catenin in ameloblastomas and tooth germs. Oral Surg Oral Med Oral Pathol Oral Radiol Endod 2010;109:425-431.

22. Souza Andrade ES, da Costa Miguel MC, Pinto LP, de Souza LB. Ameloblastoma and adenomatoid odontogenic tumor: the role of alpha2beta1, alpha3beta1, and alpha5beta1 integrins in local invasiveness and architectural characteristics. Ann Diagn Pathol 2007;11:199-205.

23. Modolo F, Martins MT, Loducca SV, de Araujo VC. Expression of integrin subunits alpha2, alpha3, alpha5, alphav, beta1, beta3 and beta4 in different histological types of ameloblastoma compared with dental germ, dental lamina and adult lining epithelium. Oral Dis 2004;10:277-282.

24. Gratzinger D, Salama ME, Poh CF, Rouse RV. Ameloblastoma, calcifying epithelial odontogenic tumor, and glandular odontogenic cyst show a distinctive immunophenotype with some myoepithelial antigen expression. J Oral Pathol Med 2008;37:177-184.

25. Altini M, Coleman H, Doglioni C, Favia G, Maiorano E. Calretinin expression in ameloblastomas. Histopathology 2000;37:27-32.

26. DeVilliers P, Liu H, Suggs C, et al. Calretinin expression in the differential diagnosis of human ameloblastoma and keratocystic odontogenic tumor. Am J Surg Pathol 2008;32:256-260.

27. Siar CH, Nakano K, Han PP, Nagatsuka H, Ng KH, Kawakami T. Differential expression of Notch receptors and their ligands in desmoplastic ameloblastoma. J Oral Pathol Med 2010;39:552-558.

28. Bologna-Molina R, Mosqueda-Taylor A, Lopez-Corella E, et al. Comparative expression of syndecan-1 and Ki-67 in peripheral and desmoplastic ameloblastomas and ameloblastic carcinoma. Pathol Int 2009;59:229-233.

29. Sauk JJ, Nikitakis NG, Scheper MA. Are we on the brink of nonsurgical treatment for ameloblastoma? Oral Surg Oral Med Oral Pathol Oral Radiol Endod 2010;110:68-78.

30. Gardner DG. A pathologist's approach to the treatment of ameloblastoma. J Oral Maxillofac Surg 1984;42:161-166.

31. Gardner DG. Some current concepts on the pathology of ameloblastomas. Oral Surg Oral Med Oral Pathol Oral Radiol Endod 1996;82:660-669.

32. Carlson ER, Marx RE. The ameloblastoma: primary, curative surgical management. J Oral Maxillofac Surg 2006;64:484-494.

33. Leibovitch I, Schwarcz RM, Modjtahedi S, Selva D, Goldberg RA. Orbital invasion by recurrent maxillary ameloblastoma. Ophthalmology 2006;113:1227-1230.

34. Waldron CA. Ameloblastoma in perspective. J Oral Surg 1966;24:331-333.

35. Sehdev MK, Huvos AG, Strong EW, Gerold FP, Willis GW. Proceedings: Ameloblastoma of maxilla and mandible. Cancer 1974;33:324-333.

36. Gardner DG, Pecak AM. The treatment of ameloblastoma based on pathologic and anatomic principles. Cancer 1980;46:2514-2519.

37. Adebayo ET, Fomete B, Adekeye EO. Delayed soft tissue recurrence after treatment of ameloblastoma in a black African: case report and review of the literature. J Craniomaxillofac Surg 2011;39:615-618.

38. Adekeye EO, Lavery KM. Recurrent ameloblastoma of the maxillo-facial region. Clinical features and treatment. J Maxillofac Surg 1986;14:153-157.

39. Hong J, Yun PY, Chung IH, et al. Long-term follow up on recurrence of 305 ameloblastoma cases. Int J Oral Maxillofac Surg 2007;36:283-288.

40. Nakamura N, Mitsuyasu T, Higuchi Y, Sandra F, Ohishi M. Growth characteristics of ameloblastoma involving the inferior alveolar nerve: a clinical and histopathologic study. Oral Surg Oral Med Oral Pathol Oral Radiol Endod 2001;91:557-562.

41. Hatada K, Noma H, Katakura A, et al. Clinicostatistical study of ameloblastoma treatment. Bull Tokyo Dent Coll 2001;42:87-95.

42. Williams TP. Management of ameloblastoma: a changing perspective. J Oral Maxillofac Surg 1993;51:1064-1070.

43. Hatada K, Noma H, Katakura A, et al. Clinicostatistical study of ameloblastoma treatment. Bull Tokyo Dent Col 2001;42:87-95.

44. Gortzak RA, Latief BS, Lekkas C, Slootweg PJ. Growth characteristics of large mandibular ameloblastomas: report of 5 cases with implications for the approach to surgery. Int J Oral Maxillofac Surg 2006;35:691-695.

45. Nakamura N, Higuchi Y, Mitsuyasu T, Sandra F, Ohishi M. Comparison of long-term results between different approaches to ameloblastoma. Oral Surg Oral Med Oral Pathol Oral Radiol Endod 2002;93:13-20.

46. Martins WD, Favaro DM. Recurrence of an ameloblastoma in an autogenous iliac bone graft. Oral Surg Oral Med Oral Pathol Oral Radiol Endod 2004;98:657-659.

47. Gardner DG. Critique of the 1995 review by Reichart et al. of the biologic profile of 3677 ameloblastomas. Oral Oncol 1999;35:443-449.

48. Robinson L, Martinez MG. Unicystic ameloblastoma: a prognostically distinct entity. Cancer 1977;40:2278-2285.

49. Patel H, Rees RT. Unicystic ameloblastoma presenting in Gardner's syndrome: a case report. Br Dent J 2005;198:747-748.

50. Qureshi SS, Qureshi SS, Medhi SS, Kane SV. Unicystic ameloblastoma of the mandible masquerading as carcinoma of the oral cavity in a 10-year-old girl. Am J Surg 2008;196:e7-9.

51. Ramesh RS, Manjunath S, Ustad TH, Pais S, Shivakumar K. Unicystic ameloblastoma of the mandible—an unusual case report and review of literature. Head Neck Oncol 2010;2:1.

52. Bisinelli JC, Ioshii S, Retamoso LB, Moyses ST, Moyses SJ, Tanaka OM. Conservative treatment of unicystic ameloblastoma. Am J Orthod Dentofacial Orthop 2010;137:396-400.

53. Philipsen HP, Reichart PA. Unicystic ameloblastoma. A review of 193 cases from the literature. Oral Oncol 1998;34:317-325.

54. Gardner DG. Plexiform unicystic ameloblastoma: a diagnostic problem in dentigerous cysts. Cancer 1981;47:1358-1363.

55. Gardner DG, Corio RL. The relationship of plexiform unicystic ameloblastoma to conventional ameloblastoma. Oral Surg Oral Med Oral Pathol 1983;56:54-60.

56. Gardner DG, Corio RL. Plexiform unicystic ameloblastoma. A variant of ameloblastoma with a low-recurrence rate after enucleation. Cancer 1984;53:1730-1735.

57. Gardner DG, Morton TH Jr, Worsham JC. Plexiform unicystic ameloblastoma of the maxilla. Oral Surg Oral Med Oral Pathol 1987;63:221-223.

58. Ackermann GL, Altini M, Shear M. The unicystic ameloblastoma: a clinicopathological study of 57 cases. J Oral Pathol 1988;17:541-546.

59. Damm DD. Enlarging pericoronal radiolucency of the posterior mandible. Unicystic ameloblastoma. Gen Dent 2008;56:760, 763.

60. Paikkatt VJ, Sreedharan S, Kannan VP. Unicystic ameloblastoma of the maxilla: a case report. J Indian Soc Pedod Prev Dent 2007;25:106-110.

61. Konouchi H, Asaumi J, Yanagi Y, et al. Usefulness of contrast enhanced-MRI in the diagnosis of unicystic ameloblastoma. Oral Oncol 2006;42:481-486.

62. Vickers RA, Gorlin RJ. Ameloblastoma: Delineation of early histopathologic features of neoplasia. Cancer 1970;26:699-710.

63. Sivapathasundharam B, Einstein A. Unicystic ameloblastoma with the presence of dentin. Indian J Dent Res 2007;18:128-130.

64. Yoon JH, Ahn SG, Kim SG. Mucous cell differentiation in a unicystic ameloblastoma. Int J Oral Maxillofac Surg 2009;38:95-97.

65. Coleman H, Altini M, Ali H, Doglioni C, Favia G, Maiorano E. Use of calretinin in the differential diagnosis of unicystic ameloblastomas. Histopathology 2001;38:312-317.

66. Eversole LR, Leider AS, Strub D. Radiographic characteristics of cystogenic ameloblastoma. Oral Surg Oral Med Oral Pathol 1984;57:572-577.

67. Ackermann GL, Altini M, Shear M. The unicystic ameloblastoma: a clinicopathological study of 57 cases. J Oral Pathol 1988;17:541-546.

68. Yavagal C, Anegundi RT, Shetty S. Unicystic plexiform ameloblastoma: an insight for pediatric dentists. J Indian Soc Pedod Prev Dent 2009;27:70-74.

69. Lau SL, Samman N. Recurrence related to treatment modalities of unicystic ameloblastoma: a systematic review. Int J Oral Maxillofac Surg 2006;35:681-690.

70. Covani U, Barone A. Piezosurgical treatment of unicystic ameloblastoma. J Periodontol 2007;78:1342-1347.

71. Gorlin RJ, Chaudhry AP. Adenoameloblastoma. Oral Surg Oral Med Oral Pathol 1958;11:762-768.

72. Philipsen HP, Reichart PA, Siar CH, et al. An updated clinical and epidemiological profile of the adenomatoid odontogenic tumour: a collaborative retrospective study. J Oral Pathol Med 2007;36:383-393.

73. Effiom OA, Odukoya O. Adenomatoid odontogenic tumour: a clinico-pathological analysis and melanin pigmentation study of 31 Nigerian cases. Niger Postgrad Med J 2005;12:131-135.

74. Philipsen HP, Reichart PA. Adenomatoid odontogenic tumour: facts and figures. Oral Oncol 1999;35:125-131.

75. Curran AE, Miller EJ, Murrah VA. Adenomatoid odontogenic tumor presenting as periapical disease. Oral Surg Oral Med Oral Pathol Oral Radiol Endod 1997;84:557-560.

76. el-Labban NG. The nature of the eosinophilic and laminated masses in the adenomatoid odontogenic tumor: a histochemical and ultrastructural study. J Oral Pathol Med 1992;21:75-81.

77. Jivan V, Altini M, Meer S. Secretory cells in adenomatoid odontogenic tumour: tissue induction or metaplastic mineralisation? Oral Dis 2008;14:445-449.

78. Philipsen HP, Reichart PA. The adenomatoid odontogenic tumour: ultrastructure of tumour cells and non-calcified amorphous masses. J Oral Pathol Med 1996;25:491-496.

79. Leon JE, Mata GM, Fregnani ER, et al. Clinicopathological and immunohistochemical study of 39 cases of adenomatoid odontogenic tumour: a multicentric study. Oral Oncol 2005;41:835-842.

80. Modolo F, Biz MT, Martins MT, Machado de Sousa SO, de Araujo NS. Expression of extracellular matrix proteins in adenomatoid odontogenic tumor. J Oral Pathol Med 2010;39:230-235.

81. Vera Sempere FJ, Artes Martinez MJ, Vera Sirera B, Bonet Marco J. Follicular adenomatoid odontogenic tumor: immunohistochemical study. Med Oral Patol Oral Cir Bucal 2006;11:E305-308.

82. Hicks MJ, Flaitz CM, Batsakis JG. Adenomatoid and calcifying epithelial odontogenic tumors. Ann Otol Rhinol Laryngol 1993;102:159-161.

83. Franklin CD, Pindborg JJ. The calcifying epithelial odontogenic tumor. A review and analysis of 113 cases. Oral Surg Oral Med Oral Pathol 1976;42:753-765.

84. Neville BW, Damm DD, Allen CM, Bouquot JE. Odontogenic cysts and tumors. In: Oral and maxillofacial pathology, 3rd ed. St. Louis, MO: Saunders Elsevier; 2009:678-740.

85. Anavi Y, Kaplan I, Citir M, Calderon S. Clearcell variant of calcifying epithelial odontogenic tumor: clinical and radiographic characteristics. Oral Surg Oral Med Oral Pathol Oral Radiol Endod 2003;95:332-339.

86. Houston GD, Fowler CB. Extraosseous calcifying epithelial odontogenic tumor: report of two cases and review of the literature. Oral Surg Oral Med Oral Pathol Oral Radiol Endod 1997;83:577-583.

87. Philipsen HP, Reichart PA. Calcifying epithelial odontogenic tumour: biological profile based on 181 cases from the literature. Oral Oncol 2000;36:17-26.

88. Gopalakrishnan R, Simonton S, Rohrer MD, Koutlas IG. Cystic variant of calcifying epithelial odontogenic tumor. Oral Surg Oral Med Oral Pathol Oral Radiol Endod 2006;102:773-777.

89. Gupta R, Singh S, Jain S, Mandal AK. Recurrent calcifying epithelial odontogenic tumor of the maxilla: report of a case with cytologic diagnosis. Acta Cytol 2006;50:545-547.

90. Wang YP, Lee JJ, Wang JT, et al. Non-calcifying variant of calcifying epithelial odontogenic tumor with Langerhans cells. J Oral Pathol Med 2007;36:436-439.

91. Kawano K, Ono K, Yada N, et al. Malignant calcifying epithelial odontogenic tumor of the mandible: report of a case with pulmonary metastasis showing remarkable response to platinum derivatives. Oral Surg Oral Med Oral Pathol Oral Radiol Endod 2007;104:76-81.

92. Cheng YS, Wright JM, Walstad WR, Finn MD. Calcifying epithelial odontogenic tumor showing microscopic features of potential malignant behavior. Oral Surg Oral Med Oral Pathol Oral Radiol Endod 2002;93:287-295.

93. Gratzinger D, Salama ME, Poh CF, Rouse RV. Ameloblastoma, calcifying epithelial odontogenic tumor, and glandular odontogenic cyst show a distinctive immunophenotype with some myoepithelial antigen expression. J Oral Pathol Med 2008;37:177-184.

94. Poomsawat S, Punyasingh J. Calcifying epithelial odontogenic tumor: an immunohistochemical case study. J Mol Histol 2007;38:103-109.

95. Murphy CL, Kestler DP, Foster JS, et al. Odontogenic ameloblast-associated protein nature of the amyloid found in calcifying epithelial odontogenic tumors and unerupted tooth follicles. Amyloid 2008;15:89-95.

96. Solomon A, Murphy CL, Weaver K, et al. Calcifying epithelial odontogenic (Pindborg) tumor-associated amyloid consists of a novel human protein. J Lab Clin Med 2003;142:348-355.

97. Perdigao PF, Carvalho VM, DE Marco L, Gomez RS. Mutation of ameloblastin gene in calcifying epithelial odontogenic tumor. Anticancer Res 2009;29:3065-3067.

98. Peacock ZS, Cox D, Schmidt BL. Involvement of PTCH1 mutations in the calcifying epithelial odontogenic tumor. Oral Oncol 2010;46:387-392.

99. Hong YS, Wang J, Liu J, Zhang B, Hou L, Zhong M. [Expression of HOX C13 in odontogenic tumors.] Shanghai Kou Qiang Yi Xue 2007;16:587-591. [Chinese]

100. Barnes L, Eveson JW, Reichart P, Sidransky D, eds. World Health Organization Classification of Tumours. Pathology and genetics of head and neck tumours. Lyon: IARC Press; 2005.

101. Agaram NP, Collins BM, Barnes L, et al. Molecular analysis to demonstrate that odontogenic keratocysts are neoplastic. Arch Pathol Lab Med 2004;128:313-317.

102. Gaitán-Cepeda LA, Quezada-Rivera D, Tenorio-Rocha F, Leyva-Huerta ER. Reclassification of odontogenic keratocyst as tumour. Impact on the odontogenic tumours prevalence. Oral Dis. 2010;16:185-7.

103. Shear M. The aggressive nature of the odontogenic keratocyst: is it a benign cystic neoplasm? Part 2. Proliferation and genetic studies. Oral Oncol 2002;38:323-331.

104. Shear M. The aggressive nature of the odontogenic keratocyst: is it a benign cystic neoplasm? Part 1. Clinical and early experimental evidence of aggressive behaviour. Oral Oncol 2002;38:219-226.

105. Macdonald-Jankowski DS, Li TK. Keratocystic odontogenic tumour in a Hong Kong community: the clinical and radiological features. Dentomaxillofac Radiol 2010;39:167-175.

106. Worrall SF. Recurrent odontogenic keratocyst within the temporalis muscle. Br J Oral Maxillofac Surg 1992;30:59-62.

107. Rud J, Pindborg JJ. Odontogenic keratocysts: a follow-up study of 21 cases. J Oral Surg 1969;27:323-330.

108. Shear M. The aggressive nature of the odontogenic keratocyst: is it a benign cystic neoplasm? Part 3. Immunocytochemistry of cytokeratin and other epithelial cell markers. Oral Oncol 2002;38:407-415.

109. Shear M. Odontogenic keratocysts: natural history and immunohistochemistry. Oral Maxillofac Surg Clin North Am 2003;15:347-362.

110. Scharffetter K, Balz-Herrmann C, Lagrange W, Koberg W, Mittermayer C. Proliferation kinetics-study of the growth of keratocysts. Morpho-functional explanation for recurrences. J Craniomaxillofac Surg 1989;17:226-233.

111. de Oliveira MG, Lauxen Ida S, Chaves AC, Rados PV, Sant'Ana Filho M. Immunohistochemical analysis of the patterns of p53 and PCNA expression in odontogenic cystic lesions. Med Oral Patol Oral Cir Bucal 2008;13:E275-280.

112. Gadbail AR, Chaudhary M, Patil S, Gawande M. Actual proliferating index and p53 protein expression as prognostic marker in odontogenic cysts. Oral Dis 2009;15:490-498.

113. Poomsawat S, Punyasingh J, Vejchapipat P. Immuno-histochemical expression of p53 protein and iNOS in odontogenic cysts. J Med Assoc Thai 2009;92:952-960.

114. Mitrou GK, Tosios KI, Kyroudi A, Sklavounou A. Odontogenic keratocyst expresses vascular endothelial growth factor: an immunohistochemical study. J Oral Pathol Med 2009;38:470-475.

115. de Vicente JC, Torre-Iturraspe A, Gutierrez AM, Lequerica-Fernandez P. Immunohistochemical comparative study of the odontogenic keratocysts and other odontogenic lesions. Med Oral Patol Oral Cir Bucal 2010;15:e109-115.

116. Mendes RA, Carvalho JF, van der Waal I. A comparative immunohistochemical analysis of COX-2, p53, and Ki-67 expression in keratocystic odontogenic tumors. Oral Surg Oral Med Oral Pathol Oral Radiol Endod 2011;111:333-339.

117. Kuroyanagi N, Sakuma H, Miyabe S, et al. Prognostic factors for keratocystic odontogenic tumor (odontogenic keratocyst): analysis of clinico-pathologic and immunohistochemical findings in cysts treated by enucleation. J Oral Pathol Med 2009;38:386-392.

118. Freier K, Pungs S, Flechtenmacher C, Hofele C. [Activation of sonic hedgehog signaling in keratocystic odontogenic tumors.] HNO 2009;57:345-350. [German]

119. Vered M, Peleg O, Taicher S, Buchner A. The immunoprofile of odontogenic keratocyst (keratocystic odontogenic tumor) that includes expression of PTCH, SMO, GLI-1 and bcl-2 is similar to ameloblastoma but different from odontogenic cysts. J Oral Pathol Med 2009;38:597-604.

120. Grachtchouk M, Liu J, Wang A, et al. Odontogenic keratocysts arise from quiescent epithelial rests and are associated with deregulated hedgehog signaling in mice and humans. Am J Pathol 2006;169:806-814.

121. Okamoto E, Kikuchi K, Miyazaki Y, et al. Significance of podoplanin expression in keratocystic odontogenic tumor. J Oral Pathol Med 2010;39:110-114.

122. Mateus GC, Lanza GH, de Moura PH, Marigo Hde A, Horta MC. Cell proliferation and apoptosis in keratocystic odontogenic tumors. Med Oral Patol Oral Cir Bucal 2008;13:E697-702.

123. Andric M, Dozic B, Popovic B, et al. Survivin expression in odontogenic keratocysts and correlation with cytomegalovirus infection. Oral Dis 2010;16:156-159.

124. Rangiani A, Motahhary P. Evaluation of bax and bcl-2 expression in odontogenic keratocysts and orthokeratinized odontogenic cysts: A comparison of two cysts. Oral Oncol 2009;45:e41-44.

125. Suyama Y, Kubota Y, Yamashiro T, Ninomiya T, Koji T, Shirasuna K. Expression of keratinocyte growth factor and its receptor in odontogenic keratocysts. J Oral Pathol Med 2009;38:476-480.

126. Hakim SG, Kosmehl H, Sieg P, et al. Altered expression of cell-cell adhesion molecules β-catenin/E-cadherin and related Wnt-signaling pathway in sporadic and syndromal keratocystic odontogenic tumors. Clin Oral Investig 2011;15:321-328.

127. Donoff RB, Harper E, Guralnick WC. Collagenolytic activity in keratocysts. J Oral Surg 1972;30:879-884.

128. Harris M. Odontogenic cyst growth and prostaglandin-induced bone resorption. Ann R Coll Surg Engl 1978;60:85-91.

129. Pitak-Arnnop P, Chaine A, Oprean N, Dhanuthai K, Bertrand JC, Bertolus C. Management of odontogenic keratocysts of the jaws: a ten-year experience with 120 consecutive lesions. J Craniomaxillofac Surg 2010;38:358-364.

130. Clark P, Marker P, Bastian HL, Krogdahl A. Expression of p53, Ki-67, and EGFR in odontogenic keratocysts before and after decompression. J Oral Pathol Med 2006;35:568-572.

131. Stoelinga PJ. Long-term follow-up on keratocysts treated according to a defined protocol Int J Oral Maxillofac Surg 2001;30:14-25.

132. Stoelinga PJ. The treatment of odontogenic keratocysts by excision of the overlying, attached mucosa, enucleation, and treatment of the bony defect with carnoy solution. J Oral Maxillofac Surg 2005;63:1662-1666.

133. Bataineh AB, al Qudah M. Treatment of mandibular odontogenic keratocysts. Oral Surg Oral Med Oral Pathol Oral Radiol Endod 1998;86:42-47.

134. Chapelle KA, Stoelinga PJ, de Wilde PC, Brouns JJ, Voorsmit RA. Rational approach to diagnosis and treatment of ameloblastomas and odontogenic keratocysts. Br J Oral Maxillofac Surg 2004;42:381-390.

135. Dammer R, Niederdellmann H, Dammer P, Nuebler-Moritz M. Conservative or radical treatment of keratocysts: a retrospective review. Br J Oral Maxillofac Surg 1997;35:46-48.

136. Marker P, Brondum N, Clausen PP, Bastian HL. Treatment of large odontogenic keratocysts by decompression and later cystectomy: a long-term follow-up and a histologic study of 23 cases. Oral Surg Oral Med Oral Pathol Oral Radiol Endod 1996;82:122-131.

137. Jackson IT, Potparic Z, Fasching M, Schievink WI, Tidstrom K, Hussain K. Penetration of the skull base by dissecting keratocyst. J Cranio-maxillofac Surg 1993;21:319-325.

138. Gorlin RJ, Goltz RW. Multiple nevoid basal-cell epithelioma, jaw cysts and bifid rib. A syndrome. N Engl J Med 1960;262:908-912.

139. Gorlin RJ, Yunis JJ, Tuna N. Multiple nevoid basal cell carcinoma, odontogenic keratocysts and skeletal anomalies. A syndrome. Acta Derm Venereol 1963;43:39-55.

140. Gorlin RJ, Vickers RA, Kellen E, Williamson JJ. Multiple basal-cell nevi syndrome. an analysis of a syndrome consisting of multiple nevoid basal-cell carcinoma, jaw cysts, skeletal anomalies, medulloblastoma, and hyporesponsiveness to parathormone. Cancer 1965;18:89-104.

141. Gorlin RJ, Sedano HO. The multiple nevoid basal cell carcinoma syndrome revisited. Birth Defects Orig Artic Ser 1971;7:140-148.

142. Gorlin RJ. Nevoid basal cell carcinoma (Gorlin) syndrome: unanswered issues. J Lab Clin Med 1999;134:551-552.

143. Li TJ, Sun LS, Luo HY, et al. [Studies on keratocystic odontogenic tumors.] Beijing Da Xue Xue Bao 2009;41:16-20. [Chinese]

144. Gorlin RJ. Nevoid basal-cell carcinoma syndrome. Medicine (Baltimore) 1987;66:98-113.

145. Leonardi R, Caltabiano M, Lo Muzio L, et al. Bilateral hyperplasia of the mandibular coronoid processes in patients with nevoid basal cell carcinoma syndrome: an undescribed sign. Am J Med Genet 2002;110:400-403.

146. Shanley S, Ratcliffe J, Hockey A, et al. Nevoid basal cell carcinoma syndrome: review of 118 affected individuals. Am J Med Genet 1994;50:282-290.

147. Dowling PA, Fleming P, Saunders ID, Gorlin RJ, Napier SS. Odontogenic keratocysts in a 5-year-old: initial manifestations of nevoid basal cell carcinoma syndrome. Pediatr Dent 2000;22(1):53-55.

148. Brannon RB. The odontogenic keratocyst. A clinicopathologic study of 312 cases. Part I. Clinical features. Oral Surg Oral Med Oral Pathol 1976;42:54-72.

149. Gorlin RJ. Nevoid basal cell carcinoma (Gorlin) syndrome. Genet Med 2004;6:530-539.

150. Bale AE, Gailani MR, Leffell DJ. Nevoid basal cell carcinoma syndrome. J Invest Dermatol 1994;103(Suppl):126S-130S.

151. Bale AE. The nevoid basal cell carcinoma syndrome: genetics and mechanism of carcinogenesis. Cancer Invest 1997;15:180-186.

152. Figueroa A, Correnti M, Avila M, Andea A, DeVilliers P, Rivera H. Keratocystic odontogenic tumor associated with nevoid basal cell carcinoma syndrome: similar behavior to sporadic type? Otolaryngol Head Neck Surg 2010;142:179-183.

153. Lam EW, Lee L, Perschbacher SE, Pharoah MJ. The occurrence of keratocystic odontogenic tumours in nevoid basal cell carcinoma syndrome. Dentomaxillofac Radiol 2009;38:475-479.

154. Pullon PA, Shafer WG, Elzay RP, Kerr DA, Corio RL. Squamous odontogenic tumor. Report of six cases of a previously undescribed lesion. Oral Surg Oral Med Oral Pathol 1975;40:616-630.

155. Goldblatt LI, Brannon RB, Ellis GL. Squamous odontogenic tumor. Report of five cases and review of the literature. Oral Surg Oral Med Oral Pathol 1982;54:187-196.

156. Philipsen HP, Reichart PA. Squamous odontogenic tumor (SOT): a benign neoplasm of the periodontium. A review of 36 reported cases. J Clin Periodontol 1996;23:922-926.

157. Lin YL, White DK. Squamous odontogenic tumor. Oral Maxillofac Surg Clin North Am 2004;16:355-357.

158. Ruhin B, Raoul G, Kolb F, et al. Aggressive maxillary squamous odontogenic tumour in a child: histological dilemma and adaptative surgical behaviour. Int J Oral Maxillofac Surg 2007;36:864-866.

159. Simon JH, Jensen JL. Squamous odontogenic tumor-like proliferations in periapical cysts. J Endod 1985;11:446-448.

160. Unal T, Gomel M, Gunel O. Squamous odontogenic tumor-like islands in a radicular cyst: report of a case. J Oral Maxillofac Surg 1987;45:346-349.

161. Olivera JA, Costa IM, Loyola AM. Squamous odontogenic tumor-like proliferation in residual cyst: case report. Braz Dent J 1995;6:59-64.

162. Schwartz-Arad D, Lustmann J, Ulmansky M. Squamous odontogenic tumor. Review of the literature and case report. Int J Oral Maxillofac Surg 1990;19:327-330.

7 MESENCHYMAL ODONTOGENIC NEOPLASMS

ODONTOGENIC MYXOMA

Definition. *Odontogenic myxoma* is an uncommon benign neoplasm that recapitulates the mesenchymal portion of the tooth-forming unit, the dental papillae.

Clinical Features. Odontogenic myxomas occur most often in the posterior tooth-bearing areas of both upper and lower jaws, and more often in the mandible than the maxilla. Most tumors are identified during the second or third decade of life. There is no identified sex predilection. As with other odontogenic neoplasms, there is usually a smooth, bony hard expansion of the buccal aspect of the alveolus (1–5). In some instances, odontogenic myxomas form outside the body of the mandible, in which case they present as a smooth-surfaced, soft tissue enlargement (6).

Dezotti et al. (7) reviewed seven myxomas, four in males and three in females, diagnosed in patients ranging from 9 to 60 years of age. All the lesions were asymptomatic. Four cases involved tooth displacement but no cases of root resorption were noted.

Li et al. (8) evaluated 25 odontogenic myxomas, 13 in males and 12 in females, with ages ranging from 6 to 66 years. Twelve tumors involved the mandible and 13 occurred in the maxilla, with a predilection for posterior areas. The posterior maxillary tumors frequently involved the maxillary sinus.

In an evaluation of 62 odontogenic myxomas, Martinez-Mata et al. (9) reported an age range of 9 to 71 years and a female predominance of about 2 to 1. The mandible was affected in 37 cases and the maxilla in 25.

Radiographic Features. As with other odontogenic neoplasms, a unilocular or multilocular radiolucency is seen (fig. 7-1). Most lesions have a well-demarcated corticated border. Residual or reactive bone may give a somewhat mixed radiopaque/radiolucent appearance. Conventional or cone beam computerized tomography (CT) may be helpful (10,11). In an evaluation of 62 cases, 39 were multilocular and 23 unilocular

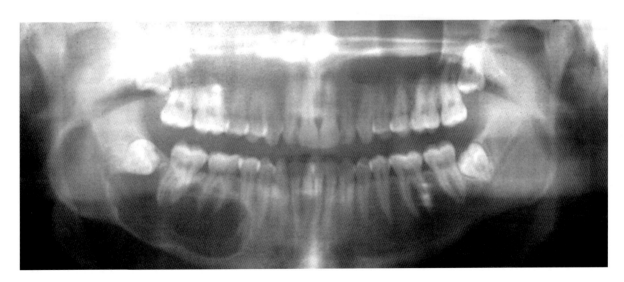

Figure 7-1

ODONTOGENIC MYXOMA

A well-demarcated, corticated radiolucency involves the right body of the mandible. The lesion is displacing the third molar.

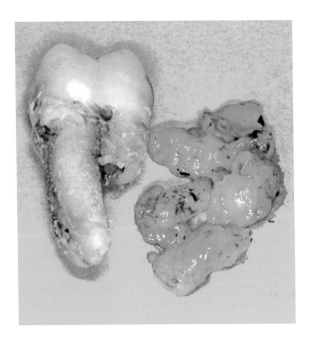

Figure 7-2

ODONTOGENIC MYXOMA

Gelatinous soft tissue and a molar tooth with root resorption are seen in the gross specimen.

(9). The lesions ranged from 1 to 13 cm; 37 multilocular (54.8 percent) and 6 unilocular lesions (26 percent) were larger than 4 cm. In an evaluation of 23 cases, 22 were multilocular (8).

When residual bone is somewhat organized, the radiographic appearance looks like a honeycomb or tennis racket strings (12). In a comparison of the radiographic and microscopic features of 30 cases, the radiographic septa were either reorientated cortical bone or sheets of dense fibrous connective tissue (13).

Gross Findings. Odontogenic myxomas consist of very loose, sometimes gelatinous, fibrovascular connective tissue with varying amounts of collagen formation (fig. 7-2). Their gross appearance is based primarily on the amount of collagen, which adds integrity to the otherwise gelatinous tissue.

Microscopic Findings. Odontogenic myxomas have an acellular, acid mucopolysaccharide, pale basophilic mesenchymal matrix with prominent, thin walled, slit-like vascular channels (fig. 7-3). The cells are well demarcated and show a spindle or stellate morphology. Nuclei are small and uniform in size. Mitosis is rare.

Mast cells and macrophages are sometimes seen. Occasional strands and cords of odontogenic epithelial cells are present in a minority of neoplasms, but are not necessary for the diagnosis (9). Some tumors may be more collagenous/fibromatous (fig. 7-4). Spherical mineralized bodies have been reported (14)

Immunohistochemical Findings. The cells of the odontogenic epithelial rests, when present, are positive for bcl-2, p53, AE1/AE3, cytokeratins 5, 7, 14, and 19, and MIB-1. The stromal cells are very positive for MIB-1. There is low expression of bc1-2 and Ki-67 proteins. Myofibroblastic differentiation has been shown (9,15).

Nonaka et al. (16) evaluated 12 odontogenic myxomas for expression of extracellular matrix metalloproteinases (MMP) 1, 2, and 9 as compared to dental germ papillae. MMP-2 was expressed only in myxomas. MMP-1 was detected in most myxomas at a proportion similar to that observed in dental papillae.

Treatment and Prognosis. Due to the loose gelatinous nature of the tumor, surgical enucleation can be difficult. Some surgeons recommend enucleation followed by chemical cauterization as the therapeutic management of choice. The goal of treatment should center on removal of medullary bone past the radiographic tumor borders although some surgeons prefer resection, especially for larger lesions. Recurrence rates vary significantly from case to case and often show a direct correlation with the size of the lesion at initial diagnosis.

In the Dezotti et al. (7) study of seven odontogenic myxomas, four were available for follow-up of 9 to 19 months: there were no recurrences. Of 25 myxomas studied by Li et al. (8), 5 were treated conservatively by enucleation and the remaining 20 by radical procedures, including block/segmental resection and partial or total maxillectomy or mandibulectomy. Follow-up data were available on 22 patients and only 1 patient initially treated by enucleation had a recurrence.

CENTRAL ODONTOGENIC FIBROMA

Definition. The *central odontogenic fibroma* is a rare benign odontogenic neoplasm of mesenchymal origin characterized by a mixture of cellular fibrous or collagenous connective tissue. There are varying numbers of odontogenic

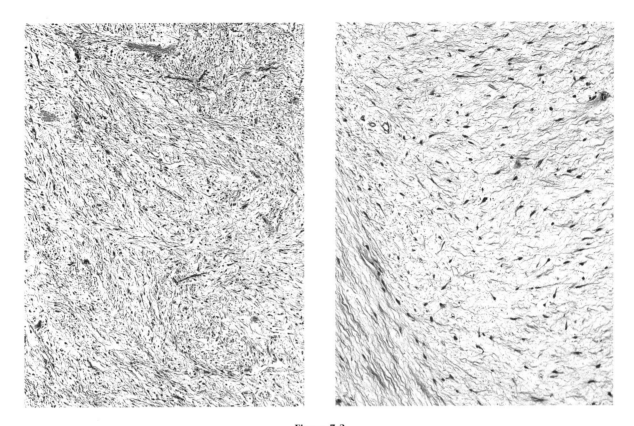

Figure 7-3

ODONTOGENIC MYXOMA

Left: There is a loose arrangement of spindle and stellate cells, with thin-walled, slit-like vascular channels.

Right: The spindle cells have ovoid nuclei and are associated with light, wavy collagen strands in a haphazard arrangement.

Figure 7-4

ODONTOGENIC MYXOMA

Increased collagen matrix characterizes this myxoma.

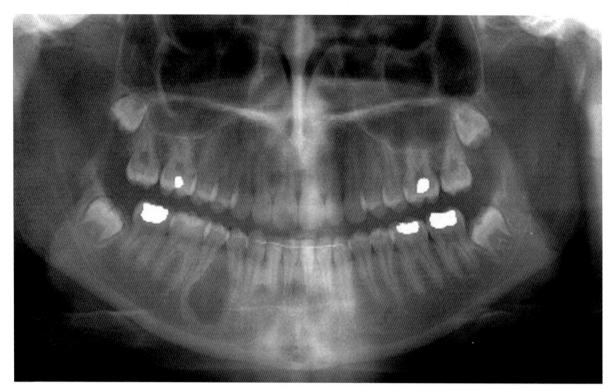

Figure 7-5

CENTRAL ODONTOGENIC FIBROMA

A well-demarcated radiolucency separates the roots of the premolars in the right mandible.

epithelial rests and strands. The lesion accounts for less than 1 percent of odontogenic neoplasms (17,18). The tumor has been described as a component of tuberous sclerosis (19).

Clinical Features. Central odontogenic fibromas have a slight female predilection and occur at essentially any age, with reports ranging from the first through the ninth decades. Tumors seem to occur more frequently in the anterior maxilla. As with other odontogenic neoplasms and cysts, this is an asymptomatic, slowly progressive buccal or palatal expansion (20–25).

Radiographic Features. Radiographically, most odontogenic fibromas present as unilocular radiolucencies with thin corticated borders demarcating the tumor from the surrounding normal bone (fig. 7-5). Larger lesions have a multilocular appearance. Rarely, tumors show evidence of mineralization (26). Because of their slow growth, they have a tendency to displace normal anatomy, including teeth, but occasional examples also show resorption.

Microscopic Findings. Central odontogenic fibromas are separated into two variants based primarily on the presence or absence of epithelial rests. This separation is of no prognostic significance. The *simple central odontogenic fibroma* consists of dense cellular or collagenous fibrous connective tissue (fig. 7-6). The lesion may be predominantly fibroblastic or generally acellular. A few odontogenic rests may be present. The second subtype, the *World Health Organization (WHO) type*, shows a similar cellular or collagenous connective tissue background admixed with numerous rests and cords of odontogenic epithelial cells (figs. 7-7, 7-8). The rests and cords show no evidence of peripheral columnar cells with polarized nuclei and no central areas resembling stellate reticulum. In some tumors, the tissue immediately surrounding the islands shows a homogenous, eosinophilic induction effect (fig. 7-9). Although mineralization is not a prominent feature in most tumors it has been reported (fig. 7-10) (27).

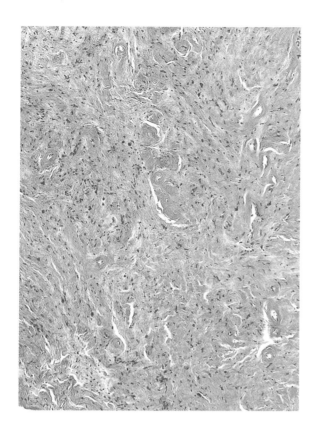 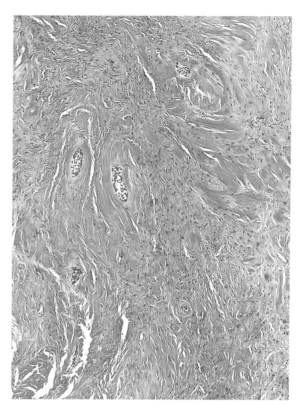

Figure 7-6

CENTRAL ODONTOGENIC FIBROMA

Left: The cellular, fibrovascular connective tissue has no discernable pattern or specific features.
Right: The cellular, fibrovascular connective tissue has a few odontogenic epithelial rests.

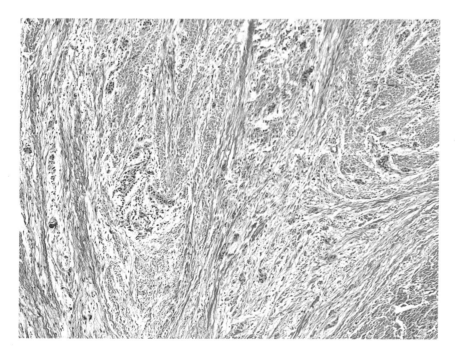

Figure 7-7

CENTRAL ODONTOGENIC FIBROMA, WHO TYPE

This tumor has a very collagenous background with numerous epithelial rests.

Figure 7-8

**CENTRAL
ODONTOGENIC FIBROMA**

Numerous rests and cords of
epithelial cells are present in a
cellular fibrovascular connective
tissue background.

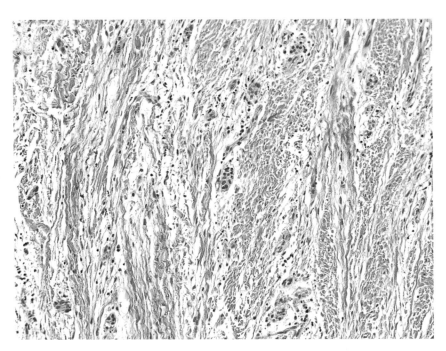

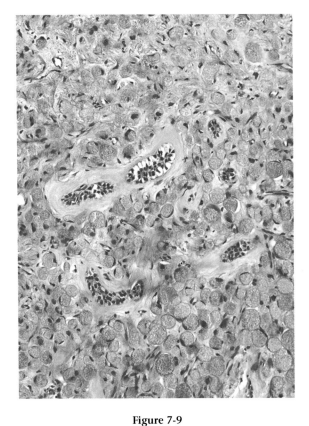

Figure 7-9

CENTRAL ODONTOGENIC FIBROMA

In this granular cell variant, sheets of ovoid cells with
granular cytoplasm surround typical odontogenic epithelial
rests. Induction is present at the periphery.

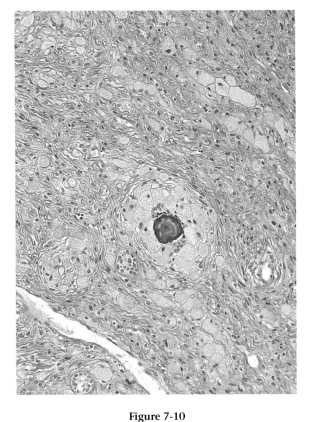

Figure 7-10

CENTRAL ODONTOGENIC FIBROMA

Cellular fibroblasts predominate, along with epithelial
rests, granular cells, and central lamellar mineralization.

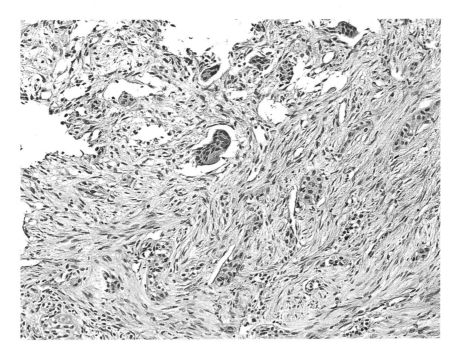

Figure 7-11

CENTRAL ODONTOGENIC FIBROMA/CENTRAL GIANT CELL LESION

The connective tissue contains numerous epithelial rests (lower right). Multiple giant cells are seen at the upper left.

Additional histopathologic variations include tumors with areas of multinucleated giant cells. These "hybrid" lesions have been reported as a possible collision tumor formed from a central odontogenic fibroma and a giant cell lesion (fig. 7-11) (28–30). Another histopathologic variant is a rarely reported tumor with numerous granular cells (31).

Treatment and Prognosis. Central odontogenic fibromas, regardless of the histopathologic subtype, are characteristically managed with conservative enucleation and curettage. Recurrent lesions are uncommon (32,33). Aggressive lesions requiring additional surgery have been reported (34).

CEMENTOBLASTOMA

Definition. *Cementoblastoma* is a benign neoplasm that occurs exclusively in direct association with the roots of teeth. These neoplasms are virtually identical to osteoblastomas microscopically, but are separated by their clinical and radiographic presentation. Cementoblastomas represent less than 6 percent of odontogenic tumors (35).

Clinical Features. Most cementoblastomas occur in the posterior body of the mandible. There is a slight male predilection and most lesions are diagnosed initially in the third decade.

As with other odontogenic neoplasms and cysts, they are characteristically asymptomatic. While most lesions involve erupted teeth (36–40), there are reports of cementoblastomas involving unerupted teeth (41). Rarely, they involve multiple teeth (42).

Brannon et al. (43) evaluated 44 cases of cementoblastoma from the Armed Forces Institute of Pathology (AFIP) archives and compared those to 74 cases previously published. The mean age at diagnosis was 21 years and 71 percent occurred in the mandible, most often in association with the first molar.

Radiographic Features. Radiographically, cementoblastomas present as a homogenous radiopacity expanding from the root(s) of a primary or permanent tooth (fig. 7-12) (43). The homogenous radiopacity is characteristically separated from surrounding normal bone by a thin radiolucent line. The degree of opacity may preclude visualization of the tooth roots, but in some instances, root resorption is seen.

Gross Findings. Because cementoblastomas are fused to the roots of teeth, tooth extraction or root resection is characteristically accomplished along with excision of the lesion. On gross examination, the root or roots of the tooth are enveloped in white, bony hard homogenous mineralized material (figs. 7-13, 7-14). There is

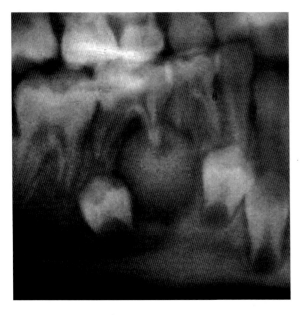

usually very little soft tissue. Lesions that are 1 to 2 cm in diameter often take more than 48 hours to demineralize.

Microscopic Findings. With proper sectioning, dense, irregular trabeculae and islands of cementum-like hard tissue fused to the residual root structure are seen (fig. 7-15). Centrally, few cementoblasts are identified; at the peripheral margins, however, plump cementoblasts rim the mineralizing tissue (figs. 7-16, 7-17). Cementoblasts are often angular with dark staining nuclei, identical to osteoblasts.

Treatment and Prognosis. Management of a cementoblastoma includes complete enucleation from its surrounding bone. As noted above, this usually requires tooth extraction or root amputation. In an evaluation of 35 AFIP cases followed for an average of 5.5 years by Brannon et al. (43), 13 (37 percent) recurred.

Figure 7-12

CEMENTOBLASTOMA

A homogeneous radiopacity is associated with the root of a primary mandibular molar and displaces both erupting premolars.

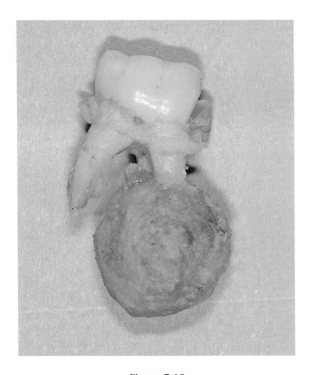

Figure 7-13

CEMENTOBLASTOMA

An intact tumor is fused to the root of the molar tooth.

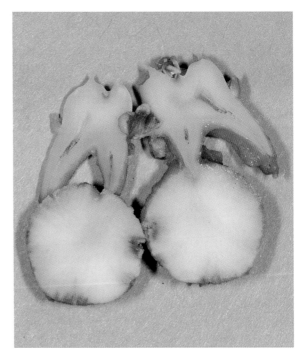

Figure 7-14

CEMENTOBLASTOMA

The sectioned tumor shows homogeneous, smooth mineralized material confluent with the molar root.

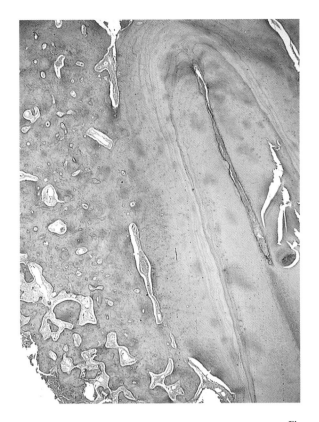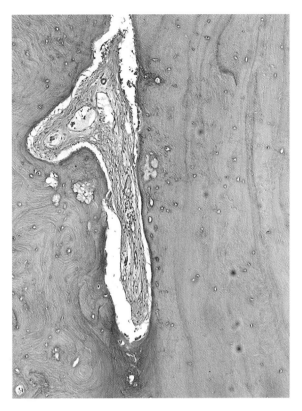

Figure 7-15

CEMENTOBLASTOMA

Left: At low power, the tooth root is seen at the right and irregular tumor cementum at the left.

Right: At higher power, normal cementum of the tooth root is at the left and irregular neoplastic appositional lines of cementum at the right.

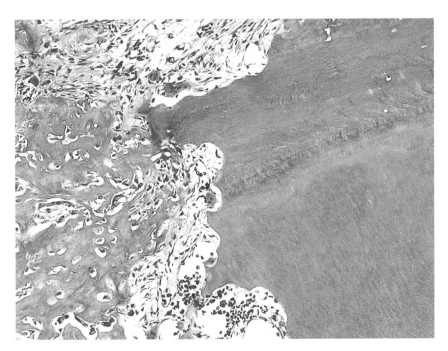

Figure 7-16

CEMENTOBLASTOMA

Large, polyhedral cementoblasts and multinucleated giant cells are seen adjacent to a tooth root undergoing resorption.

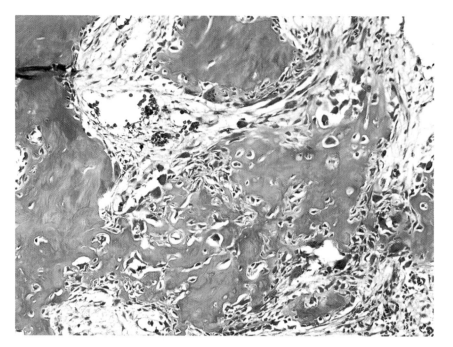

Figure 7-17

CEMENTOBLASTOMA

At the tumor periphery, large, angular cementoblasts produce irregular masses of cementum.

REFERENCES

1. Brannon RB. Central odontogenic fibroma, myxoma (odontogenic myxoma, fibromyxoma), and central odontogenic granular cell tumor. Oral Maxillofac Surg Clin North Am 2004;16:359-374.

2. Fenton S, Slootweg PJ, Dunnebier EA, Mourits MP. Odontogenic myxoma in a 17-month-old child: a case report. J Oral Maxillofac Surg 2003;61:734-736.

3. Mehrotra D, Kamboj M. Recurrent odontogenic myxofibroma of the mandible in a 12 year old: an illustrative case report. J Clin Pediatr Dent 2008;32:309-312.

4. Simon EN, Merkx MA, Vuhahula E, Ngassapa D, Stoelinga PJ. Odontogenic myxoma: a clinicopathological study of 33 cases. Int J Oral Maxillofac Surg 2004;33:333-337.

5. Mortellaro C, Berrone M, Turatti G, et al. Odontogenic tumors in childhood: a retrospective study of 86 treated cases. Importance of a correct histopathologic diagnosis. J Craniofac Surg 2008;19:1173-1176.

6. Aytac-Yazicioglu D, Eren H, Gorgun S. Peripheral odontogenic myxoma located on the maxillary gingiva: report of a case and review of the literature. Oral Maxillofac Surg 2008;12:167-171.

7. Dezotti MS, Azevedo LR, Fontao FN, Capelozza AL, Sant'ana E. Odontogenic myxoma—a case report and clinico-radiographic study of seven tumors. J Contemp Dent Pract 2006;7:117-124.

8. Li TJ, Sun LS, Luo HY. Odontogenic myxoma: a clinicopathologic study of 25 cases. Arch Pathol Lab Med 2006;130:1799-1806.

9. Martinez-Mata G, Mosqueda-Taylor A, Carlos-Bregni R, et al. Odontogenic myxoma: clinico-pathological, immunohistochemical and ultrastructural findings of a multicentric series. Oral Oncol 2008;44:601-607.

10. Araki M, Kameoka S, Matsumoto N, Komiyama K. Usefulness of cone beam computed tomography for odontogenic myxoma. Dentomaxillofac Radiol 2007;36:423-427.

11. Koseki T, Kobayashi K, Hashimoto K, et al. Computed tomography of odontogenic myxoma. Dentomaxillofac Radiol 2003;32:160-165.

12. Zhang J, Wang H, He X, Niu Y, Li X. Radiographic examination of 41 cases of odontogenic myxomas on the basis of conventional radiographs. Dentomaxillofac Radiol 2007;36:160-167.

13. Noffke CE, Raubenheimer EJ, Chabikuli NJ, Bouckaert MM. Odontogenic myxoma: review of the literature and report of 30 cases from South Africa. Oral Surg Oral Med Oral Pathol Oral Radiol Endod 2007;104:101-109.

14. Oygur T, Dolanmaz D, Tokman B, Bayraktar S. Odontogenic myxoma containing osteocement-like spheroid bodies: report of a case with an unusual histopathological feature. J Oral Pathol Med 2001;30:504-506.

15. Iezzi G, Piattelli A, Rubini C, Artese L, Fioroni M, Carinci F. MIB-1, Bcl-2 and p53 in odontogenic myxomas of the jaws. Acta Otorhinolaryngol Ital 2007;27:237-242.

16. Nonaka CF, Augusto Vianna Goulart Filho J, Cristina da Costa Miguel M, Batista de Souza L, Pereira Pinto L. Immunohistochemical expression of matrix metalloproteinases 1, 2, and 9 in odontogenic myxoma and dental germ papilla. Pathol Res Pract 2009;205:458-465.

17. Daniels JS. Central odontogenic fibroma of mandible: a case report and review of the literature. Oral Surg Oral Med Oral Pathol Oral Radiol Endod 2004;98:295-300.

18. Daskala I, Kalyvas D, Kolokoudias M, Vlachodimitropoulos D, Alexandridis C. Central odontogenic fibroma of the mandible: a case report. J Oral Sci 2009;51:457-461.

19. Swarnkar A, Jungreis CA, Peel RL. Central odontogenic fibroma and intracranial aneurysm associated with tuberous sclerosis. Am J Otolaryngol 1998;19:66-69.

20. Bueno S, Berini L, Gay C. Central odontogenic fibroma: a review of the literature and report of a new case. Med Oral 1999;4:422-434.

21. Ramer M, Buonocore P, Krost B. Central odontogenic fibroma—report of a case and review of the literature. Periodontal Clin Investig 2002;24:27-30.

22. Brannon RB, Goode RK, Eversole LR, Carr RF. The central granular cell odontogenic tumor: report of 5 new cases. Oral Surg Oral Med Oral Pathol Oral Radiol Endod 2002;94:614-621.

23. Dezotti MS, Azevedo LR, Fontao FN, Capelozza AL, Sant'ana E. Odontogenic myxoma—a case report and clinico-radiographic study of seven tumors. J Contemp Dent Pract 2006;7:117-124.

24. Cicconetti A, Bartoli A, Tallarico M, Maggiani F, Santaniello S. Central odontogenic fibroma interesting the maxillary sinus. A case report and literature survey. Minerva Stomatol 2006;55:229-239.

25. Hollowell M, Gang D, Pantanowitz L. Odontogenic fibroma. Ear Nose Throat J 2010;89:214-215.

26. Araki M, Nishimura S, Matsumoto N, Ohnishi M, Ohki H, Komiyama K. Central odontogenic fibroma with osteoid formation showing atypical radiographic appearance. Dentomaxillofac Radiol 2009;38:426-430.

27. Raubenheimer EJ, Noffke CE. Central odontogenic fibroma-like tumors, hypodontia, and enamel dysplasia: review of the literature and report of a case. Oral Surg Oral Med Oral Pathol Oral Radiol Endod 2002;94:74-77.

28. de Lima Mde D, de Aquino Xavier FC, Vanti LA, de Lima PS, de Sousa SC. Hybrid central giant cell granuloma and central odontogenic fibroma-like lesion of the mandible. Otolaryngol Head Neck Surg 2008;139:867-868.

29. Tosios KI, Gopalakrishnan R, Koutlas IG. So-called hybrid central odontogenic fibroma/central giant cell lesion of the jaws. A report on seven additional cases, including an example in a patient with cherubism, and hypotheses on the pathogenesis. Head Neck Pathol 2008;2:333-338.

30. Younis RH, Scheper MA, Lindquist CC, Levy B. Hybrid central odontogenic fibroma with giant cell granuloma-like component: case report and review of literature. Head Neck Pathol 2008;2:222-226.

31. Vincent SD, Hammond HL, Ellis GL, Juhlin JP. Central granular cell odontogenic fibroma. Oral Surg Oral Med Oral Pathol 1987;63:715-721.

32. Brazao-Silva MT, Fernandes AV, Durighetto-Junior AF, Cardoso SV, Loyola AM. Central odontogenic fibroma: a case report with long-term follow-up. Head Face Med 2010;6:20.

33. Covani U, Crespi R, Perrini N, Barone A. Central odontogenic fibroma: a case report. Med Oral Patol Oral Cir Bucal 2005;10(Suppl 2):E154-157.

34. Drebber U, Scheer M, Zoller JE, Dienes HP. [The central odontogenic fibroma. A rare tumor.] Pathologe 2003;24:136-140. [German]

35. Slimani F, Elbouihi M, Oukerroum A, et al. [Maxillary cementoblastoma. A case report.] Rev Med Brux 2009;30(3):185-188. [French]

36. Barker GL, Begley A, Balmer C. Cementoblastoma in the maxilla: a case report. Prim Dent Care 2009;16:154-156.

37. Hirai E, Yamamoto K, Kounoe T, Kondo Y, Yonemasu H, Kurokawa H. Benign cementoblastoma of the anterior maxilla. J Oral Maxillofac Surg 2010;68:671-674.

38. Huber AR, Folk GS. Cementoblastoma. Head Neck Pathol 2009;3:133-135.

39. Neves FS, Falcao AF, Dos Santos JN, Dultra FK, Rebello IM, Campos PS. Benign cementoblastoma: case report and review of the literature. Minerva Stomatol 2009;58:55-59.

40. Pattyn E, Mermuys K, Lateur L. Cementoblastoma. JBR-BTR 2007;90:306.

41. Zaitoun H, Kujan O, Sloan P. An unusual recurrent cementoblastoma associated with a developing lower second molar tooth: a case report. J Oral Maxillofac Surg 2007;65:2080-2082.

42. de Amorim RF, Silveira EJ, Franca MN, Guimaraes Mdo C, Lima Junior N, de Carvalho DR. A case of extensive maxillary benign cementoblastoma. J Contemp Dent Pract 2010;11:56-62.

43. Brannon RB, Fowler CB, Carpenter WM, Corio RL. Cementoblastoma: an innocuous neoplasm? A clinicopathologic study of 44 cases and review of the literature with special emphasis on recurrence. Oral Surg Oral Med Oral Pathol Oral Radiol Endod 2002;93:311-320.

8 MIXED EPITHELIAL/ MESENCHYMAL NEOPLASMS

AMELOBLASTIC FIBROMA

Definition. *Ameloblastic fibroma* is a benign odontogenic neoplasm characterized by the proliferation of immature odontogenic epithelium and mesenchyme, both of which are characteristic of the developing tooth. Unlike ameloblastic fibro-odontoma or the variants of odontoma, complex or compound, ameloblastic fibromas do not produce enamel, dentin, or cementum.

Using age, sex, and site of occurrence of various lesions, Slootweg (1) concluded that ameloblastic fibromas represent a separate entity that does not develop into a more differentiated odontogenic tumor. In a review of 123 cases, Chen et al. (2) showed that 88 occurred in the first two decades of life and 30 occurred in patients over the age of 22 years. These data support the view that most ameloblastic fibromas diagnosed in adults are true neoplasms. The authors suggested that a small but unknown number of these tumors, which occur in childhood, may represent the primitive stage of a developing odontoma (2).

In young patients, developing odontomas have little if any mineralization and are histopathologically indistinguishable from an ameloblastic fibroma. Separating these early developing odontomas from an ameloblastic fibroma is impossible (3–8).

Clinical Features. The tumor can be found in any tooth-bearing site, but most often occurs in the premolar-molar region of the mandible. There is no gender predilection, but the lesion is usually identified in a bimodal age distribution. Most lesions are diagnosed before age 20, although another smaller occurrence cluster is noted during the fourth and fifth decades.

As with other odontogenic neoplasms, the lesion is slow growing and asymptomatic unless secondarily inflamed. A firm expansion of the buccal cortical plate of the mandible or maxilla is the most common clinical finding.

Radiographic Features. Ameloblastic fibroma, similar to other odontogenic neoplasms, appears radiographically as a well-demarcated, well-corticated radiolucency. Depending on the size of the tumor, the radiolucency appears unilocular or multilocular. It may be associated with the crown of an unerupted tooth.

Microscopic Findings. Ameloblastic fibroma is characterized by the proliferation of odontogenic epithelial islands in a background of primitive cellular mesenchyme (fig. 8-1). The latter component is cellular, young basophilic fibromyxoid tissue suggestive of developing tooth pulp or dental papillae. The cells appear stellate or spindled. Admixed within this mesenchymal background are islands, cords, and strands of ovoid, cuboidal, and occasionally columnar epithelium. Small islands may show a central area of stellate epithelial cells characteristic of stellate reticulum. These islands may be identical to the neoplastic cells seen in follicular ameloblastoma but the surrounding young cellular mesenchymal tissue is the differentiating feature. Mitoses are rare. Occasional islands have a peripheral rim of eosinophilic acellular material representing an induction effect; however, there is no evidence of mineralization. If mineralization is seen, the lesion is actually an ameloblastic fibro-odontoma.

Immunohistochemical Findings. In an evaluation of HOXC13 mRNA expression in odontogenic tumors, all odontogenic epithelium was positive except for the epithelial islands in ameloblastic fibromas (9). The positive rates for HOXC13 mRNA expression were 97.9 percent in ameloblastomas, 100 percent in calcifying cystic odontogenic tumors and calcifying odontogenic tumors, 70.0 percent in keratocystic odontogenic tumors, 42.9 percent in the normal oral mucosa, and 0 percent in ameloblast fibroma. The authors concluded that HOXC13 mRNA expression may be a marker that can be used

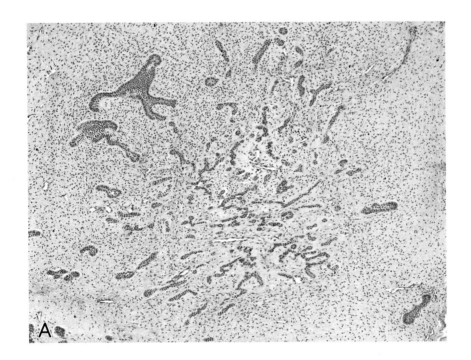

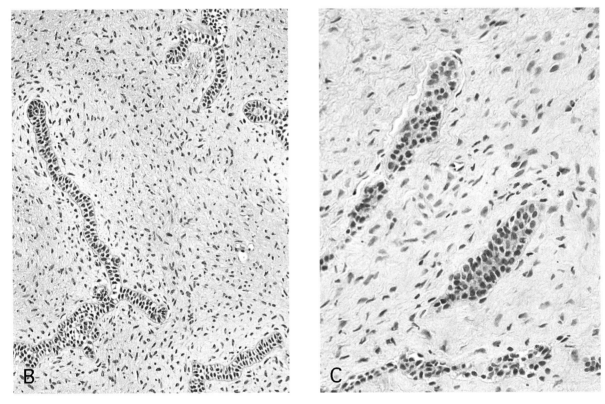

Figure 8-1

AMELOBLASTIC FIBROMA

A: Nests and cords of epithelial cells are present in a background of cellular mesenchymal tissue resembling dental papillae.
B: Double-stranded cords of odontogenic epithelial cells have a cellular mesenchymal background.
C: Islands and strands of ovoid epithelial cells are seen in a cellular mesenchymal background.

to distinguish cases of ameloblastic fibroma and ameloblastoma. Immunohistochemical analysis for *MIB-1* genes, important in the regulation of apoptosis, showed the labeling indices in the mesenchymal component of the rare, recurrent ameloblastic fibroma are high in contrast with the nonrecurrent ameloblastic fibroma (10).

Treatment and Prognosis. Conservative surgical enucleation of the tumor is the treatment of choice for all small unilocular lesions. The tumor does not have the infiltrative margins characteristic of an ameloblastoma and therefore recurrence rates are low. With early detection and removal, the long-term prognosis is favorable. Larger multilocular lesions, however, may be destructive and reports of recurrence of 40 percent were reported in a 1972 article from a series of cases at the Armed Forces Institute of Pathology (11).

Chen et al. (2), studying 123 cases, suggested that the age of the patients is an important consideration when choosing therapeutic methods and that aggressive surgery should not be employed for the treatment of younger patients. Because a significant number of the rare ameloblastic fibrosarcomas reportedly develop from ameloblastic fibromas, long-term follow-up is recommended (12).

AMELOBLASTIC FIBRO-ODONTOMA

Definition. *Ameloblastic fibro-odontoma* is an odontogenic tumor that has caused a degree controversy in the literature regarding its appropriate classification. Some have classified the tumor as an early developmental stage of odontoma (hamartoma). Others define this tumor as an ameloblastic fibroma that also produces enamel and dentin. There are reports of large, progressively destructive ameloblastic fibro-odontomas, which clearly indicate that at least some of these tumors are neoplastic rather than hamartomatous (3).

General Features. Ameloblastic fibro-odontomas are usually located in the posterior jaws with about equal frequency in the maxilla and mandible. Most patients are young adults, with a mean age of 10 years. Whether these data are skewed from improper inclusion of maturing odontomas is difficult to assess. There is no significant gender predilection.

Clinical Features. As with all odontogenic tumors, ameloblastic fibro-odontomas are usually asymptomatic. Some tumors cause significant cortical plate expansion. Most are identified during radiographic studies for other reasons or when a tooth has failed to erupt (13,14).

Radiographic Features. The tumor usually presents as a well-circumscribed unilocular or multilocular radiolucency that often shows radiopaque portions corresponding to the apposition of enamel, dentin, and cementum. The mineralized material can appear as small radiopacities or as large homogeneous radiopacities, identical to complex or compound odontomas. The amount of mineralization varies widely, and some lesions have no evidence of radiopacity.

Microscopic Findings. The histopathologic features of an ameloblastic fibro-odontoma are characterized by the proliferation of both epithelial and induced mesenchymal elements described previously in tooth germ formation (fig. 8-2). The mesenchymal component presents as basophilic or eosinophilic fibromyxoid tissue suggestive of developing tooth pulp or dental papillae, focally identical to ameloblastic fibromas. Admixed within the mesenchymal background are islands, cords, and strands of ovoid, cuboidal, and columnar ameloblastic epithelial cells with areas resembling stellate reticulum (fig. 8-3). Other cells include columnar odontoblasts. Mitoses are infrequent. Mineralized and premineralized elements include enamel, enamel matrix, amorphous and tubular dentin, and cementum (15–17). Areas of apposition may or may not appear morphologically similar to a forming tooth.

In an evaluation of five cases with electron microscopy, Slootweg (1) noted that the ultrastructure of the tumors was identical to normally developing odontogenic tissues, with the exception that some mesenchymal cells failed to develop into tall columnar odontoblasts. Nestin, an intermediate filament constituting the cytoskeleton, adheres to the dentin tubules in ameloblastic fibro-odontomas (18).

Treatment and Prognosis. Small ameloblastic fibro-odontomas are generally treated with simple enucleation. Multilocular lesions should be treated with curettage/peripheral ostectomy. Recurrences have been reported but are rare (17,19)

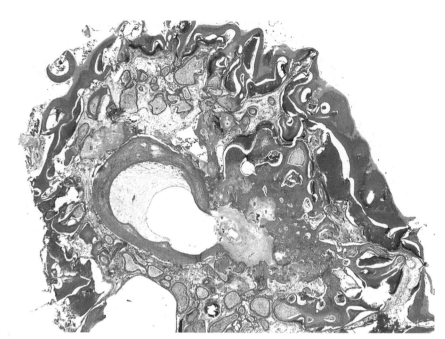

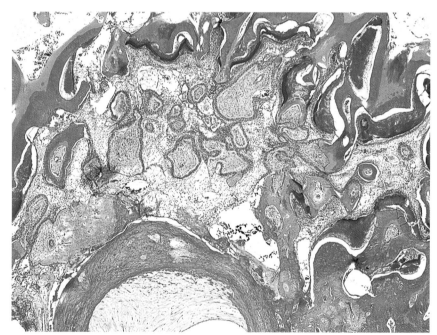

Figure 8-2

AMELOBLASTIC FIBRO-ODONTOMA

Top: Foci of eosinophilic dentin, cementum, and basophilic enamel matrix are seen.

Bottom: The cellular soft tissue consists of ameloblasts with adjacent stellate reticulum-like tissue and columnar odontoblasts.

ODONTOMA

Definition. *Odontomas* are the most commonly diagnosed odontogenic tumor. They are considered by many to be hamartomas rather than true neoplasms. Odontomas are subdivided into two types: complex and compound. *Complex odontomas*, when fully developed, consist almost entirely of sheets of enamel, enamel matrix, dentin, and cementum arranged in a haphazard manner. *Compound odontomas* consist of the same mineralized materials, with greater organization forming multiple small, malformed teeth. Complex and compound odontomas occur with equal frequency and some cases show features of both subtypes.

General Features. Odontomas occur more frequently in the maxilla than the mandible. The compound variant is found more often in

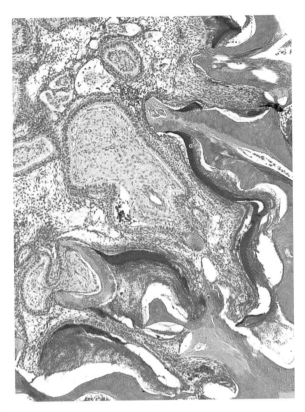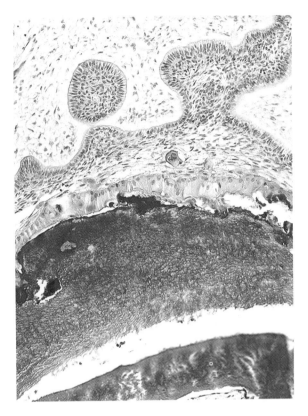

Figure 8-3

AMELOBLASTIC FIBRO-ODONTOMA

Left: A haphazard arrangement of ameloblasts, odontoblasts, and stellate cells with tubular dentin, cementum, and enamel matrix.

Right: A row of tall, columnar ameloblasts is adjacent to basophilic enamel matrix.

the anterior maxilla and the complex variant occurs more often in the posterior maxilla. Most odontomas are initially diagnosed within the first two decades of life.

Clinical Features. While some larger odontomas cause clinically evident expansion of the mandible or maxilla, most are identified on radiographs made for other reasons. They are always asymptomatic unless secondarily inflamed by trauma or continuity with the surface. They range in size from less than 1 cm to more than 6 cm in diameter. They may cause morphologic problems with developing teeth and may delay eruption (20,21).

Radiographic Features. Both complex and compound odontomas show a well-demarcated radiolucency with a uniform corticated border delineating the lesion from the surrounding bone. Centrally, the lesion shows increasing evidence of homogeneous radiopacity as min-

eralization of the tooth matrix material progresses. In compound odontomas, the radiopaque material eventually appears multilobular, like a cluster of grapes, coinciding with the formation of multiple, poorly formed tooth-like structures (fig. 8-4). Compared with compound lesions, the radiopaque material of complex odontomas appears more homogeneous and is usually more opaque than the surrounding normal bone (fig. 8-5).

Gross Findings. Compound odontomas usually appear as a cluster of small, white, bony hard, smooth-surfaced nodules of varying sizes and shapes. By contrast, complex odontomas appear as homogeneous, white, bony hard tumors that have often been fractured or sectioned during removal by the surgeon (fig. 8-6). Both are accompanied by varying amounts of nondescript, tan soft tissue. For large complex odontomas measuring more that 2 to 3 cm, demineralization prior to processing may take

103

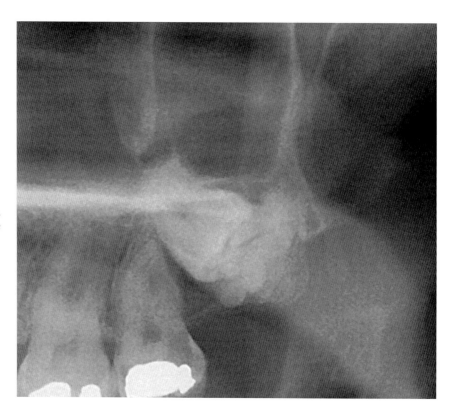

Figure 8-4

COMPOUND ODONTOMA

Multiple radiopaque lobules are noted in the follicular space of a maxillary third molar.

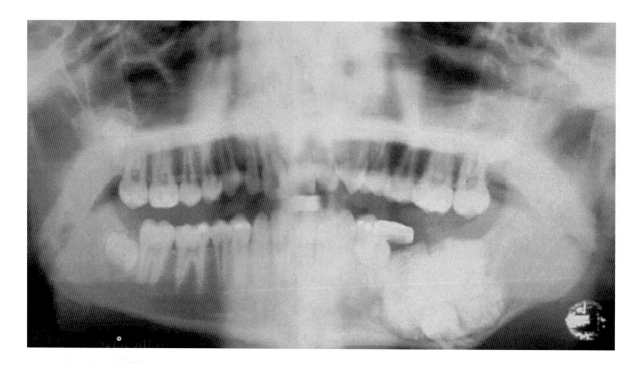

Figure 8-5

COMPLEX ODONTOMA

A homogeneous well-circumscribed radiopacity has displaced a molar tooth to the inferior border of the mandible.

up to 72 hours due to slow penetration of the solution into the dense mineralized tumor.

Microscopic Findings. Compound odontomas consist of dentin, cementum, and enamel matrix arranged so as to suggest the formation of teeth (fig. 8-7). Complex odontomas, when mature, consist almost entirely of a conglomeration of dentin, cementum, and enamel arranged in a haphazard manner (figs. 8-8). During the demineralization process necessary for routine microscopic sectioning, the enamel portion of complex and compound odontomas is reduced to retracted and fragmented, homogenous, basophilic material. This is because enamel is less than 5 percent organic soft tissue when completely formed.

Some soft tissue elements may be seen adjacent to the mineralizations, including reduced enamel epithelium adjacent to the enamel and columns of odontoblasts and mesenchymal dental pulp adjacent to the dentin. Odontogenic rests are also seen. A variety of odontogenic cysts and tumors have occurred in association with odontomas (18,22,34).

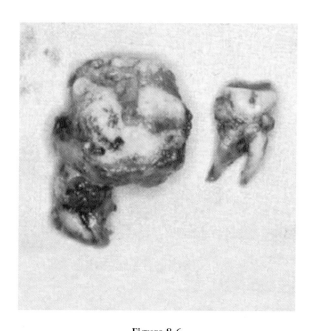

Figure 8-6

COMPLEX ODONTOMA

Grossly, the tumor from figure 8-5 is a homogeneous, bony hard, 2.5-cm mass.

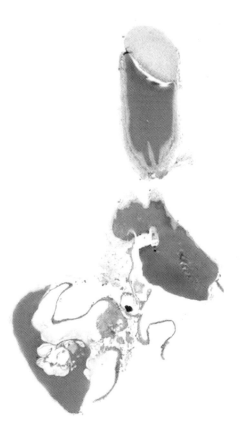

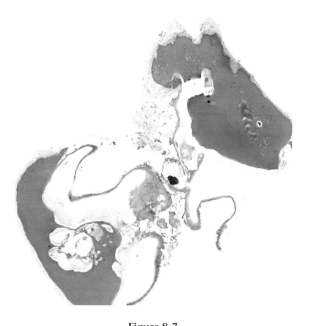

Figure 8-7

COMPOUND ODONTOMA

Left: The three irregular-shaped masses of eosinophilic tooth material include eosinophilic dentin, cellular pulp, and enamel matrix.

Above: Sheets of eosinophilic tubular dentin, basophilic enamel matrix, and reduced enamel epithelium are seen.

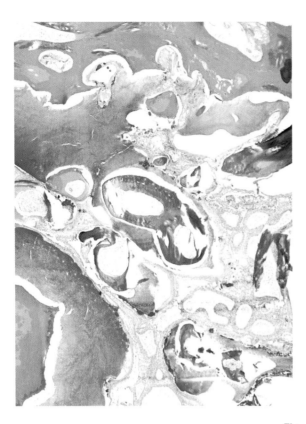 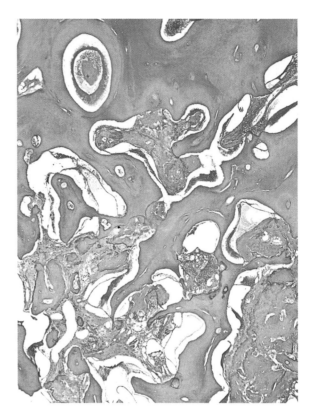

Figure 8-8

COMPLEX ODONTOMA

Left: Irregular sheets of eosinophilic tubular dentin, basophilic enamel matrix, and strands of ameloblastic epithelium are seen in this immature odontoma.

Right: A more mature complex odontoma has irregular sheets of dentin, enamel matrix, and little residual soft tissue.

Treatment and Prognosis. Complex and compound odontomas are treated with local, conservative excision although larger lesions may require a more complex surgical approach (23–25). Recurrence rates are low because the lesions are hamartomatous rather than neoplastic in origin.

CALCIFYING CYSTIC ODONTOGENIC TUMOR (CALCIFYING ODONTOGENIC CYST, GORLIN CYST, DENTINOGENIC GHOST CELL TUMOR, ODONTOGENIC GHOST CELL TUMOR)

Definition. Following the original description of *calcifying cystic odontogenic tumor* by Gorlin in 1962, the classification of odontogenic lesions characterized by ghost cells has continued to evolve (26,27). The World Health Organization (WHO) classification scheme published in 1992 reclassified calcifying odontogenic cysts as benign tumors (28). While some

classify this lesion as an epithelial odontogenic tumor, the presence of hard tissue resembling dentin in some cases indicates some degree of mesenchymal induction. The tumor is an unusual jaw lesion that can vary from a simple, central bony, epithelial-lined cyst to a complex, focally solid tumor mass. Both variants can be intraosseous or extraosseous, and often appear in association with other odontogenic tumors especially odontomas. Due to the variety of classification schemes proposed in the recent and not so recent past, both cystic and solid variants are described in this section.

Classification. As inferred by the number and variety of terms suggested for this entity, there have been a variety of classification schemes published (Table 8-1). In 1981, Praetorius et al. (29) was the first to subclassify variants into cysts and neoplasms. Included were three cystic variants: 1) a simple unilocular

Table 8-1

**CALCIFYING CYSTIC ODONTOGENIC
TUMOR CLASSIFICATIONS**

Praetorius et al.: 1981 (29)[a]
  Type 1: Cystic
      Simple unicystic
      Odontoma-producing type
      Ameloblastomatous-proliferating type
  Type 2: Neoplastic (dentinogenic ghost cell tumor)

Hong et al: 1991 (30)
  Type 1: Cystic
      Nonproliferative
      Proliferative
      Ameloblastomatous
      With odontoma
  Type 2: Neoplastic
      Ameloblastomatous ex coc
      Peripheral ghost cell tumor
      Central ghost cell tumor

Buchner: 1991 (31)
  Peripheral (extraosseous)
    Cystic
    Neoplastic, solid
  Central (intraosseous)
    Cystic: Simple
          With odontoma
          With other odontogenic tumors
          Clear cell and pigmented variants
    Neoplastic: Dentinogenic and/or epithelial
            odontogenic ghost cell tumors

Toida: 1998 (33)
  Cyst: Calcifying odontogenic ghost cell cyst
  Neoplasm:
    Benign
      Calcifying ghost cell odontogenic tumor,
          cystic variant
      Calcifying ghost cell odontogenic tumor,
          solid variant
    Malignant calcifying ghost cell odontogenic tumor
    Multiple lesions from all categories above associ-
        ated with other odontogenic tumors including
        odontomas and ameloblastomas

Ledesma–Montes et al: 2008 (32)
  Calcifying cystic odontogenic tumor
    Simple cystic
    Odontoma associated
    Ameloblastomatous proliferative
    Associated with benign odontogenic tumors
        other than odontoma
  Dentinogenic ghost cell tumor
    Type 1: Central
    Type 2: Peripheral
  Ghost cell odontogenic carcinoma (GCOC)
    arising de novo
    ex calcifying odontogenic tumor
    ex dentinogenic ghost cell tumor

[a]Numbers in parentheses are references.

variant with moderate mural proliferations of epithelium and little or no mineralization; 2) a unilocular variant in combination with a luminal compound or complex odontoma or an intramural ameloblastic fibroma; and 3) a unilocular cyst with extensive luminal as well as mural ameloblastoma-like proliferations. The neoplastic variant, termed *dentinogenic ghost cell tumor*, showed ameloblastoma-like strands and islands of epithelium with varying numbers of ghost cells and mineralization that closely resembles dentin.

In 1991, Hong et al. (30) proposed a new classification scheme consisting of four cystic and three neoplastic variants. The cystic variants included: 1) nonproliferative type, characterized by a simple unicystic structure; 2) a proliferative type, characterized by a cystic structure with multiple daughter cysts, extensive ghost cell formations, and increased mineralizations; 3) an ameloblastomatous type, characterized by an ameloblastoma-like cyst lining epithelium with ghost cells and mineralizations; and 4) an odontoma-associated type. The neoplastic variants included: 1) ameloblastoma ex calcifying odontogenic cyst, which showed unifocal and multifocal intraluminal and intramural ameloblastoma proliferating from the cyst; 2) peripheral epithelial odontogenic ghost cell tumor, which occurred in the gingiva and resembled peripheral ameloblastoma except for clustered ghost cells in the central portion of epithelial islands and dentinoid; and 3) central epithelial odontogenic ghost cell tumor, which showed ameloblastomatous or adenomatoid odontogenic tumor-like epithelial clusters with ghost cell formation and dentinoid.

Also in 1991, Buchner (31) proposed a classification which separated peripheral cysts and neoplasms from their central bony counterparts. Subsequent alternative classification schemes have been proposed by Toida in 1998 and Ledesma-Montes in 2008 (32,33).

General Features. The origin of calcifying cystic odontogenic tumor is probably the early dental lamina. This is supported by the fact that pituitary craniopharyngiomas and calcifying epitheliomas of Malherbe often mimic calcifying cystic odontogenic tumors. As with other odontogenic neoplasms and cysts, the lesion occurs in any tooth-bearing site. In an evaluation

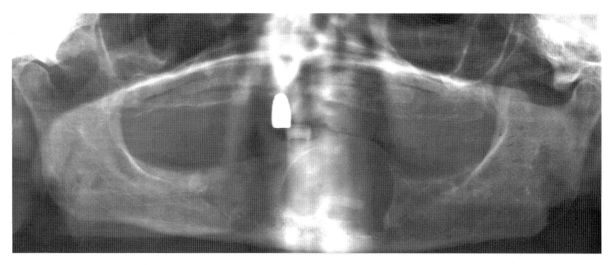

Figure 8-9

CALCIFYING CYSTIC ODONTOGENIC TUMOR

The panoramic radiograph shows a corticated radiolucency of the anterior mandible.

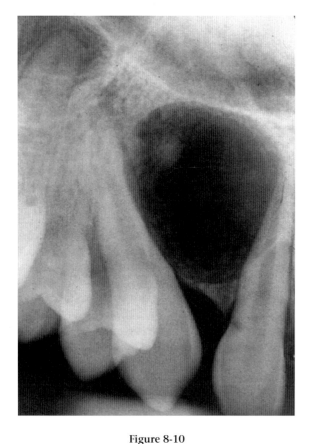

Figure 8-10

CALCIFYING CYSTIC ODONTOGENIC TUMOR

A well-demarcated radiolucency with small "snowflake" radiopacities is displacing the roots of the maxillary right canine and lateral incisor.

of 1,088 odontogenic tumors excluding odontomas as hamartomas, 6.5 percent were calcifying cystic odontogenic tumors (34).

The lesion has been diagnosed in individuals under 10 and over 80 years of age although the peak incidence is in the second and third decades. There is essentially equal distribution between females and males when all types are considered. Lesions in young adults are often associated with odontomas. The anterior portion of the jaws are more commonly involved than posterior regions. There may be a slight maxillary predominance over the mandible (32,35,36).

Clinical Features. For central bony lesions, the most common clinical finding is the firm expansion of the buccal cortical plate. The mucosa over the expansion is usually normal in appearance and there is seldom perforation of these slowly growing tumors. The lesions are asymptomatic unless secondarily inflamed.

Radiographic Features. The intraosseous lesions show radiographic features similar to other odontogenic tumors and cysts (figs. 8-9, 8-10). The borders are well demarcated and corticated. The lesion may be unilocular or multilocular, depending on size. The slow growth tends to displace normal anatomic structures, including teeth, although resorption can be seen (fig. 8-11). Mineralizations found within the lesion appear as small homogeneous radiopacities (fig. 8-10).

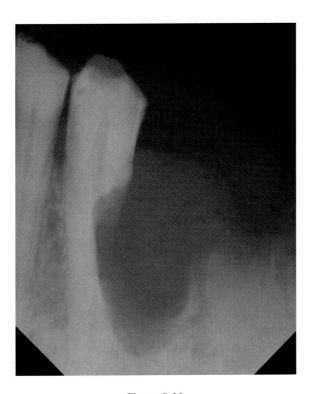

Figure 8-11

CALCIFYING CYSTIC ODONTOGENIC TUMOR

A well-demarcated radiolucency of the left mandible is causing resorption of the canine root.

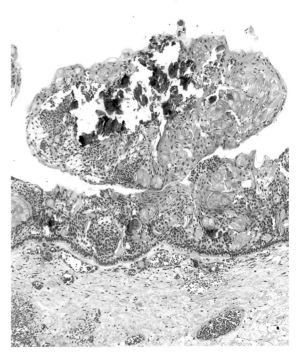

Figure 8-12

CALCIFYING CYSTIC ODONTOGENIC TUMOR

A cystic variant shows a uniform basal cell layer, stellate cells, and sheets of eosinophilic ghost cells.

Gross Findings. The gross appearance varies greatly based on the cystic or tumoral growth pattern. Depending on the amount of mineralization present, some lesions need to be demineralized and others can be processed without delay.

Microscopic Findings. Calcifying cystic odontogenic tumors may grossly and microscopically appear cystic, multicystic, or solid. Cystic lesions are lined by a focally thickened layer of stratified squamous epithelium. Some areas show a well-defined basal layer consisting of cuboidal or columnar cells that resemble ameloblasts (figs. 8-12–8-14). The more superficial layers of epithelium appear stellate or fusiform, suggesting stellate reticulum. Ghost cells similar to those found in pilomatricoma (calcifying epithelioma of Malherbe) are found individually or in sheets and are an important factor in differentiating the lesion from an ameloblastoma. In some tumors, the ghost cells are numerous, forming sheets of lamellar, eosinophilic material which often undergoes dystrophic mineraliza-

tion. Other foci of mineralization resembling dentin or cementum are often found. Solid tumors consist of a haphazard arrangement of cells showing the same features without the cystic lumen (fig. 8-15). Some tumors have sheets and islands of clear, glycogen-containing epithelial cells, separated by a thin fibrous connective tissue stroma (37).

Immunohistochemical Findings. On the basis of the histopathologic features and the negative reaction to polyclonal antikeratin antibody, it was suggested that the ghost cells are the result of coagulation necrosis (30). Subsequent studies, however, have shown that these cells in both adamantinomatous craniopharyngiomas and calcifying cystic odontogenic tumor variants stain for high and low molecular weight cytokeratins and involucrin, characteristic of terminally differentiated keratinocytes (38). Based on a positive reaction of polyclonal antibodies to type I acidic and type II neutral basic hard alpha keratins and monoclonal antibody to type II neutral/basic hard alpha keratins,

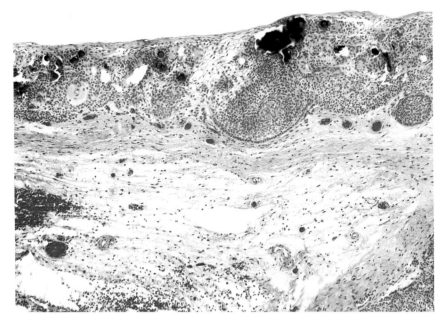

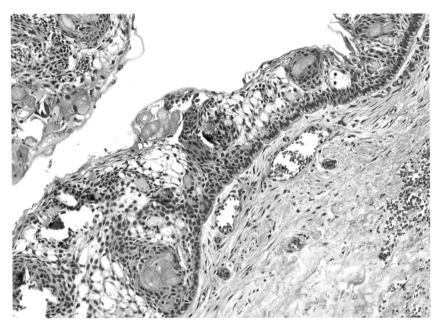

Figure 8-13

CALCIFYING CYSTIC ODONTOGENIC TUMOR

Top: Numerous mineralizations are present within the stellate epithelium of this cystic variant.

Bottom: The cystic variant shows columnar basal cells, stellate and spindle epithelial cells, and groups of eosinophilic ghost cells.

ghost cell keratinization may be similar to hair (39). Keratin expression in calcifying cystic odontogenic tumor appears similar to stratified squamous epithelium, with the basal layer expressing keratin (K)14 and the more superficial cells expressing K10/13 (40). Cytokeratins 8, 14, and 19; AE1/AE3 and 34betaE12; bcl-2; and Mel-CAM have also been demonstrated (41). The biologic properties of some of the eosinophilic amorphous material is suggestive of poorly calcified osteodentin (42).

Evaluations of Wnt-beta-catenin-TCF-Lef immunohistochemical profiles in pilomatricomas, craniopharyngiomas, and calcifying cystic odontogenic tumors indicate dysfunction of the cellular adhesion complex, contributing to tumorigenesis (43–45). The presence of beta-catenin mutations differentiates calcifying cystic odontogenic tumor from ameloblastoma (46). Proliferative activity, as measured by Ki-67, is greater in the epithelium of stand-alone central bony calcifying cystic odontogenic tumors

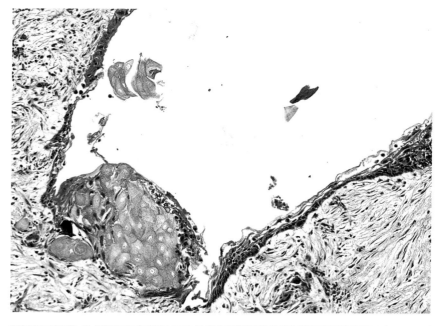

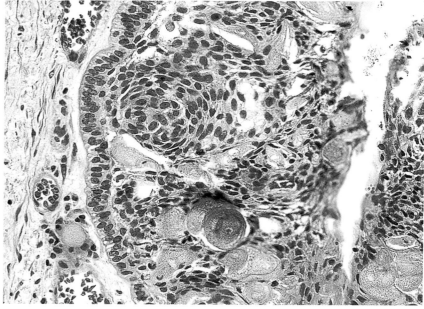

Figure 8-14

CALCIFYING CYSTIC ODONTOGENIC TUMOR

Top: The tumor is lined by thin, nonkeratinizing stratified squamous epithelium and there is a single focus of eosinophilic ghost cells.

Bottom: The lining of a cystic variant shows a columnar basal cell layer with stellate and spindle epithelial cells, and nests of ghost cells.

compared to those associated with odontomas and peripheral lesions (41).

Treatment and Prognosis. The initial treatment can be controversial, but most central bony tumors are adequately managed with simple enucleation of unilocular lesions and enucleation with bony curettage for multilocular lesions. Radiographic follow-up is prudent.

In a series of 21 intraosseous calcifying cystic odontogenic tumors, two patients experienced multiple recurrences following conservative surgery (47). One case was identified as a malignant tumor arising from a previously benign calcifying cystic odontogenic tumor. Sun et al. (48) evaluated the therapy provided for seven patients with calcifying cystic odontogenic tumors with follow-up ranging from 7 to 105 months and recommended resection of tumors with 0.5 cm clear margins followed by long-term follow-up.

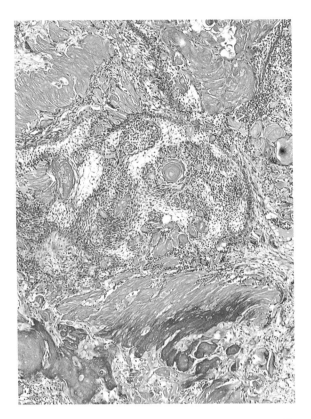 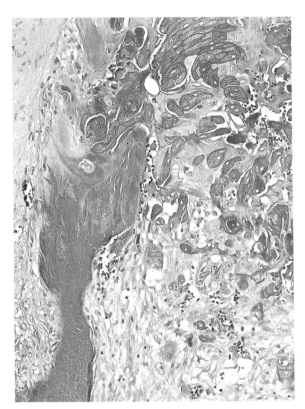

Figure 8-15

CALCIFYING CYSTIC ODONTOGENIC TUMOR

Left: The solid variant has strands and cords of columnar and stellate epithelial cells and sheets of ghost cells.
Right: A solid variant shows numerous ghost cells and an island of eosinophilic mineralized tissue resembling dentin.

REFERENCES

1. Slootweg PJ. An analysis of the interrelationship of the mixed odontogenic tumors—ameloblastic fibroma, ameloblastic fibro-odontoma, and the odontomas. Oral Surg Oral Med Oral Pathol 1981;51:266-276.
2. Chen Y, Wang JM, Li TJ. Ameloblastic fibroma: a review of published studies with special reference to its nature and biological behavior. Oral Oncol 2007;43:960-969.
3. Gardner DG. The mixed odontogenic tumors. Oral Surg Oral Med Oral Pathol 1984;58:166-168.
4. Cohen DM, Bhattacharyya I. Ameloblastic fibroma, ameloblastic fibro-odontoma, and odontoma. Oral Maxillofac Surg Clin North Am 2004;16:375-384.
5. Chen SH, Katayanagi T, Osada K, et al. Ameloblastoma and its relationship to ameloblastic fibroma: their histogenesis based on an unusual case and review of the literature. Bull Tokyo Dent Coll 1991;32:51-56.
6. Martin-Granizo López R, Ortega L, González Corchón MA, Berguer Sández A. Ameloblastic fibroma of the mandible. Report of two cases. Med Oral 2003;8:150-153.
7. Miller AS, Lopez CF, Pullon PA, Elzay RP. Ameloblastic fibro-odontoma. Report of seven cases. Oral Surg Oral Med Oral Pathol 1976;41:354-356.
8. Tomich CE. Benign mixed odontogenic tumors. Semin Diagn Pathol 1999;16:308-316.

9. Hong YS, Wang J, Liu J, Zhang B, Hou L, Zhong M. [Expression of HOX C13 in odontogenic tumors.] Shanghai Kou Qiang Yi Xue 2007;16:587-591. [Chinese]

10. Takeda Y. Ameloblastic fibroma and related lesions: current pathologic concept. Oral Oncol 1999;35:535-540.

11. Trodahl JN. Ameloblastic fibroma. A survey of cases from the Armed Forces Institute of Pathology. Oral Surg Oral Med Oral Pathol 1972;33:547-558.

12. Muller S, Parker DC, Kapadia SB, Budnick SD, Barnes EL. Ameloblastic fibrosarcoma of the jaws. A clinicopathologic and DNA analysis of five cases and review of the literature with discussion of its relationship to ameloblastic fibroma. Oral Surg Oral Med Oral Pathol Oral Radiol Endod 1995;79:469-477.

13. De Rui G, Meloni SM, Contini M, Tullio A. Ameloblastic fibro-odontoma. Case report and review of the literature. J Craniomaxillofac Surg 2010;38:141-144.

14. Sivapathasundharam B, Manikandhan R, Sivakumar G, George T. Ameloblastic fibro odontoma. Indian J Dent Res 2005;16:19-21.

15. Tomich CE. Benign mixed odontogenic tumors. Semin Diagn Pathol 1999;16:308-316.

16. Cohen DM, Bhattacharyya I. Ameloblastic fibroma, ameloblastic fibro-odontoma, and odontoma. Oral Maxillofac Surg Clin North Am 2004;16:375-384.

17. Oghli AA, Scuto I, Ziegler C, Flechtenmacher C, Hofele C. A large ameloblastic fibro-odontoma of the right mandible. Med Oral Patol Oral Cir Bucal 2007;12:E34-37.

18. Fujita S, Hideshima K, Ikeda T. Nestin expression in odontoblasts and odontogenic ectomesenchymal tissue of odontogenic tumours. J Clin Pathol 2006;59:240-245.

19. Reis SR, de Freitas CE, do Espirito Santo AR. Management of ameloblastic fibro-odontoma in a 6-year-old girl preserving the associated impacted permanent tooth. J Oral Sci 2007;49:331-335.

20. Budnick SD. Compound and complex odontomas. Oral Surg Oral Med Oral Pathol 1976;42:501-506.

21. Philipsen HP, Reichart PA, Praetorius F. Mixed odontogenic tumours and odontomas. Considerations on interrelationship. Review of the literature and presentation of 134 new cases of odontomas. Oral Oncol 1997;33:86-99.

22. Bhattacharyya I. Case of the month. Ameloblastic fibro-odontoma. Todays FDA 2010;22:21-23.

23. Korpi JT, Kainulainen VT, Sandor GK, Oikarinen KS. Removal of large complex odontoma using Le Fort I osteotomy. J Oral Maxillofac Surg 2009;67:2018-2021.

24. Scolozzi P, Lombardi T. Removal of large complex odontoma using Le Fort I osteotomy. J Oral Maxillofac Surg 2010;68:950-951; author reply 951.

25. Chrcanovic BR, Jaeger F, Freire-Maia B. Two-stage surgical removal of large complex odontoma. Oral Maxillofac Surg 2010;14:247-252.

26. Gorlin RJ, Pindborg JJ, Odont, Clausen FP, Vickers RA. The calcifying odontogenic cyst—a possible analogue of the cutaneous calcifying epithelioma of Malherbe. An analysis of fifteen cases. Oral Surg Oral Med Oral Pathol 1962;15:1235-1243.

27. Gorlin RJ, Pindborg JJ, Redman RS, Williamson JJ, Hansen LS. The calcifying odontogenic cyst. A new entity and possible analogue of the cutaneous calcifying epithelioma of Malherbe. Cancer 1964;17:723-729.

28. Kramer IR, Pindborg JJ, Shear M. The WHO Histological Typing of Odontogenic Tumours. A commentary on the second edition. Cancer 1992;70:2988-2994.

29. Praetorius F, Hjorting-Hansen E, Gorlin RJ, Vickers RA. Calcifying odontogenic cyst. Range, variations and neoplastic potential. Acta Odontol Scand 1981;39:227-240.

30. Hong SP, Ellis GL, Hartman KS. Calcifying odontogenic cyst. A review of ninety-two cases with reevaluation of their nature as cysts or neoplasms, the nature of ghost cells, and subclassification. Oral Surg Oral Med Oral Pathol 1991;72:56-64.

31. Buchner A. The central (intraosseous) calcifying odontogenic cyst: an analysis of 215 cases. J Oral Maxillofac Surg 1991;49:330-339.

32. Ledesma-Montes C, Gorlin RJ, Shear M, et al. International collaborative study on ghost cell odontogenic tumours: calcifying cystic odontogenic tumour, dentinogenic ghost cell tumour and ghost cell odontogenic carcinoma. J Oral Pathol Med 2008;37:302-308.

33. Toida M. So-called calcifying odontogenic cyst: review and discussion on the terminology and classification. J Oral Pathol Med 1998;27:49-52.

34. Buchner A, Merrell PW, Carpenter WM. Relative frequency of central odontogenic tumors: a study of 1,088 cases from Northern California and comparison to studies from other parts of the world. J Oral Maxillofac Surg 2006;64:1343-1352.

35. Ellis GL. Odontogenic ghost cell tumor. Semin Diagn Pathol 1999;16:288-292.

36. Cheng Y, Long X, Li X, Bian Z, Chen X, Yang X. Clinical and radiological features of odontogenic ghost cell carcinoma: review of the literature and report of four new cases. Dentomaxillofac Radiol 2004;33:152-157.

37. Yoon JH, Ahn SG, Kim SG, Kim J. Odontogenic ghost cell tumour with clear cell components: clear cell odontogenic ghost cell tumour? J Oral Pathol Med 2004;33:376-379.

38. Badger KV, Gardner DG. The relationship of adamantinomatous craniopharyngioma to ghost cell ameloblastoma of the jaws: a histopathologic and immunohistochemical study. J Oral Pathol Med 1997;26:349-355.

39. Kusama K, Katayama Y, Oba K, et al. Expression of hard alpha-keratins in pilomatrixoma, craniopharyngioma, and calcifying odontogenic cyst. Am J Clin Pathol 2005;123:376-381.

40. Crivelini MM, Felipini RC, Coclete GA, Soubhia AM. Immunoexpression of keratins in the calcifying cystic odontogenic tumor epithelium. J Oral Pathol Med 2009;38:393-396.

41. Fregnani ER, Pires FR, Quezada RD, Shih I, Vargas PA, de Almeida OP. Calcifying odontogenic cyst: clinicopathological features and immunohistochemical profile of 10 cases. J Oral Pathol Med 2003;32:163-170.

42. Mori M, Kasai T, Nakai M, et al. Dentinogenic ghost cell tumor: histologic aspects, immunohistochemistry, lectin binding profiles, and biophysical studies. Oral Oncol 2000;36:134-143.

43. Kim J, Lee EH, Yook JI, Han JY, Yoon JH, Ellis GL. Odontogenic ghost cell carcinoma: a case report with reference to the relation between apoptosis and ghost cells. Oral Surg Oral Med Oral Pathol Oral Radiol Endod 2000;90:630-635.

44. Hassanein AM, Glanz SM, Kessler HP, Eskin TA, Liu C. Beta-catenin is expressed aberrantly in tumors expressing shadow cells. Pilomatricoma, craniopharyngioma, and calcifying odontogenic cyst. Am J Clin Pathol 2003;120:732-736.

45. Ahn SG, Kim SA, Kim SG, Lee SH, Kim J, Yoon JH. Beta-catenin gene alterations in a variety of so-called calcifying odontogenic cysts. APMIS 2008;116:206-211.

46. Sekine S, Sato S, Takata T, et al. Beta-catenin mutations are frequent in calcifying odontogenic cysts, but rare in ameloblastomas. Am J Pathol 2003;163:1707-1712.

47. Li TJ, Yu SF. Clinicopathologic spectrum of the so-called calcifying odontogenic cysts: a study of 21 intraosseous cases with reconsideration of the terminology and classification. Am J Surg Pathol 2003;27:372-384.

48. Sun G, Huang X, Hu Q, Yang X, Tang E. The diagnosis and treatment of dentinogenic ghost cell tumor. Int J Oral Maxillofac Surg 2009;38:1179-1183.

9 MALIGNANT ODONTOGENIC NEOPLASMS

MALIGNANT AMELOBLASTOMA

Definition. *Malignant ameloblastomas* are neoplasms with benign clinical, radiographic, and microscopic features, yet they metastasize, indicating clear malignant behavior. Both primary and metastatic tumors appear cytologically benign. Since the diagnosis can only be made following the identification of metastasis, the lesion has also been referred to as *metastasizing ameloblastoma* (1).

Clinical Features. In many cases, the metastases are delayed, up to many years. The lung is the most common site but cervical lymph nodes are also involved (2–8).

Kunze et al. (9) presented a case and reviewed 25 previously published cases. The lung was the most frequent metastatic site (88 percent), followed by the regional lymph nodes. Metastases were also reported in bone, brain, kidney, small intestine, and liver. The interval between the diagnosis of the primary tumor and the identification of metastases can be long, with so-called disease-free intervals ranging from 9 to 11 years. The average survival time following the identification of metastasis in reported cases is only 2 to 3 years (10).

Microscopic Findings. The primary tumor and metastatic deposits show no features of anaplasia (9). Most cases reported have the features of follicular or plexiform ameloblastoma in both the primary and metastatic tumor sites (figs. 9-1, 9-2).

Treatment and Prognosis. Because the diagnosis of malignancy cannot be made prior to the identification of metastasis, treatment often involves radiation and chemotherapy. Long-term outcomes are difficult to predict due to the paucity of cases reported (8,11,12). Laughlin (10) indicated that disseminated ameloblastoma responds poorly to chemotherapy.

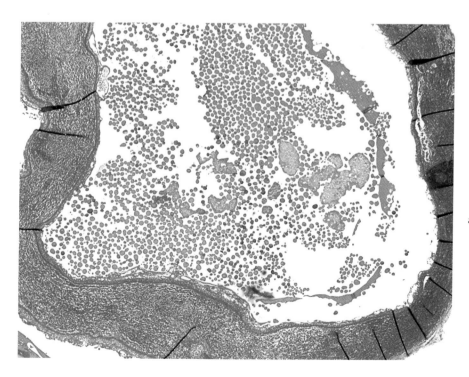

Figure 9-1

MALIGNANT AMELOBLASTOMA

A cyst-like tumor is seen in a cervical lymph node.

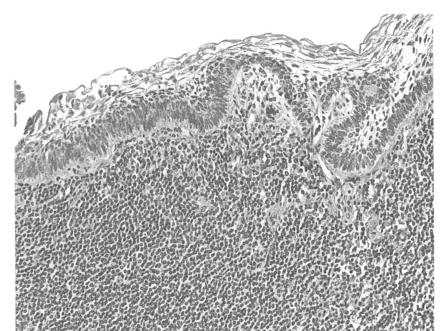

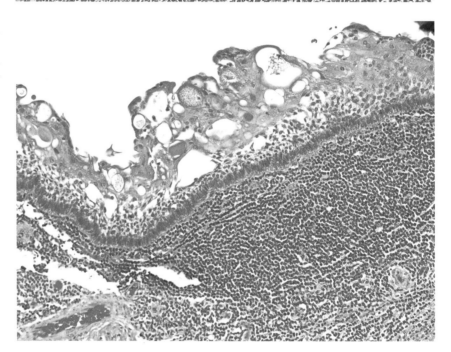

Figure 9-2

MALIGNANT AMELOBLASTOMA

Top: Ameloblastoma in a cervical lymph node has a uniform, columnar basal cell layer and luminal epithelium characteristic of the follicular primary tumor.

Bottom: Ameloblastoma with acanthomatous features in a lymph node.

AMELOBLASTIC CARCINOMA

Definition. *Ameloblastic carcinoma*, in contrast to malignant ameloblastoma, shows the microscopic features characteristic of malignancy, including cellular pleomorphism, focal tissue necrosis, increased mitotic activity, atypical mitoses, and an increased nuclear to cytoplasmic ratio. These are very rare lesions.

Clinical Features. In 1987 Corio et al. (13) described eight cases from the Armed Forces Institute of Pathology (AFIP) files. The mean age of patients was 30.1 years, with no sex predilection noted. Seven cases involved the mandible and one involved the maxilla, with the posterior regions favored. The most common signs and symptoms were swelling, pain, trismus, and dysphonia.

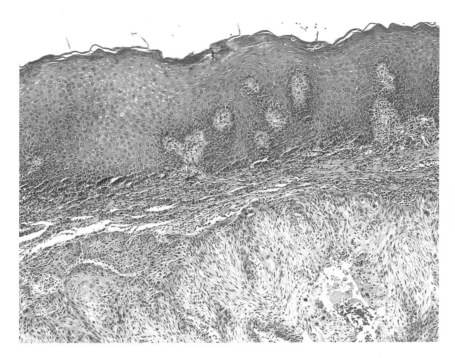

Figure 9-3

AMELOBLASTIC CARCINOMA

Perforation of the cortical plate has allowed the malignant tumor to infiltrate the gingival connective tissue, seen here subjacent to the oral mucosa.

Benlyazid et al. (14) reviewed 66 cases of ameloblastic carcinoma. The median age was 44 years, with a predominance of men (42 of 66). Mandibular lesions outnumbered maxillary lesions 2 to 1.

In a literature review of 26 cases, Kruse et al. (15) found a mean age at diagnosis of 54 years and a male to female ratio of almost 3 to 1. Nine patients had pulmonary metastasis and one had cervical lymph node involvement. Two cases slowed no microscopic evidence of malignancy of the primary tumor, while the metastatic tumors showed clear malignant features.

Yoon et al. (16) added six cases to the literature. The average age at the time of diagnosis was 61 years. The male to female ratio and the mandible to maxilla ratio were both almost 2 to 1. Most cases (70 percent) involved the posterior portion of the jaw. Two patients (33.3 percent) had metastatic lesions in the regional lymph nodes without distant metastasis.

Radiographic Features. Most ameloblastic carcinomas have the radiographic features common to rapidly growing, malignant neoplasms. These include poorly demarcated borders, destruction of anatomic structures including tooth roots, cortical plate perforation, and radiopaque bony sequestra (13).

Microscopic Findings. At low power, the features are those of one or more variants of amelo-blastoma, including epithelial tumor cell islands with peripheral columnar cells showing centrally polarized nuclei (figs. 9-3, 9-4). At higher power, however, the cytopathologic features associated with malignancy include increased mitotic activity, increased nuclear to cytoplasmic ratio, nuclear pleomorphism, vascular invasion, and foci of necrosis (figs. 9-5, 9-6) (16,17).

Immunohistochemical Findings. Yoon et al. (16) in their report of six cases found positive immunostaining for cytokeratins 5, 14, and 18, features not identified in previous reports (18). There is a marked increase in argyrophilic nuclear organizing regions (AgNORs) in ameloblastic carcinomas compared to ameloblastomas, and the malignant tumor cells show evidence of alpha-smooth muscle actin (SMA), another feature not seen in ameloblastomas (19,20).

An evaluation for bcl-2, syndecan-1, and Ki-67 helps distinguish benign from malignant tumors (21,22). Notch 1 signaling peptide may contribute to cell cycle arrest in ameloblastic carcinoma (23). Abiko et al. (24) reported a case of ameloblastic carcinoma ex ameloblastoma. Direct sequencing showed no genetic mutation of exons 5-8 of the *p53* gene. Hypermethylation of CpG islands of the *p16* gene was detected in the malignant parts of the tumor, suggesting that such hypermethylation may be involved in malignant transformation.

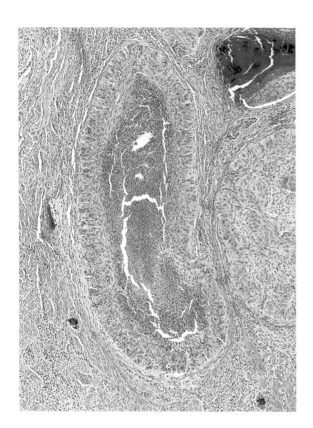 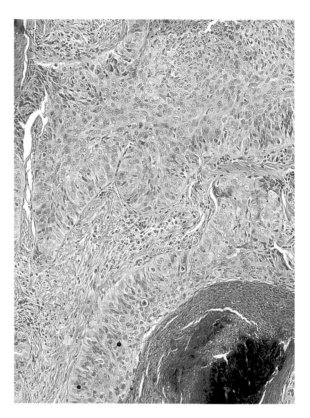

Figure 9-4

AMELOBLASTIC CARCINOMA

Left: An anaplastic epithelial island is seen with central necrosis.
Right: The islands of epithelium show pleomorphism and foci of columnar cells characteristic of ameloblastoma.

Figure 9-5

AMELOBLASTIC CARCINOMA

Mitotic figures, cellular pleomorphism, and tall columnar cells are seen.

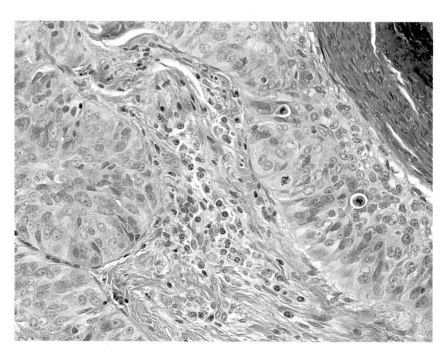

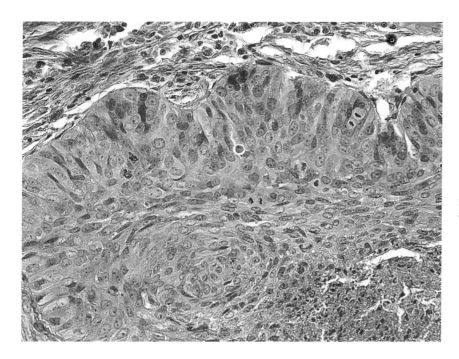

Figure 9-6

AMELOBLASTIC CARCINOMA

Foci of necrosis, cellular pleomorphism, and tall columnar anaplastic ameloblasts are seen.

Treatment and Prognosis. Based on 14 cases reported by Hall et al. (17), aggressive surgical intervention provides the best chance for survival. Patients treated otherwise had recurrences that substantially reduced 5-year survival rates.

In a review of 98 cases in the literature, Yoon et al. (16) found the recurrence rate in patients treated with surgical resection was 28.3 percent, whereas the recurrence rate in cases treated conservatively was 92.3 percent. Metastatic lesions were detected in 22 percent of patients during follow-up, and the lung was the most common area of distant metastasis. The 5- and 10-year survival rates were 72.9 and 56.8 percent, respectively.

Simko et al. (25) described an unusual case of a mandibular ameloblastic carcinoma in a 64-year-old female. There was no regional or distant metastasis at the time of initial treatment with surgical resection; however, 11 months postsurgery, the patient developed pulmonary metastasis and died of widespread disease at 28 months.

In an evaluation of 26 patients with ameloblastic carcinoma of the maxilla, 9 had pulmonary metastasis and 1 had cervical lymph node spread (15). Two had primary tumors with benign features while the metastasis showed clear features of anaplasia. Six patients died of disease. In a review of 66 cases, 15 patients died with metastatic spread in the lung, brain, and bones (14). The survival rate was 68.7 percent at 5 years.

AMELOBLASTIC FIBROSARCOMA

Definition. *Ameloblastic fibrosarcoma* is a rare malignancy apparently arising from a preexisting odontogenic myxoma or an odontogenic mixed tumor such as an ameloblastic fibro-odontoma or ameloblastic fibroma (26).

General Features. Only about 68 cases have been reported worldwide (27). Most cases are initially diagnosed at a later age compared to ameloblastic fibromas (28,29). Some cases that involved malignant transformation of ameloblastic fibromas were initially diagnosed years after initial treatment or showed evidence of progressive anaplasia in sequential recurrences (30,31).

A peripheral case was reported in an 89-year-old patient with a previous history of peripheral ameloblastoma (32). One odontogenic carcinosarcoma with both epithelial and mesenchymal components showed clear signs of malignancy in the primary tumor, recurrences, and metastases (33).

Microscopic Findings. Microscopic evaluation of these aggressive lesions shows evidence of typical odontogenic epithelium, usually in a follicular pattern. Peripheral columnar cells with centrally polarized nuclei surround areas of stellate reticulum–like cells, typical of follicular ameloblastoma (fig. 9-7). The surrounding mesenchymal tissue, however, is hypercellular with

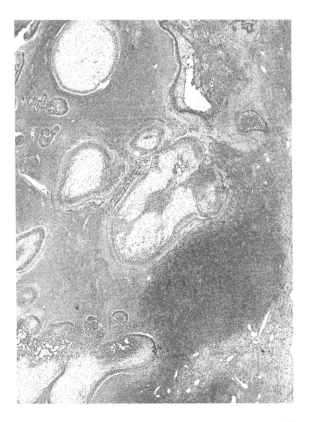 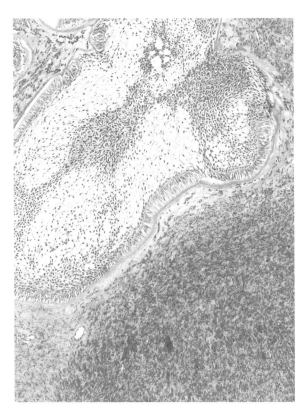

Figure 9-7

AMELOBLASTIC FIBROSARCOMA

Left: Islands of typical follicular ameloblastoma are seen in a cellular background.

Right: The peripheral columnar cells with centrally polarized nuclei typical of ameloblastoma are adjacent to pleomorphic spindle cells.

marked nuclear pleomorphism and increased mitotic activity (fig. 9-8). The fibroblastic cells are often arranged in a haphazard pattern, although streaming and a herringbone pattern can be identified focally.

Studies have shown evidence of fibroblastic, fibrohistiocytic, myofibroblastic, and osteoblastic differentiation in these sarcomas (34–36). Occasional foci of mineralization suggest dentin, enamel matrix, or cementum (figs. 9-9, 9-10) (37–39).

Immunohistochemical Findings. The mesenchymal component of ameloblastic fibrosarcoma stains for higher levels of Ki-67, proliferating cell nuclear antigen (PCNA), p53, and CD34 compared to ameloblastic fibroma (35,40–42). In an evaluation of six cases for PCNA, the mesenchymal component of ameloblastic fibrosarcoma stained at a significantly higher rate (41 percent) than ameloblastic fibroma

(3 percent) (43). In addition, MIB-1 labeling is higher in ameloblastic fibrosarcomas and recurrent ameloblastic fibromas (44). Aneuploidy is present in a minority of ameloblastic sarcomas and this feature has not been shown to correlate with histologic grade (28).

Treatment and Prognosis. Treatment for these rare neoplasms is often similar to that for other sarcomas: radical surgery and chemotherapy (36).

PRIMARY INTRAOSSEOUS CARCINOMA

Definition. *Primary intraosseous carcinomas* are rare squamous cell or undifferentiated epithelial malignancies arising centrally within the maxilla or the mandible. It is presumed that these lesions arise from odontogenic epithelial rests. In order to establish the diagnosis of this rare lesion there should be no evidence of anaplasia in the adjacent surface mucosa, or

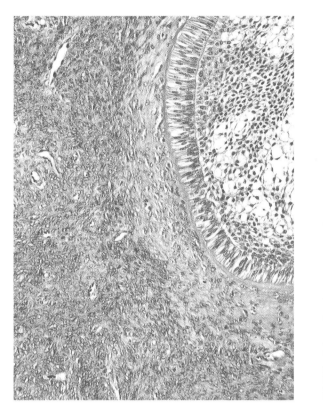 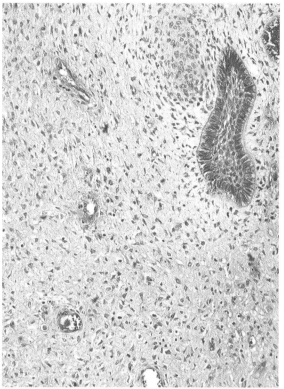

Figure 9-8

AMELOBLASTIC FIBROSARCOMA

Left: The spindle cells exhibit pleomorphism and numerous mitotic figures.
Right: Amorphous matrix material is adjacent to the pleomorphic spindle cells.

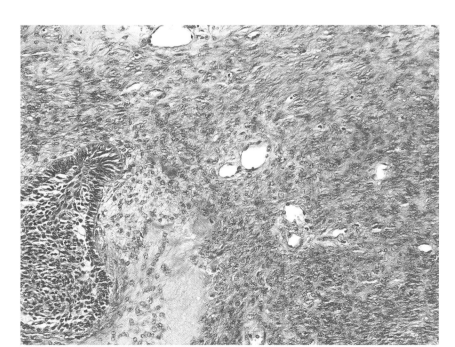

Figure 9-9

AMELOBLASTIC FIBROSARCOMA

Homogeneous eosinophilic dentin-like matrix is adjacent to the pleomorphic spindle cells and follicle of ameloblastoma.

121

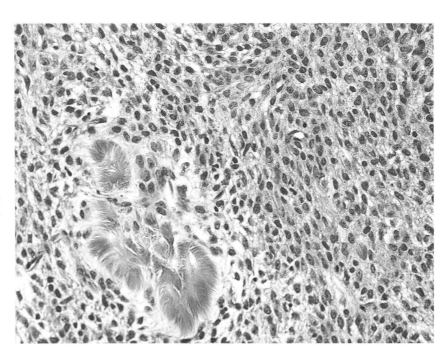

Figure 9-10

AMELOBLASTIC FIBROSARCOMA

Pleomorphic spindle cells and mitotic figures are seen along with eosinophilic dysplastic dentin-like material.

evidence to suggest an origin from an adjacent major or minor salivary gland. In addition, metastatic lesions to the jaws need to be excluded. While most primary intraosseous carcinomas are squamous cell carcinomas, central mucoepidermoid and adenoid cystic carcinomas are also seen (45–48).

Clinical Features. Usually, there is a submucosal enlargement with evidence of progression and occasional pain either related to neurologic involvement or secondary inflammation (49,50). Huang et al. (51) evaluated 39 cases of primary intraosseous squamous cell carcinoma in 26 men and 13 women. The age at diagnosis ranged from 24 to 82 years. The tumors occurred predominantly in the posterior mandible.

Of 50 central mucoepidermoid carcinomas of the jaws evaluated by Browand and Waldron (45), 34 occurred in the mandible and 16 in the maxilla. Most were in females and most were initially diagnosed in the fourth or fifth decade, although ages ranged from 1 to 85 years. Radiographically they resembled benign odontogenic tumors or cysts. Following initial treatment, 13 tumors recurred and four patients died as a result of their tumors.

Radiographic Features. These lesions are extremely variable radiographically, ranging from features suggestive of slow growth identical to most odontogenic tumors and cysts to features characteristic of rapidly growing central bony lesions. These features include ragged poorly defined margins and destruction of adjacent normal anatomy including multidirectional resorption of tooth roots. Widened periodontal ligament spaces, often a feature of central bony malignancies, are the result of rapid spread and expansion of tumor cells along the path of least resistance, which in this case includes the soft tissues of the periodontal ligament.

Microscopic Findings. The microscopic findings are identical to those of malignancies originating from epithelium of surface mucosa or salivary gland. Primary carcinomas show islands and cords of anaplastic epithelium with cellular pleomorphism, increased mitotic activity, atypical mitoses, individual cell keratinization, and keratin pearls (fig. 9-11). Mucoepidermoid carcinomas or other salivary gland malignancies show the cytologic and morphologic features characteristic of their extramedullary counterparts.

Ikeda et al. (47) described a central mandibular mucoepidermoid carcinoma composed of epidermoid cells, clear cells, mucous cells, and intermediate cells, which were surrounded by cellular-rich collagenous stroma. Immunohistochemistry was positive for myoepithelial markers in the trabecular portion of the tumor.

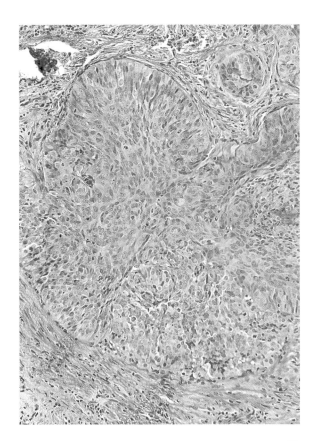 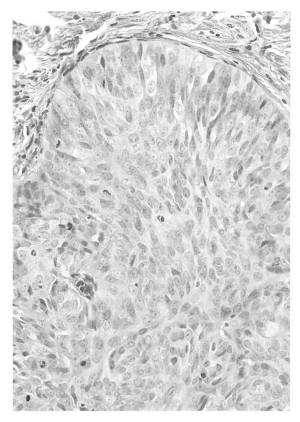

Figure 9-11

PRIMARY INTRAOSSEOUS CARCINOMA

Left: There are large and small islands of pleomorphic epithelium.
Right: Features include cellular pleomorphism, mitotic figures, and hyperchromasia.

Mohamed et al. (48) described a multilocular, mandibular lesion in a 53-year-old woman that showed epithelial cells with both cribriform and tubular growth patterns, areas of cystic degeneration, and localized formations of aberrant dental hard tissue. The case was diagnosed as a central adenoid cystic carcinoma with a comment regarding the pluripotent nature of oral ectoderm.

Treatment and Prognosis. Therapeutic management is usually based on staging criteria identical to those of extramedullary epithelial malignancies and often involves radical surgery with adjacent lymph node dissection followed by radiation and, if appropriate, chemotherapy. In an evaluation of 39 patients with primary intraosseous squamous cell carcinoma, the overall survival rates were 69.8 percent at 2 years and 36.3 percent at 5 years (51).

CARCINOMA ARISING FROM KERATOCYSTIC ODONTOGENIC TUMORS AND ODONTOGENIC CYSTS

Definition. The 2005 World Health Organization (WHO) classification of odontogenic head and neck tumors includes special reference to carcinomas that arise from keratocystic odontogenic tumors and nonkeratinizing odontogenic cysts. These rare squamous malignancies arise from a variety of odontogenic cysts, including most frequently dentigerous cysts but also radicular, residual, and lateral periodontal cysts (52–56), and from keratocystic odontogenic tumors (57,58). The malignancy most often reported is squamous cell carcinoma, although examples of mucoepidermoid carcinoma and other salivary gland carcinomas have also been reported (59). Although extremely rare, patient work-up should also include assessment

123

for possible metastatic spread into the walls of odontogenic cysts (60).

Clinical Features. The clinical features vary from those of a slowly progressive, asymptomatic enlargement to a rapidly enlarging submucosal tumor with pain due to secondary inflammation or peripheral nerve involvement. Most tumors are reported in patients over 60 years old. There is a 2 to 1 mandibular to maxilla predilection.

Brookstone and Huvos (61) reviewed 11 primary intraosseous salivary gland malignancies including mucoepidermoid carcinomas, adenoid cystic carcinomas, and adenocarcinomas not otherwise specified (NOS). Patients ranged in age from 10 to 67 years. Only 1 case involved the maxilla. Eight were associated with an odontogenic cyst.

Radiographic Features. Malignant neoplasms arising in odontogenic cysts or benign tumors often show no radiographic features suggesting malignancy (58). Usually there is a well-demarcated radiolucency with corticated borders. The clinician seldom suspects the presence of a malignancy before or during initial surgery.

Microscopic Findings. A diagnosis of malignancy arising from an odontogenic cyst or benign cystic neoplasm requires clear documentation of transition from a benign epithelial-lined cavity to carcinoma. Anaplastic epithelium may be identified focally in the cyst lining.

Treatment and Prognosis. The treatment is based entirely on the staging of the malignancy identified. Protocols vary slightly among various institutions but almost always involve radical surgery, lymph node dissection, and radiation or chemotherapy for the most aggressive lesions.

Zachariades et al. (62) reported a case of squamous cell carcinoma arising from the wall of a keratocystic odontogenic tumor treated with wide resection and radical neck dissection. No positive lymph nodes were found. The malignancy recurred locally and the patient died 2 years later with pulmonary metastasis.

CLEAR CELL ODONTOGENIC CARCINOMA

Definition. *Clear cell odontogenic carcinoma* is a malignant epithelial neoplasm characterized by a predominance of cells with glycogen-rich cytoplasm. Some tumors consist entirely of these clear cells while others occur in associa-

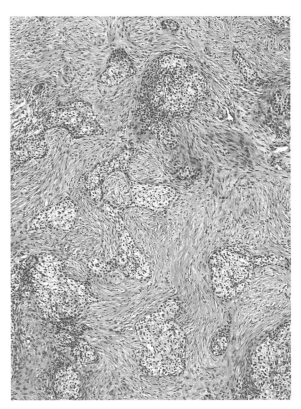

Figure 9-12

CLEAR CELL ODONTOGENIC CARCINOMA

The islands of epithelial cells have clear cytoplasm.

tion with other odontogenic tumor cell types including ameloblastomas and calcifying cystic odontogenic tumors. Braunshtein et al. (63) reviewed the reported features of clear cell odontogenic carcinoma and clear cell ameloblastoma and suggested that they represented a continuum of the same neoplasm.

Clinical Features. While few cases have been reported, over 75 percent occur in the mandible, with a distinct female predilection. Most cases are diagnosed in patients over 40 years of age (64,65).

Microscopic Findings. The cells of this neoplasm are often arranged in islands or cords surrounded by loose or densely hyalinized fibrovascular connective tissue (fig. 9-12). Peripheral island cells may show focal evidence of central nuclear polarization, suggestive of follicular ameloblastoma (66). The nuclei may be bland in some tumors, but substantial pleomorphism is noted in others (figs. 9-13–9-15). The cytoplasm

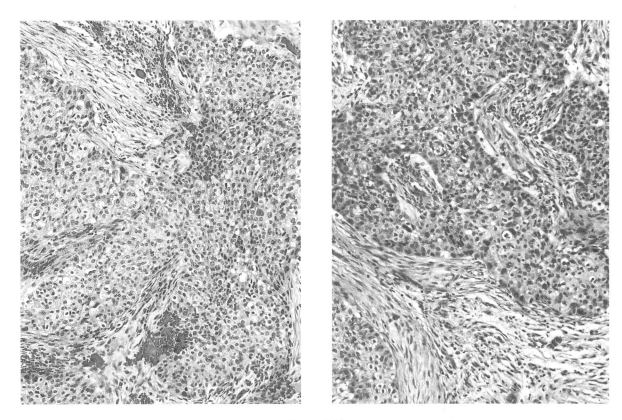

Figure 9-13

CLEAR CELL ODONTOGENIC CARCINOMA

Left: An island of polygonal cells, many with clear cytoplasm and others showing extensive pleomorphism. Hyperchromasia is seen.

Right: An island of pleomorphic cells with hyperchromatic nuclei and increased mitotic activity; numerous cells have clear cytoplasm.

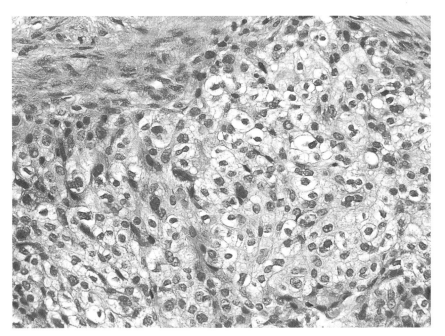

Figure 9-14

CLEAR CELL ODONTOGENIC CARCINOMA

Pleomorphic nuclei and polygonal cells with clear cytoplasm are seen.

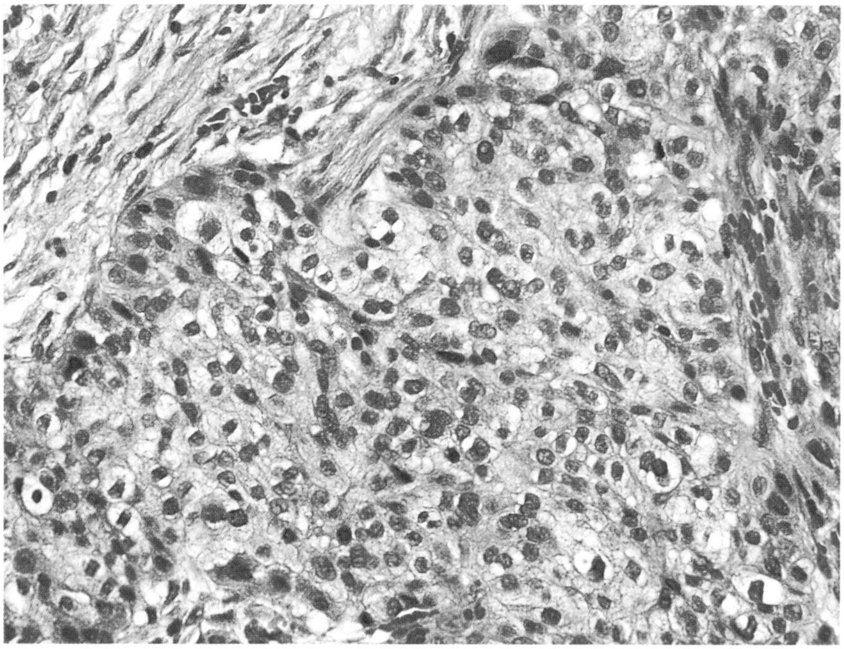

Figure 9-15

CLEAR CELL ODONTOGENIC CARCINOMA

Cellular pleomorphism, hyper-chromatic nuclei, and cells with clear cytoplasm clear are seen.

appears clear with hematoxylin and eosin (H&E) staining and is periodic acid–Shiff (PAS) positive, diastase labile, and resistant to staining with alcian blue. Some tumors contain foci of ghost cells and mineralized material resembling dentin or cementum (67,68).

Immunohistochemical Findings. Carinci et al. (69) used complementary DNA microarrays to identify several genes in clear cell odontogenic carcinomas that were differentially regulated compared to non-neoplastic tissue. Clear cell odontogenic carcinomas react to cytokeratins AE1/AE3, 8, 14, 18, and 19; epithelial membrane antigen, and S-100 protein (70,71). Low labeling indices for the proliferation markers Ki-67, PCNA, and p53 protein suggest that this malignancy is less aggressive than other odontogenic malignancies (71).

Treatment and Prognosis. Because of the few cases reported, therapeutic management protocols vary widely. Due to reports of pulmonary and lymphatic metastases, staging procedures similar to those for primary intraosseous carcinoma are often followed (65).

August et al. (64) reviewed the treatment of 36 patients with clear cell odontogenic tumors. All were treated with resection and 1 patient had postoperative radiation. Average follow-up was 2 years. There was no evidence of recurrent disease. Brandwein et al. (72) reported a case of an

81-year-old woman who had three locoregional recurrences within 21 months of resection. In an analysis of 43 cases, Ebert et al. (73) found local recurrence rates of 80 percent following curettage and 43 percent following resection. Patient age and sex, and tumor site could not be used as risk predictors. The authors recommended surgery to include lymph node dissection and adjuvant radiation treatment for selected cases.

ODONTOGENIC GHOST CELL CARCINOMA

Odontogenic ghost cell carcinoma is a rare malignancy of the jaws that is thought to arise de novo or from a preexisting calcifying cystic odontogenic tumor. As indicated by the name, this malignancy features many of the same microscopic features as calcifying cystic odontogenic tumor, including ghost cells (fig. 9-16). Few cases have been reported and some authors feel this lesion is better characterized as a variant of ameloblastoma (74–79).

In 2009, Li and Gao (80) described a case of dentinogenic ghost cell tumor that transformed into a ghost cell odontogenic carcinoma at the fifth recurrence over a span of 21 years. The carcinoma showed more obvious atypia, necrosis, and numerous mitoses. Ghost cells were far less frequent than in the original neoplasm. In another reported transformation case, cellular atypia, mitotic activity, Ki-67 labeling index,

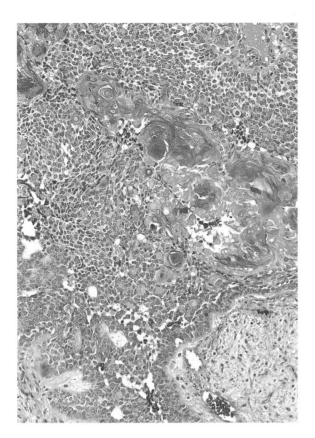 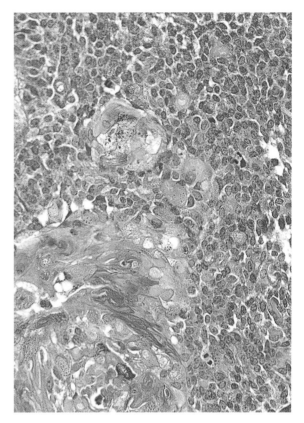

Figure 9-16

ODONTOGENIC GHOST CELL CARCINOMA

Left: The spindle- and ovoid-shaped epithelial cells have a hyperchromatic nuclear border typical eosinophilic ghost cells.

Right: Pleomorphic epithelial cells with hyperchromatic nuclei show evidence of mitotic activity. They are adjacent to eosinophilic ghost cells.

and p53 positivity were all increased in comparison with the initially resected specimen (81).

Staining for matrix metallopeptidase 9 (MMP-9) protein is significantly stronger in the stromal cells of all ghost cell odontogenic carcinomas compared to calcifying cystic odontogenic tumors, and may be associated with invasiveness (82). Proliferative activity as measured by Ki-67 staining is higher in ghost cell odontogenic carcinoma than in calcifying cystic odontogenic tumor (82).

In an evaluation of 26 cases, Gong et al. (83) concluded that NF-kappaB and MMP-9 may play a key role in the local invasion of both calcifying cystic odontogenic tumor and ghost cell odontogenic carcinoma. Tartrate-resistant acid phosphatase (TRAP) and vitronectin receptor are expressed in the ghost cells, suggesting that the cytokines produced by ghost cells may play an important role in bone resorption (84).

Because of the low number of cases reported, therapeutic management protocols vary widely. Staging procedures similar to those for primary intraosseous carcinoma and soft tissue carcinoma with bone invasion are often followed.

REFERENCES

1. Jundt G, Reichart PA. [Malignant odontogenic tumors.] Pathologe 2008;29:205-213. [German]
2. Slootweg PJ, Muller H. Malignant ameloblastoma or ameloblastic carcinoma. Oral Surg Oral Med Oral Pathol 1984;57:168-176.
3. Duffey DC, Bailet JW, Newman A. Ameloblastoma of the mandible with cervical lymph node metastasis. Am J Otolaryngol 1995;16:66-73.
4. Newman L, Howells GL, Coghlan KM, DiBiase A, Williams DM. Malignant ameloblastoma revisited. Br J Oral Maxillofac Surg 1995;33:47-50.
5. Ameerally P, McGurk M, Shaheen O. Atypical ameloblastoma: report of 3 cases and a review of the literature. Br J Oral Maxillofac Surg 1996;34:235-239.
6. Dao TV, Bastidas JA, Kelsch R, Kraut RA. Malignant ameloblastoma: a case report of a recent onset of neck swelling in a patient with a previously treated ameloblastoma. J Oral Maxillofac Surg 2009;67:2685-2689.
7. Reid-Nicholson M, Teague D, White B, Ramalingam P, Abdelsayed R. Fine needle aspiration findings in malignant ameloblastoma: a case report and differential diagnosis. Diagn Cytopathol 2009;37:586-591.
8. Ricard AS, Majoufre-Lefebvre C, Siberchicot F, Laurentjoye M. A multirecurrent ameloblastoma metastatic to the lung. Rev Stomatol Chir Maxillofac 2010;111:98-100.
9. Kunze E, Donath K, Luhr HG, Engelhardt W, De Vivie R. Biology of metastasizing ameloblastoma. Pathol Res Pract 1985;180:526-535.
10. Laughlin EH. Metastasizing ameloblastoma. Cancer 1989;64:776-780.
11. Newman L, Howells GL, Coghlan KM, DiBiase A, Williams DM. Malignant ameloblastoma revisited. Br J Oral Maxillofac Surg 1995;33:47-50.
12. Senra GS, Pereira AC, Murilo dos Santos L, Carvalho YR, Brandao AA. Malignant ameloblastoma metastasis to the lung: a case report. Oral Surg Oral Med Oral Pathol Oral Radiol Endod 2008;105:e42-46.
13. Corio RL, Goldblatt LI, Edwards PA, Hartman KS. Ameloblastic carcinoma: a clinicopathologic study and assessment of eight cases. Oral Surg Oral Med Oral Pathol 1987;64:570-576.
14. Benlyazid A, Lacroix-Triki M, Aziza R, Gomez-Brouchet A, Guichard M, Sarini J. Ameloblastic carcinoma of the maxilla: case report and review of the literature. Oral Surg Oral Med Oral Pathol Oral Radiol Endod 2007;104:e17-24.
15. Kruse AL, Zwahlen RA, Gratz KW. New classification of maxillary ameloblastic carcinoma based on an evidence-based literature review over the last 60 years. Head Neck Oncol 2009;1:31.
16. Yoon HJ, Hong SP, Lee JI, Lee SS, Hong SD. Ameloblastic carcinoma: an analysis of 6 cases with review of the literature. Oral Surg Oral Med Oral Pathol Oral Radiol Endod 2009;108:904-913.
17. Hall JM, Weathers DR, Unni KK. Ameloblastic carcinoma: an analysis of 14 cases. Oral Surg Oral Med Oral Pathol Oral Radiol Endod 2007;103:799-807.
18. Lau SK, Tideman H, Wu PC. Ameloblastic carcinoma of the jaws. A report of two cases. Oral Surg Oral Med Oral Pathol Oral Radiol Endod 1998;85:78-81.
19. Bello IO, Alanen K, Slootweg PJ, Salo T. Alpha-smooth muscle actin within epithelial islands is predictive of ameloblastic carcinoma. Oral Oncol 2009;45:760-765.
20. Kamath KP, Vidya M, Shetty N, Karkera BV, Jogi H. Nucleolar organizing regions and alpha-smooth muscle actin expression in a case of ameloblastic carcinoma. Head Neck Pathol 2010;4:157-162.
21. Angiero F, Borloni R, Macchi M, Stefani M. Ameloblastic carcinoma of the maxillary sinus. Anticancer Res 2008;28:3847-3854.
22. Bologna-Molina R, Mosqueda-Taylor A, Lopez-Corella E, et al. Comparative expression of syndecan-1 and Ki-67 in peripheral and desmoplastic ameloblastomas and ameloblastic carcinoma. Pathol Int 2009;59:229-233.
23. Nakano K, Siar CH, Tsujigiwa H, Nagatsuka H, Nagai N, Kawakami T. Notch signaling in benign and malignant ameloblastic neoplasms. Eur J Med Res 2008;13:476-480.
24. Abiko Y, Nagayasu H, Takeshima M, et al. Ameloblastic carcinoma ex ameloblastoma: report of a case-possible involvement of CpG island hypermethylation of the p16 gene in malignant transformation. Oral Surg Oral Med Oral Pathol Oral Radiol Endod 2007;103:72-76.
25. Simko EJ, Brannon RB, Eibling DE. Ameloblastic carcinoma of the mandible. Head Neck 1998;20:654-659.
26. Pindborg JJ. Ameloblastic sarcoma in the maxilla. Report of a case. Cancer 1960;13:917-920.
27. Pontes HA, Pontes FS, Silva BS, et al. Immunoexpression of Ki67, proliferative cell nuclear antigen, and Bcl-2 proteins in a case of ameloblastic fibrosarcoma. Ann Diagn Pathol 2010;14:447-452.
28. Muller S, Parker DC, Kapadia SB, Budnick SD, Barnes EL. Ameloblastic fibrosarcoma of the jaws. A clinicopathologic and DNA analysis of five cases and review of the literature with discussion of its relationship to ameloblastic fibroma. Oral Surg Oral Med Oral Pathol Oral Radiol Endod 1995;79:469-477.

29. Kobayashi K, Murakami R, Fujii T, Hirano A. Malignant transformation of ameloblastic fibroma to ameloblastic fibrosarcoma: case report and review of the literature. J Craniomaxillofac Surg 2005;33:352-355.

30. Hayashi Y, Tohnai I, Ueda M, Nagasaka T. Sarcomatous overgrowth in recurrent ameloblastic fibrosarcoma. Oral Oncol 1999;35:346-348.

31. Guthikonda B, Hanna EY, Skoracki RJ, Prabhu SS. Ameloblastic fibrosarcoma involving the anterior and middle skull base with intradural extension. J Craniofac Surg 2009;20:2087-2090.

32. Dufau JP, Paume P, Soulard R, Gros P. [Peripheral ameloblastic fibrosarcoma]. Ann Pathol 2002;22:310-313. [French]

33. Kunkel M, Ghalibafian M, Radner H, Reichert TE, Fischer B, Wagner W. Ameloblastic fibrosarcoma or odontogenic carcinosarcoma: a matter of classification? Oral Oncol 2004;40:444-449.

34. Nasu M, Matsubara O, Yamamoto H. Ameloblastic fibrosarcoma: an ultrastructural study of the mesenchymal component. J Oral Pathol 1984;13:178-187.

35. Wang L, Lu Y, Takashi T, et al. [Ameloblastic fibrosarcoma: an immunohistochemical and ultrastructural study of the mesenchymal component]. Hua Xi Yi Ke Da Xue Xue Bao 1999;30:318-320, 323. [Chinese]

36. Dallera P, Bertoni F, Marchetti C, Bacchini P, Campobassi A. Ameloblastic fibrosarcoma of the jaw: report of five cases. J Craniomaxillofac Surg 1994;22:349-354.

37. Takeda Y, Kuroda M, Suzuki A. Ameloblastic odontosarcoma (ameloblastic fibro-odontosarcoma) in the mandible. Acta Pathol Jpn 1990;40:832-837.

38. Tajima Y, Utsumi N, Suzuki S, Fujita K, Takahashi H. Ameloblastic fibrosarcoma arising de novo in the maxilla. Pathol Int 1997;47:564-568.

39. Zabolinejad N, Hiradfar M, Anvari K, Razavi AS. Ameloblastic fibrosarcoma of the maxillary sinus in an infant: a case report with long-term follow-up. J Pediatr Surg 2008;43:e5-8.

40. Huguet P, Castellvi J, Avila M, et al. Ameloblastic fibrosarcoma: report of a case. Immunohistochemical study and review of the literature. Med Oral 2001;6:173-179.

41. Batista de Paula AM, da Costa Neto JQ, da Silva Gusmao E, Guimaraes Santos FB, Gomez RS. Immunolocalization of the p53 protein in a case of ameloblastic fibrosarcoma. J Oral Maxillofac Surg 2003;61:256-258.

42. Lee OJ, Kim HJ, Lee BK, Cho KJ. CD34 expressing ameloblastic fibrosarcoma arising in the maxilla: a new finding. J Oral Pathol Med 2005;34:318-320.

43. Lu Y, Takata T, Wang L, et al. [An immunohistochemical study of the proliferating activity of ameloblastic fibroma and ameloblastic fibrosarcoma]. Hua Xi Yi Ke Da Xue Xue Bao 1998;29:390-393. [Chinese]

44. Sano K, Yoshida S, Ninomiya H, et al. Assessment of growth potential by MIB-1 immunohistochemistry in ameloblastic fibroma and related lesions of the jaws compared with ameloblastic fibrosarcoma. J Oral Pathol Med 1998;27:59-63.

45. Browand BC, Waldron CA. Central mucoepidermoid tumors of the jaws. Report of nine cases and review of the literature. Oral Surg Oral Med Oral Pathol 1975;40:631-643.

46. Waldron CA, Koh ML. Central mucoepidermoid carcinoma of the jaws: report of four cases with analysis of the literature and discussion of the relationship to mucoepidermoid, sialodontogenic, and glandular odontogenic cysts. J Oral Maxillofac Surg 1990;48:871-877.

47. Ikeda T, Fujita S, Hayashi T, et al. Intraosseous carcinoma of the mandible composed of cells expressing myoepithelial cell-associated antigens. Pathol Int 2008;58:427-431.

48. Mahomed F, Altini M, Meer S, Rikhotso E, Pearl C. Central adenoid cystic carcinoma of the mandible with odontogenic features: report of a case. Head Neck 2009;31:975-980.

49. Shamim T. Primary intraosseous squamous cell carcinoma of the mandible arising de novo. J Coll Physicians Surg Pak 2009;19:454-455.

50. Yamada T, Ueno T, Moritani N, Mishima K, Hirata A, Matsumura T. Primary intraosseous squamous cell carcinomas: five new clinicopathologic case studies. J Craniomaxillofac Surg 2009;37:448-453.

51. Huang JW, Luo HY, Li Q, Li TJ. Primary intraosseous squamous cell carcinoma of the jaws. Clinicopathologic presentation and prognostic factors. Arch Pathol Lab Med 2009;133:1834-1840.

52. Chretien PB, Carpenter DF, White NS, Harrah JD, Lightbody PM. Squamous carcinoma arising in a dentigerous cyst. Presentation of a fatal case and review of four previously reported cases. Oral Surg Oral Med Oral Pathol 1970;30:809-816.

53. Baker RD, D'Onofrio ED, Corio RL, Crawford BE, Terry BC. Squamous-cell carcinoma arising in a lateral periodontal cyst. Oral Surg Oral Med Oral Pathol 1979;47:495-499.

54. Gingell JC, Beckerman T, Levy BA, Snider LA. Central mucoepidermoid carcinoma. Review of the literature and report of a case associated with an apical periodontal cyst. Oral Surg Oral Med Oral Pathol 1984;57:436-440.

55. Copete MA, Cleveland DB, Orban RE Jr, Chen SY. Squamous carcinoma arising from a dentigerous cyst: report of a case. Compend Contin Educ Dent 1996;17:202-204.

56. Charles M, Barr T, Leong I, Ngan BY, Forte V, Sándor GK. Primary intraosseous malignancy originating in an odontogenic cyst in a young child. J Oral Maxillofac Surg 2008;66:813-819.

57. Dabbs DJ, Schweitzer RJ, Schweitzer LE, Mantz F. Squamous cell carcinoma arising in recurrent odontogenic keratocyst: case report and literature review. Head Neck 1994;16:375-378.

58. Falaki F, Delavarian Z, Salehinejad J, Saghafi S. Squamous cell carcinoma arising from an odontogenic keratocyst: a case report. Med Oral Patol Oral Cir Bucal 2009;14:E171-174.

59. Waldron CA, Mustoe TA. Primary intraosseous carcinoma of the mandible with probable origin in an odontogenic cyst. Oral Surg Oral Med Oral Pathol 1989;67:716-724.

60. Eichhorn W, Wehrmann M, Blessmann M, et al. Metastases in odontogenic cysts: literature review and case presentation. Oral Surg Oral Med Oral Pathol Oral Radiol Endod 2010;109:582-586.

61. Brookstone MS, Huvos AG. Central salivary gland tumors of the maxilla and mandible: a clinicopathologic study of 11 cases with an analysis of the literature. J Oral Maxillofac Surg 1992;50:229-236.

62. Zachariades N, Markaki S, Karabela-Bouropoulou V. Squamous cell carcinoma developing in an odontogenic keratocyst. Arch Anat Cytol Pathol 1995;43:350-353.

63. Braunshtein E, Vered M, Taicher S, Buchner A. Clear cell odontogenic carcinoma and clear cell ameloblastoma: a single clinicopathologic entity? A new case and comparative analysis of the literature. J Oral Maxillofac Surg 2003;61:1004-1010.

64. August M, Faquin W, Troulis M, Kaban L. Clear cell odontogenic carcinoma: evaluation of reported cases. J Oral Maxillofac Surg 2003;61:580-586.

65. Chera BS, Villaret DB, Orlando CA, Mendenhall WM. Clear cell odontogenic carcinoma of the maxilla: a case report and literature review. Am J Otolaryngol 2008;29:284-290.

66. Yamamoto H, Inui M, Mori A, Tagawa T. Clear cell odontogenic carcinoma: a case report and literature review of odontogenic tumors with clear cells. Oral Surg Oral Med Oral Pathol Oral Radiol Endod 1998;86:86-89.

67. Ariyoshi Y, Shimahara M, Miyauchi M, Nikai H. Clear cell odontogenic carcinoma with ghost cells and inductive dentin formation—report of a case in the mandible. J Oral Pathol Med 2002;31:181-183.

68. Berho M, Huvos AG. Central hyalinizing clear cell carcinoma of the mandible and the maxilla a clinicopathologic study of two cases with an analysis of the literature. Hum Pathol 1999;30:101-105.

69. Carinci F, Volinia S, Rubini C, et al. Genetic profile of clear cell odontogenic carcinoma. J Craniofac Surg 2003;14:356-362.

70. Muramatsu T, Hashimoto S, Inoue T, Shimono M, Noma H, Shigematsu T. Clear cell odontogenic carcinoma in the mandible: histochemical and immunohistochemical observations with a review of the literature. J Oral Pathol Med 1996;25:516-521.

71. Xavier FC, Rodini CO, Ramalho LM, Sarmento VA, Nunes FD, de Sousa SC. Clear cell odontogenic carcinoma: case report with immunohistochemical findings adding support to the challenging diagnosis. Oral Surg Oral Med Oral Pathol Oral Radiol Endod 2008;106:403-410.

72. Brandwein M, Said-Al-Naief N, Gordon R, Urken M. Clear cell odontogenic carcinoma: report of a case and analysis of the literature. Arch Otolaryngol Head Neck Surg 2002;128:1089-1095.

73. Ebert CS Jr, Dubin MG, Hart CF, Chalian AA, Shockley WW. Clear cell odontogenic carcinoma: a comprehensive analysis of treatment strategies. Head Neck 2005;27:536-542.

74. Scott J, Wood GD. Aggressive calcifying odontogenic cyst—a possible variant of ameloblastoma. Br J Oral Maxillofac Surg 1989;27:53-59.

75. Raubenheimer EJ, van Heerden WF, Sitzmann F, Heymer B. Peripheral dentinogenic ghost cell tumor. J Oral Pathol Med 1992;21:93-95.

76. McCoy BP, O Carroll MK, Hall JM. Carcinoma arising in a dentinogenic ghost cell tumor. Oral Surg Oral Med Oral Pathol 1992;74:371-378.

77. Dubiel-Bigaj M, Olszewski E, Stachura J. The malignant form of calcifying odontogenic cyst. A case report. Patol Pol 1993;44:39-41.

78. Kao SY, Pong BY, Li WY, Gallagher GT, Chang RC. Maxillary odontogenic carcinoma with distant metastasis to axillary skin, brain, and lung: case report. Int J Oral Maxillofac Surg 1995;24:229-232.

79. Alcalde RE, Sasaki A, Misaki M, Matsumura T. Odontogenic ghost cell carcinoma: report of a case and review of the literature. J Oral Maxillofac Surg 1996;54:108-111.

80. Li BB, Gao Y. Ghost cell odontogenic carcinoma transformed from a dentinogenic ghost cell tumor of maxilla after multiple recurrences. Oral Surg Oral Med Oral Pathol Oral Radiol Endod 2009;107:691-695.

81. Motosugi U, Ogawa I, Yoda T, et al. Ghost cell odontogenic carcinoma arising in calcifying odontogenic cyst. Ann Diagn Pathol 2009;13:394-397.

82. Gong Y, Wang L, Wang H, Li T, Chen X. The expression of NF-kappaB, Ki-67 and MMP-9 in CCOT, DGCT and GCOC. Oral Oncol 2009;45:515-520.

83. Gong YL, Wang L, Chen XM, Wang HK, Wang XH. [Expression of nuclear factor-kappaB, Ki-67 and matrix metalloproteinase-9 in calcifying odontogenic cyst.] Zhonghua Kou Qiang Yi Xue Za Zhi 2006;41:627-630. [Chinese]

84. Roh GS, Jeon BT, Park BW, et al. Ghost cell odontogenic carcinoma of the mandible: a case report demonstrating expression of tartrate-resistant acid phosphatase (TRAP) and vitronectin receptor. J Craniomaxillofac Surg 2008;36:419-423.

10 HYBRID TUMORS

Hybrid neoplasms, which have microscopic features of more than one tumor type, both benign and malignant, are common. The literature has numerous reports of hybrid odontogenic tumors containing various tumor combinations.

ODONTOAMELOBLASTOMA

Definition. Originally described in the 1950s, *odontoameloblastoma* has been controversial both in terms of diagnosis and therapeutic management (1,2). This neoplasm is also referred to as *ameloblastic odontoma*, the name used in the 1971 World Health Organization (WHO) classification of odontogenic head and neck tumors. Only about 50 cases have been reported in the literature (3,4).

Clinical Features. Some authors believe that only a handful of the cases reported meet the strict histologic criteria for diagnosis (5). Published tumors seem to occur more often in females, with an equal occurrence in the man-dible and maxilla. They involve the posterior regions of the jaws more often than the anterior, and have been diagnosed in patients as young as 2 and as old as 50 years.

Microscopic Findings. Most authors agree that this lesion represents a hybrid tumor consisting of an ameloblastoma and various forms of an odontoma, with the formation of dentin and enamel (figs. 10-1, 10-2). A similar lesion forming dentin, but not enamel, is termed *dentinoameloblastoma* (6). Other reports describe aggressive large tumors that are difficult to separate histologically from an "aggressive" ameloblastic fibro-odontoma (7,8).

Treatment and Prognosis. Odontoameloblastomas and ameloblastomas have the same potential to produce bone expansion and root resorption, and a similar recurrence rate following conservative treatment. A firm diagnosis is essential because recommended initial therapeutic management is parallel to that of a stand-alone ameloblastoma, followed by close follow-up (5,9).

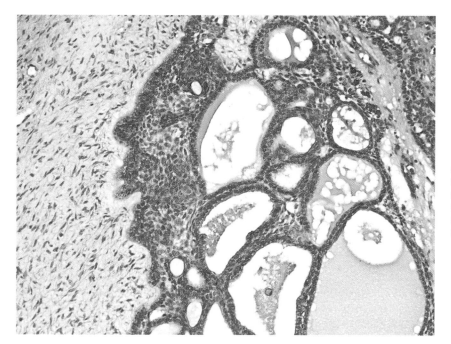

Figure 10-1

ODONTOAMELOBLASTOMA

The tumor hybrid shows evidence of an early odontoma with dental papillae (left), and double rows of columnar cells with hyperchromatic, polarized nuclei characteristic of plexiform ameloblastoma (right).

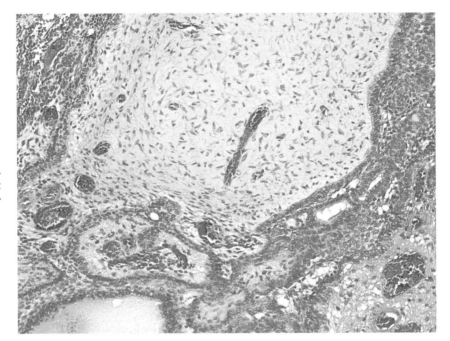

Figure 10-2

ODONTOAMELOBLASTOMA

The dental papilla of a developing odontoma is shown at the top and plexiform ameloblastoma at the bottom.

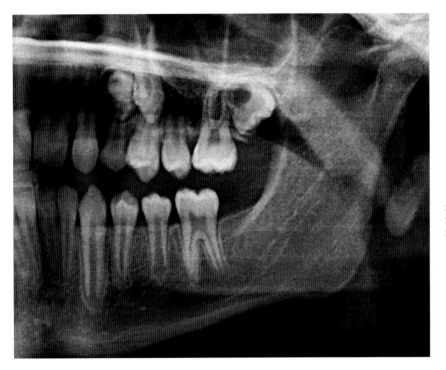

Figure 10-3

CALCIFYING CYSTIC ODONTOGENIC TUMOR AND ODONTOMA

A radiolucency containing numerous lobular radiopacities in the left maxilla displaces the impacted canine.

CALCIFYING CYSTIC ODONTOGENIC TUMOR (DENTINOGENIC GHOST CELL TUMOR) HYBRIDS

Calcifying cystic odontogenic tumors have been reported in combination with a variety of other odontogenic neoplasms including odontomas (figs. 10-3–10-5) (10,11), adenoma-

toid odontogenic tumors (12), ameloblastomas (13,14), and ameloblastic fibromas (15,16). A pigmented calcifying cystic odontogenic tumor occurred with an odontoma in the mandibular canine region of a 14-year-old boy (17). The pigment was melanin produced by dendritic melanocytes (17). Another hybrid odontogenic

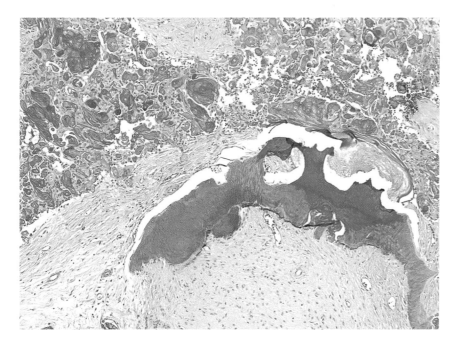

Figure 10-4

CALCIFYING CYSTIC ODONTOGENIC TUMOR AND ODONTOMA

Sheets of columnar and spindle epithelial cells with ghost cells typical of a calcifying cystic odontogenic tumor are adjacent to enamel matrix, dentin, and pulp characteristic of a compound odontoma.

Figure 10-5

CALCIFYING CYSTIC ODONTOGENIC TUMOR AND ODONTOMA

An island of columnar and stellate epithelium with ghost cells typical of a calcifying cystic odontogenic tumor is adjacent to a sheet of globular and tubular dentin forming one area of a complex odontoma.

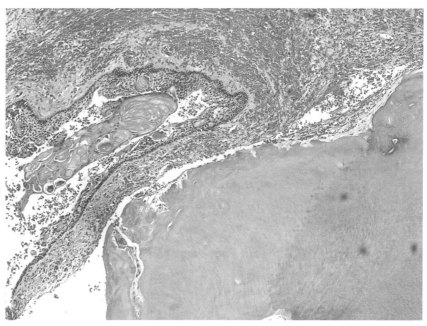

tumor with features of ameloblastic fibro-odontoma, calcifying cystic odontogenic tumor, and adenomatoid odontogenic tumor has been reported (18).

OTHER HYBRID TUMORS

Hybrid odontogenic tumors with features of adenomatoid odontogenic tumor and odontoma (8), as well as calcifying odontogenic tumor in combination with adenomatoid odontogenic tumor (7) or peripheral ameloblastoma have been reported (19).

Therapeutic management for these lesions is difficult to gage because of the paucity of reports, but treatment should be guided by the biologic behavior and recurrence rates for the most aggressive component of the hybrid.

REFERENCES

1. Frissell CT, Shafer WG. Ameloblastic odontoma; report of a case. Oral Surg Oral Med Oral Pathol 1953;6:1129-1133.
2. Silva CA. Odontoameloblastoma. Oral Surg Oral Med Oral Pathol 1956;9:545-552.
3. Martin-Granizo-López R, López-Garcia-Asenjo J, de-Pedro-Marina M, Dominguez-Cuadrado L. Odontoameloblastoma: a case report and a review of the literature. Med Oral 2004;9:340-344.
4. Mosca RC, Marques MM, Barbosa SC, Marcucci M, Oliveira JX, Lascala CA. Odontoameloblastoma: report of two cases. Indian J Dent Res 2009;20:230-234.
5. Mosqueda-Taylor A, Carlos-Bregni R, Ramirez-Amador V, Palma-Guzman JM, Esquivel-Bonilla D, Hernandez-Rojase LA. Odontoameloblastoma. Clinico-pathologic study of three cases and critical review of the literature. Oral Oncol 2002;38:800-805.
6. Slabbert H, Altini M, Crooks J, Uys P. Ameloblastoma with dentinoid induction: dentinoameloblastoma. J Oral Pathol Med 1992;21:46-48.
7. Mosqueda-Taylor A, Carlos-Bregni R, Ledesma-Montes C, Fillipi RZ, de Almeida OP, Vargas PA. Calcifying epithelial odontogenic tumor-like areas are common findings in adenomatoid odontogenic tumors and not a specific entity. Oral Oncol 2005;41:214-215.
8. Martinez A, Mosqueda-Taylor A, Marchesani FJ, Brethauer U, Spencer ML. Adenomatoid odontogenic tumor concomitant with cystic complex odontoma: case report. Oral Surg Oral Med Oral Pathol Oral Radiol Endod 2009;108:e25-29.
9. Reichart PA, Jundt G. [Benign "mixed" odontogenic tumors.] Pathologe 2008;29:189-198. [German]
10. Chindasombatjaroen J, Kakimoto N, Akiyama H, et al. Computerized tomography observation of a calcifying cystic odontogenic tumor with an odontoma: case report. Oral Surg Oral Med Oral Pathol Oral Radiol Endod 2007;104:e52-57.
11. Marques YF, Botelho TL, Xavier FC, Rangel AL, Rege IC, Mantesso A. Importance of cone beam computed tomography for diagnosis of calcifying cystic odontogenic tumour associated to odontoma. Report of a case. Med Oral Patol Oral Cir Bucal 2010;15:e490-493.
12. Buch RS, Coerdt W, Wahlmann U. [Adenomatoid odontogenic tumor in calcifying odontogenic cyst.] Mund Kiefer Gesichtschir 2003;7:301-305. [German]
13. Ide F, Obara K, Mishima K, Saito I. Ameloblastoma ex calcifying odontogenic cyst (dentinogenic ghost cell tumor). J Oral Pathol Med 2005;34:511-512.
14. Nosrati K, Seyedmajidi M. Ameloblastomatous calcifying odontogenic cyst: a case report of a rare histologic variant. Arch Iran Med 2009;12:417-420.
15. Yoon JH, Kim HJ, Yook JI, Cha IH, Ellis GL, Kim J. Hybrid odontogenic tumor of calcifying odontogenic cyst and ameloblastic fibroma. Oral Surg Oral Med Oral Pathol Oral Radiol Endod 2004;98:80-84.
16. Lin CC, Chen CH, Lin LM, et al. Calcifying odontogenic cyst with ameloblastic fibroma: report of three cases. Oral Surg Oral Med Oral Pathol Oral Radiol Endod 2004;98:451-460.
17. Han PP, Nagatsuka H, Siar CH, et al. A pigmented calcifying cystic odontogenic tumor associated with compound odontoma: a case report and review of literature. Head Face Med 2007;3:35.
18. Phillips MD, Closmann JJ, Baus MR, Torske KR, Williams SB. Hybrid odontogenic tumor with features of ameloblastic fibro-odontoma, calcifying odontogenic cyst, and adenomatoid odontogenic tumor: a case report and review of the literature. J Oral Maxillofac Surg 2010;68:470-474.
19. Etit D, Uyaroglu MA, Erdogan N. Mixed odontogenic tumor: ameloblastoma and calcifying epithelial odontogenic tumor. Indian J Pathol Microbiol 2010;53:122-124.

PERIPHERAL ODONTOGENIC NEOPLASMS AND CYSTS

PERIPHERAL ODONTOGENIC NEOPLASMS

If reactive tumors of the gingiva and alveolar mucosa, such as peripheral ossifying fibroma and peripheral giant cell granuloma, are excluded, odontogenic tumors originating outside bone are rare. Nevertheless, the remnants of the dental lamina, rests of Serres, and basal cells of the gingival mucosa retain the potential to form a variety of odontogenic cysts and neoplasms.

General Features

In an evaluation of over 90,000 oral and maxillofacial pathology accessions over a 20-year span, Buchner et al. (1) identified 45 (0.05 percent) that were classified as peripheral odontogenic neoplasms. These tumors accounted for 4 percent of all odontogenic neoplasms accessioned. Peripheral odontogenic fibroma was the most common neoplasm, with 23 cases identified, and was the only peripheral odontogenic neoplasm with a greater frequency than its central bony counterpart. Next were 13 cases of peripheral ameloblastoma, followed by 6 cases of peripheral calcifying cystic odontogenic tumor.

In an evaluation of almost 40,000 oral pathology accessions, Ide et al. (2) identified 25 peripheral odontogenic tumors. Odontogenic fibromas and ameloblastomas were the most prevalent. Also identified were 5 cases termed peripheral odontogenic hamartoma. The authors speculated that all these lesions developed from pluripotent rests of Serres.

Manor et al. (3) identified 6 peripheral odontogenic tumors out of 406 consecutive gingival enlargement biopsies. These included 2 peripheral odontogenic fibromas, 2 calcifying cystic odontogenic tumors, 1 ameloblastoma, and 1 calcifying odontogenic tumor.

Clinical Features

All peripheral odontogenic neoplasms present as slowly growing, firm, smooth-surfaced enlargements of the gingiva and alveolar mucosa. The surface mucosa is normal and there is seldom any change in hue. Continued enlargement can result in ulceration secondary to mastication trauma. The enlargements are asymptomatic unless secondarily inflamed. Although slow growing, continued growth can displace adjacent teeth crowns.

In 2008 Ide et al.(4) added 5 cases to a review of the literature that included 14 adenomatoid odontogenic tumors, 15 keratocystic odontogenic tumors, 5 ameloblastic fibromas, and 7 odontomas. Most of the adenomatoid odontogenic tumors, ameloblastic fibromas, and odontomas were initially diagnosed within the first two decades, whereas keratocystic odontogenic tumors were first diagnosed in middle-aged adults. A marked female predominance was apparent for adenomatoid odontogenic tumors, keratocystic odontogenic tumors, and ameloblastic fibromas. Approximately 90 percent of ameloblastic fibromas occurred in the maxilla. Adenomatoid odontogenic tumors and odontomas were identified most often in the incisor area, and keratocystic odontogenic tumors and ameloblastic fibromas were typically located in permanent canine/premolar and deciduous molar regions. Although most adenomatoid odontogenic tumors and keratocystic odontogenic tumors involved the buccal gingiva, odontomas showed a predilection for the lingual gingiva. With the exception of keratocystic odontogenic tumors, there were no recurrences.

Radiographic Features

It is unusual for peripheral odontogenic neoplasms to cause any change in the underlying bone. At most, a cupping-out of the periosteal surface occurs in all but the most unusual cases. Still, radiographic analysis is important to rule out peripheral extension of a central bony lesion.

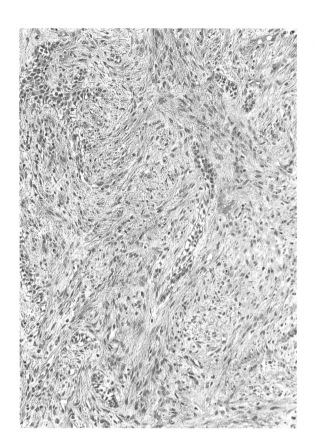 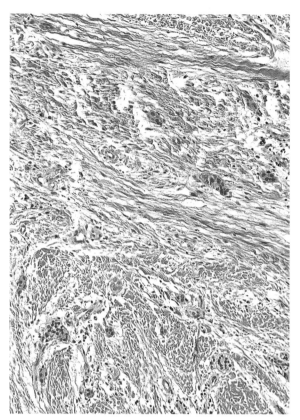

Figure 11-1

PERIPHERAL ODONTOGENIC FIBROMA

Left: Numerous rests of odontogenic epithelium are seen in a cellular fibrous connective tissue background.
Right: Odontogenic epithelial rests in a more collagenous connective tissue matrix than in the left figure.

Peripheral Odontogenic Fibroma

Peripheral odontogenic fibromas are, based on the reported cases, the most common odontogenic neoplasm of gingival soft tissues. They occur more often in females, in the posterior mandible, with a wide age range at the time of diagnosis (5). Most are asymptomatic unless secondarily inflamed. They have a slow growth rate, but like most any neoplasm, can achieve significant size if not removed (6).

Peripheral odontogenic fibromas appear microscopically identical to their central bony counterparts. Fibrous connective tissue ranges from predominantly collagenous to cellular, with numerous spindle-shaped fibroblasts (fig. 11-1). Tumors have varying numbers of epithelial rests as well as larger islands and cords of odontogenic epithelium. There should be little, if any, ameloblastic differentiation. Some cases,

similar to the central bony counterpart, show foci of granular cells (7).

This tumor should be differentiated from the more common reactive enlargement of the gingiva known as peripheral ossifying fibroma (8). These latter lesions, described below, often have a similar fibrous connective tissue background. Most, however, have few epithelial rests and are characterized instead by areas of mineralization resembling bone and cementum.

Peripheral Ameloblastoma
(Extraosseous Ameloblastoma)

Peripheral ameloblastomas present clinically as firm, smooth-surfaced soft tissue enlargements of the gingiva or alveolar mucosa (fig. 11-2). The neoplastic cells arise from epithelial rests or from the basal cells of the overlying mucosa. In an evaluation of 160 published cases, Philipsen

136

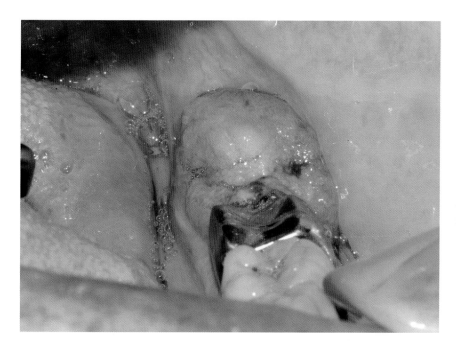

Figure 11-2

PERIPHERAL AMELOBLASTOMA

An asymptomatic, lobulated, soft tissue enlargement involves the alveolar ridge posterior to the mandibular molars.

et al. (9) found that peripheral neoplasms accounted for 2 to 10 percent of all ameloblastomas. The average age at diagnosis was 52 years, which was substantially older than for those with intraosseous lesions. The authors identified five reports of nongingival ameloblastomas but felt these most likely represented unusual salivary gland tumors (10). Like central bony tumors, peripheral ameloblastomas occurred more often in males, although in another series of 39 cases, no male bias was noted (11).

Microscopically, the tumors are identical to their central bony counterparts (figs. 11-3, 11-4) (12). In a series of 39 cases, the most predominant pattern was plexiform (11). Basal cell ameloblastomas have been misdiagnosed as basal cell carcinomas (13). By definition, these tumors do not infiltrate the underlying bone. If there is underlying bone involvement beyond the cortical plate, the lesion is an intraosseous ameloblastoma. Although rare, peripheral ameloblastomas have undergone malignant transformation (14).

Kishino et al. (15) evaluated the immunohistochemical profile of eight peripheral ameloblastomas and found positive staining for cytokeratins (CK) 13, 14, and 19 in all; CK18 in six; and CK8 in five tumors. The mean Ki-67 labeling index was significantly lower than in intraosseous ameloblastomas.

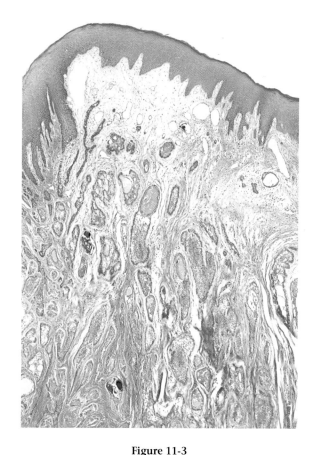

Figure 11-3

PERIPHERAL AMELOBLASTOMA

Islands of epithelial cells infiltrate the connective tissue.

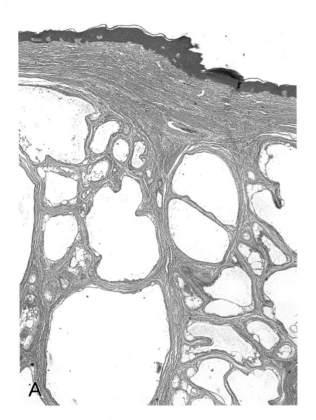

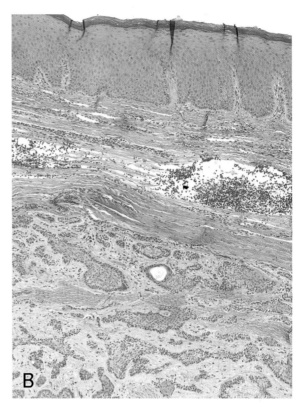

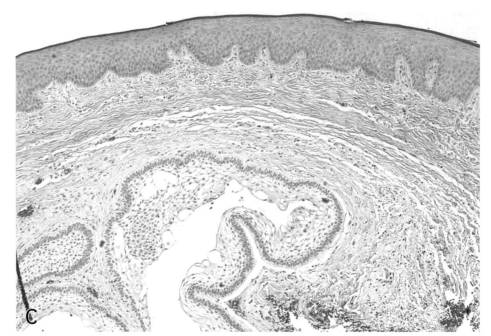

Figure 11-4

PERIPHERAL AMELOBLASTOMA

A: A follicular ameloblastoma variant with extensive cystic change is seen in the gingival connective tissue.

B: Follicles of ameloblastoma with squamous metaplasia are seen in the gingival connective tissue.

C: At high power, an island of follicular ameloblastoma is seen subjacent to the parakeratinized surface mucosa.

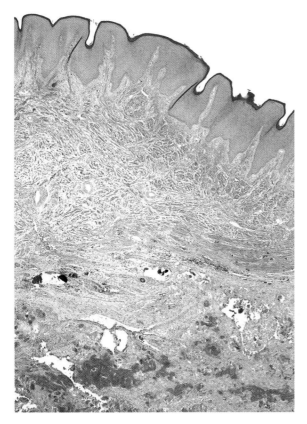

Figure 11-5

**PERIPHERAL CALCIFYING
CYSTIC ODONTOGENIC TUMOR**

Islands of epithelial cells are noted in the deep, gingival connective tissue.

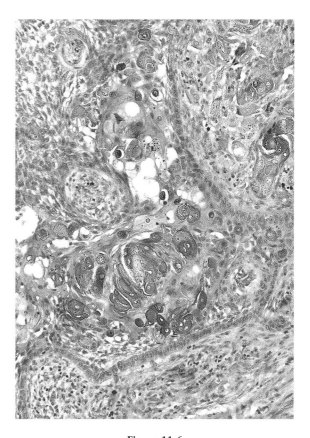

Figure 11-6

**PERIPHERAL CALCIFYING
CYSTIC ODONTOGENIC TUMOR**

The epithelium has a uniform basal cell layer, whorls of spindle cells, and typical eosinophilic ghost cells.

Peripheral Calcifying Epithelial Odontogenic Tumor

Peripheral calcifying epithelial odontogenic tumor, a rare central neoplasm, has also been reported as a peripheral soft tissue enlargement of the gingiva (16–18). Peripheral tumors show the same microscopic features as their central counterparts. Abrahao et al. (19) reported an unusual, multifocal case of peripheral calcifying epithelial odontogenic tumor involving the mandibular gingiva of a 40-year-old female.

Mesquita et al. (20) described a case involving the maxillary gingiva in a 48-year-old female. The lesion showed polyhedral and clear cells with evidence of amyloid. The tumor was positive for AE1/AE3 and CK14. There was immunoexpression of fibronectin; types I, III, and IV collagen; and laminin.

Peripheral Calcifying Cystic Odontogenic Tumor

With less than 50 cases reported in the literature, *peripheral calcifying cystic odontogenic tumor* is a rare lesion. As with other peripheral odontogenic neoplasms, these tumors present clinically as a smooth-surfaced, firm, slowly growing gingival mass that is asymptomatic unless secondarily inflamed. Most originate in gingiva anterior to the molar region and approximately 66 percent are cystic when examined microscopically (21–23).

Peripheral calcifying cystic odontogenic tumors have the same microscopic features as their central counterparts (figs. 11-5, 11-6). Because of the variable microscopic features, an incisional biopsy can lead to a misdiagnosis of ameloblastoma (24).

139

Candido et al. (25) reported a case involving the mandibular canine region in a 45-year-old male. Immunohistochemical analysis demonstrated staining for pancytokeratin and two neural markers. Dendritic cells (Langerhans cells and melanocytes) were identified within the neoplasm.

Peripheral Odontogenic Myxoma

Peripheral variants of odontogenic myxoma are rare, but have been reported to involve the mandibular and maxillary gingiva (26). As with other peripheral odontogenic tumors, peripheral myxoma is slowly growing and less aggressive than central myxoma and has a low recurrence rate.

Peripheral Keratocystic Odontogenic Tumor

While some cases of *peripheral keratocystic odontogenic tumor* in the literature probably represent simple gingival cysts, others show microscopic features identical to their central bony counterparts, and can be associated with basal cell nevus syndrome (27,28). Less than 20 cases have been reported. Faustino et al. (29) reported a case involving the posterior mandibular gingiva in a 57-year-old female which recurred 12 months after excision.

Peripheral Odontoma

Few cases of *peripheral odontoma* have been reported in the literature (30,31). Alternative terms including *ectopic tooth, ectopic soft tissue mesiodens, ectopic odontoma,* and *extraosseous tooth germ* have been used to describe this entity in various stages of development. Cases most often involve children.

Microscopically, all cases exhibit the features of compound or complex odontoma development. These include ameloblasts, enamel matrix, odontoblasts, dentin, and dental papillae.

Peripheral Ameloblastic Fibroma

Only three *peripheral ameloblastic fibromas* have been reported in the English language literature (32). As is the case with the central counterpart, especially in young patients, these lesions may be difficult to distinguish from soft tissue tooth germs, early developing ameloblastic fibro-odontomas, and complex/compound odontomas.

Treatment

Most peripheral odontogenic neoplasms are treated with simple conservative excision. Recurrences are rare even for ameloblastomas (33).

REACTIVE TUMORS OF THE GINGIVA

A variety of reactive enlargements occur with some frequency in the gingival and alveolar mucosal soft tissues. The three most commonly identified that clinically mimic soft tissue neoplasms are peripheral ossifying fibroma, peripheral giant cell granuloma, and pyogenic granuloma.

Peripheral Ossifying Fibroma

Definition. *Peripheral ossifying fibroma* is a common soft tissue enlargement thought to be reactive in nature and occurring exclusively on the gingival or alveolar mucosa. These enlargements are felt to arise from cells of the periodontal ligament. They should not be confused with peripheral odontogenic fibromas described previously which are distinct histologically and identified far less frequently.

General Features. Peripheral ossifying fibromas are most often identified in teenagers and young adults. They are found more often in females and have a slight predilection for the maxillary incisor-premolar region. In an evaluation of 207 cases, Buchner and Hansen (34) reported that almost 60 percent occurred in the maxilla; over half occurred in the incisor/canine region of both arches.

Cuisia and Brannon (35) reviewed 134 peripheral ossifying fibromas in patients ranging in age from 1 to 19 years. Tumors were found more frequently in females (60 percent) and had a predilection for the maxillary gingiva (60 percent) and the incisor/canine region. Only 2 were associated with primary teeth.

Kumar et al. (36) described an unusual case of multiple peripheral ossifying fibromas in a 49-year-old female which were felt to be the result of a genetic mutation. Silva et al. (37) reported an unusual case that included a peripheral ossifying fibroma between two mandibular incisors of a 45-year-old female, and a concurrent central odontogenic fibroma in the anterior mandible. Both were excised and there was no recurrence at 1 year follow-up.

Clinical Features. Peripheral ossifying fibromas characteristically appear as smooth, sessile

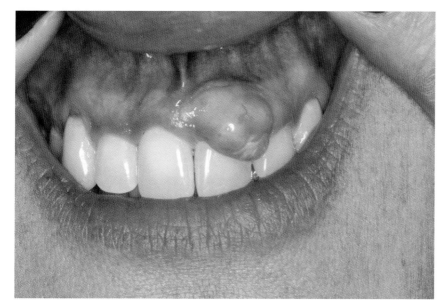

Figure 11-7

PERIPHERAL OSSIFYING FIBROMA

A smooth, asymptomatic soft tissue mass involves the gingiva of the anterior maxilla.

or pedunculated soft tissue enlargements often originating from the papillae between the teeth (fig. 11-7). Lesions are often ulcerated and secondary inflammation can result in increased erythema. They are slowly growing tumors, but continued growth can displace adjacent teeth crowns.

Microscopic Findings. Microscopically, there is cellular fibrous connective tissue with plump, spindle-shaped fibroblasts. Ulceration of the surface results in effacement of the superficial tumor by necrotic debris, neutrophils, and organizing granulation tissue. Within the tumor, varying amounts of metaplastic woven bone are identified, often depending on the age of the lesion (figs. 11-8, 11-9). Small globular mineralizations resembling cementum may also be identified. Occasional lesions have multinucleated giant cells.

Immunohistochemical Findings. An immunohistochemical analysis of four tumors revealed that the proliferating cells showed myofibroblastic characteristics and did not express estrogen or progesterone receptors (38).

Treatment and Prognosis. Treatment for peripheral ossifying fibroma involves local surgical excision. The recurrence rate ranges from 8 to 20 percent (34,35,38). Similar to other peripheral lesions, peripheral ossifying fibromas have no predilection to become aggressive, and recurrent lesions should also be removed via conservative excision.

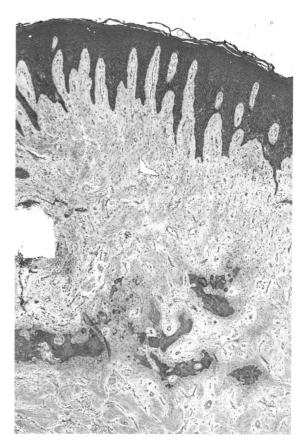

Figure 11-8

PERIPHERAL OSSIFYING FIBROMA

Parakeratinized stratified squamous epithelium surfaces cellular fibrovascular connective tissue. Foci of mineralization are seen.

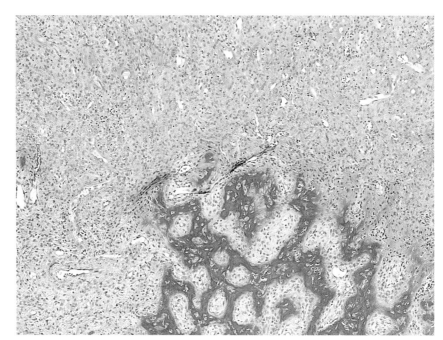

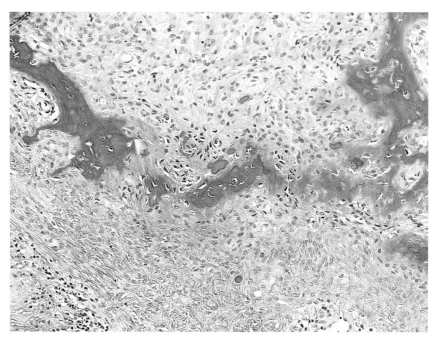

Figure 11-9

PERIPHERAL OSSIFYING FIBROMA

Top: Numerous spindle-shaped fibroblasts, collagen fibers, and islands and trabeculae of woven bone are seen.

Bottom: Plump fibroblasts surround trabeculae of woven bone and basophilic cementum-like islands.

Peripheral Giant Cell Granuloma

Definition. *Peripheral giant cell granulomas* are most likely reactive in nature but behave clinically as a benign neoplasm. The origin of the giant cells is controversial but many investigators believe they originate from the mononuclear phagocyte system. Extragnathic tumors have been reported. Unlike the central bony giant cell lesions, peripheral tumors are not usually associated with hyperparathyroidism.

General Features. An evaluation of 1,180 reported cases revealed that peripheral giant cell granulomas were found more often in females, all age groups were affected, and most tumors were first diagnosed in patients between 40 and 60 years of age (39). The mandible was more

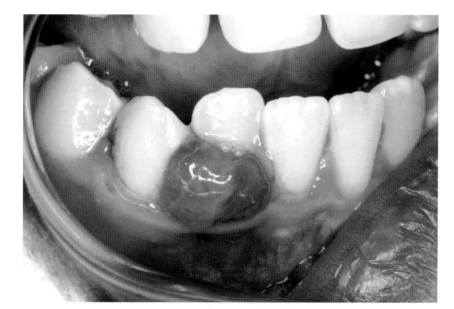

Figure 11-10

PERIPHERAL GIANT CELL GRANULOMA

A smooth, erythematous, asymptomatic soft tissue mass involves the gingiva of the anterior mandible.

Figure 11-11

PERIPHERAL GIANT CELL GRANULOMA

A surface of parakeratinized stratified squamous epithelium overlays fibrovascular connective tissue infiltrated with spindle-shaped and multinucleated giant cells.

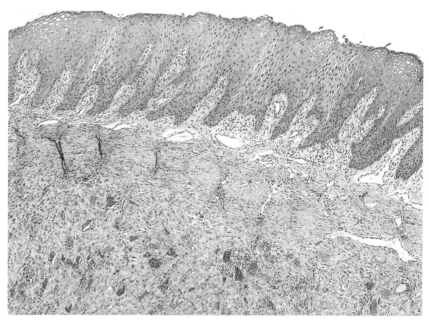

often affected than the maxilla. In a 12-year retrospective study of 575 cases by Motamedi et al. (40), patients ranged in age from 2 to 85 years. About 52 percent occurred in females and 48 percent in males. Over 80 percent were first diagnosed before age 40 and just over 60 percent involved the mandibular gingiva. In the same study, peripheral giant cell granulomas outnumbered their central bony counterparts 2 to 1.

Ozden et al. (41) reported the first case of a peripheral giant cell granuloma occurring in association with dental implants. The tumor was

removed and the implant replaced. Follow-up for 1 year revealed no recurrence.

Clinical Features. Because of a large vascular component, peripheral giant cell granulomas often appear red or blue (fig. 11-10). They have a smooth surface which is often ulcerated. These are slowly growing tumors that can displace adjacent teeth crowns.

Microscopic Findings. Microscopically, the lesions consist of plump spindle-shaped mesenchymal cells and numerous nondescript multinucleated giant cells (figs. 11-11, 11-12).

143

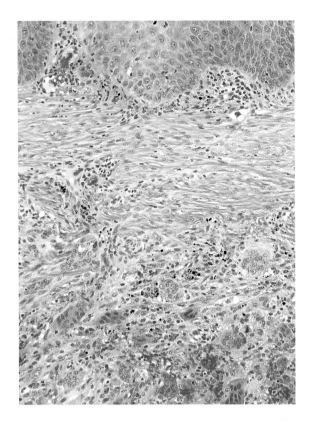
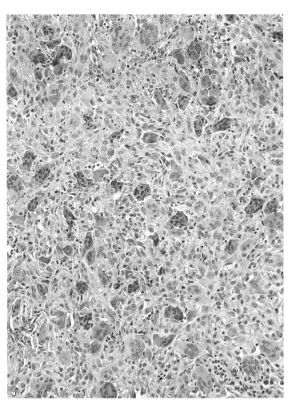

Figure 11-12

PERIPHERAL GIANT CELL GRANULOMA

Left: Numerous thin-walled vascular channels, hemorrhage, and multinucleated giant cells are seen in the connective tissue subjacent to the surface mucosa.

Right: Seen are numerous multinucleated giant cells, spindle-shaped cells, vascular channels, and hemorrhage.

Most tumors show significant hemorrhage and hemosiderin deposition. Osteoid and woven bone are often identified. Mitotic figures should not be considered a sign of malignancy. These lesions are microscopically identical to central giant cell lesions of the jaws but are not associated with primary or secondary hyperparathyroidism.

Immunohistochemical Findings. In one study, 30 peripheral giant cell lesions of the jaws and 24 extragnathic giant cell tumors (tendon sheath and salivary gland) all showed an identical cellular composition (42). Giant cell lesions at all extragnathic sites contain the same osteolytic proteases and express cytokines effective in bone metabolism. Factors indicating the differentiation and activation of osteoclasts, including RANK, macrophage colony stimulating factor (M-CSF), cathepsin K, and matrix metalloproteinase (MMP) 9 were present.

Treatment and Prognosis. Successful therapeutic management most often involves conservative excision. Recurrence rates are less than 2 percent (40). The lesions have no predilection for aggressive behavior or malignant change. Should the lesions recur, conservative excision continues to be the treatment of choice.

Pyogenic Granuloma

Definition. *Pyogenic granulomas* of the gingiva are reactive soft tissue proliferations and should be distinguished from lobular capillary hemangiomas of the skin (43). They occur frequently on the gingiva in areas of chronic inflammation. Multiple lesions are often identified as a result of hormonal changes during pregnancy (*pregnancy tumors*).

Clinical Features. When these tumors involve gingiva and sometimes other areas of the

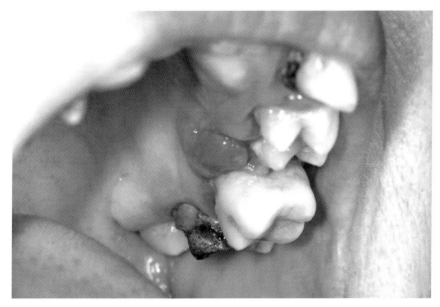

Figure 11-13

PYOGENIC GRANULOMA

An erythematous, easily bleeding soft tissue enlargement involves the gingiva of the left maxilla.

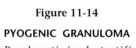
Figure 11-14

PYOGENIC GRANULOMA

Parakeratinized stratified squamous epithelium with extensive areas of ulceration overlies the vascular fibrous connective tissue.

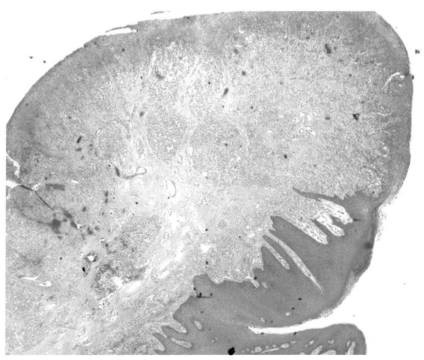

oral mucosa, they present as smooth, erythematous, often ulcerated soft tissue enlargements which bleed easily when traumatized (fig. 11-13). They often grow rapidly. Gingival inflammation and poor oral hygiene are exacerbating factors. They are found most often in young adults, but affect a wide age range (44–46). A recent report describes a tumor involving a dental implant (47).

Microscopic Findings. The typical granulation tissue features numerous endothelial-lined vascular channels surrounded by loose fibrous connective tissue and varying infiltrates of acute and chronic inflammatory cells (figs. 11-14, 11-15). Some lesions show an alarming number of mitotic figures. In ulcerated lesions, necrotic debris and neutrophils are noted near the surface. In older lesions, the granulation tissue

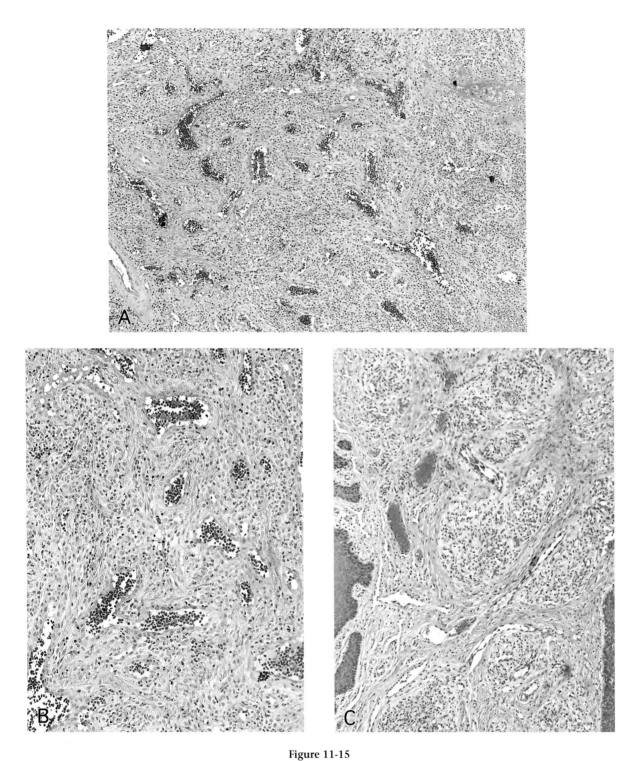

Figure 11-15

PYOGENIC GRANULOMA

A: There are numerous thin-walled vascular channels in a cellular background.

B: Numerous vascular channels are surrounded by plump endothelial cells, and an infiltrate of lymphocytes, plasma cells, and neutrophils.

C: A more mature lesion with less inflammation, more fibrous connective tissue, and groups of thin-walled vascular channels than seen in B.

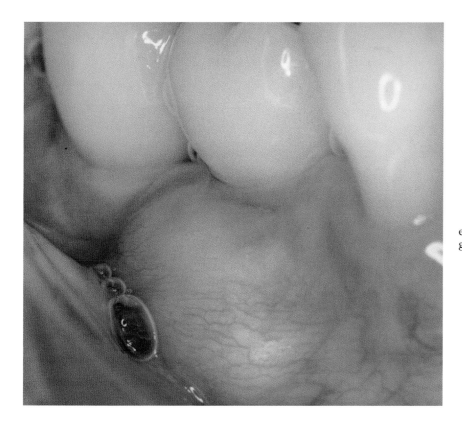

Figure 11-16

GINGIVAL CYST

A clear, fluid-filled submucosal enlargement involves the gingiva.

undergoes progressive fibrosis, leaving behind clusters of thin-walled vascular channels.

Treatment and Prognosis. Treatment of these lesions involves conservative surgical excision. Recurrences are often associated with persistence of local inflammatory or systemic hormonal factors. When these lesions occur during pregnancy, they often resolve partially or completely following delivery.

GINGIVAL CYSTS IN ADULTS

Definition. *Gingival cysts* are developmental lesions that form in the gingival and alveolar mucosal soft tissues. They develop from epithelial rests of Serres or from the basal cells of the gingiva (48,49).

Clinical Features. Gingival cysts are most frequently identified in the mandibular buccal gingiva anterior to the molar region and rarely exceed 1 cm in diameter (fig. 11-16). They are usually of normal color but may have a bluish hue. These cysts are most often identified in adults between 40 and 60 years of age (49,50). A cyst of the gingiva occurred following gingival graft surgery (51).

Radiographic Features. In most instances, radiographs reveal no underlying bony abnormalities. At the time of surgery, however, a cupping-out of the subjacent cortical plate is sometimes identified.

Microscopic Findings. Microscopically, most gingival cysts have a lining of cuboidal epithelial cells, 1 to 4 cells in thickness, resembling reduced enamel epithelium or nonkeratinized stratified squamous epithelium without rete ridges (fig. 11-17) (52). Plaque-like epithelial thickenings, similar to those identified in lateral periodontal and botryoid cysts, are sometimes present. There should be no uniformity of the basal cell layer or corrugation of the luminal surface, features of keratocystic odontogenic tumors. Multicystic or "botryoid" forms occur (49).

Treatment and Prognosis. Therapeutic management involves simple conservative excision. Recurrences are not expected.

GINGIVAL CYSTS IN INFANTS

Definition. *Gingival cysts of infants* are nonkeratinizing or keratinizing cysts that occur on the alveolar ridges of newborns. They involve

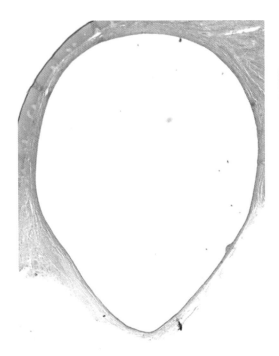

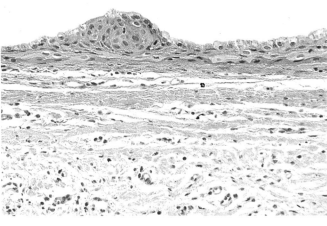

Figure 11-17

GINGIVAL CYST

Left: The gingival epithelium is separated from an underlying cystic lumen by fibrovascular connective tissue.

Below: A thin surface of squamous and cuboidal epithelium with a plaque-like thickening lines the cystic cavity.

the maxillary or mandibular gingiva and occur as a single lesion or as groups. Cysts that form in the tissues along the midline of the palate are referred to as *Epstein pearls*. A third group of soft tissue cysts form at the junction of the hard and soft palate, and these are known as *Bohn nodules* (53). Of 541 newborns, 89 percent showed gingival or median palatal cysts, or Bohn nodules (54).

Clinical Features. These soft tissue cysts present clinically as smooth-surfaced, white-yellow sessile enlargements of the gingival or palatal soft tissues.

Microscopic Findings. Microscopically, the cysts are usually lined by a thin layer of nonkeratinizing or parakeratinizing stratified squamous epithelium. The lumen contains desquamated epithelial cells or keratin debris. There should be no uniformity of the basal cell layer or corrugation of the luminal surface, features characteristic of keratocystic odontogenic tumors.

Treatment and Prognosis. Therapeutic management is often unnecessary because the cysts rupture and resolve spontaneously.

REFERENCES

1. Buchner A, Merrell PW, Carpenter WM. Relative frequency of peripheral odontogenic tumors: a study of 45 new cases and comparison with studies from the literature. J Oral Pathol Med 2006;35:385-391.

2. Ide F, Obara K, Mishima K, et al. Peripheral odontogenic tumor: a clinicopathologic study of 30 cases. General features and hamartomatous lesions. J Oral Pathol Med 2005;34:552-557.

3. Manor Y, Mardinger O, Katz J, Taicher S, Hirshberg A. Peripheral odontogenic tumours—differential diagnosis in gingival lesions. Int J Oral Maxillofac Surg 2004;33:268-273.

4. Ide F, Mishima K, Saito I, Kusama K. Rare peripheral odontogenic tumors: report of 5 cases and comprehensive review of the literature. Oral Surg Oral Med Oral Pathol Oral Radiol Endod 2008;106:e22-28.

5. Garcia BG, Johann AC, da Silveira-Junior JB, Aguiar MC, Mesquita RA. Retrospective analysis of peripheral odontogenic fibroma (WHO-type) in Brazilians. Minerva Stomatol 2007;56:115-119.

6. Lin CT, Chuang FH, Chen JH, Chen CM, Chen YK. Peripheral odontogenic fibroma in a Taiwan chinese population: a retrospective analysis. Kaohsiung J Med Sci 2008;24:415-421.

7. Rinaggio J, Cleveland D, Koshy R, Gallante A, Mirani N. Peripheral granular cell odontogenic fibroma. Oral Surg Oral Med Oral Pathol Oral Radiol Endod 2007;104:676-679.

8. Gardner DG. The peripheral odontogenic fibroma: an attempt at clarification. Oral Surg Oral Med Oral Pathol 1982;54:40-48.

9. Philipsen HP, Reichart PA, Nikai H, Takata T, Kudo Y. Peripheral ameloblastoma: biological profile based on 160 cases from the literature. Oral Oncol 2001;37:17-27.

10. Woo SB, Smith-Williams JE, Sciubba JJ, Lipper S. Peripheral ameloblastoma of the buccal mucosa: case report and review of the English literature. Oral Surg Oral Med Oral Pathol 1987;63:78-84.

11. el-Mofty SK, Gerard NO, Farish SE, Rodu B. Peripheral ameloblastoma: a clinical and histologic study of 11 cases. J Oral Maxillofac Surg 1991;49:970-974; discussion 974-975.

12. LeCorn DW, Bhattacharyya I, Vertucci FJ. Peripheral ameloblastoma: a case report and review of the literature. J Endod 2006;32:152-154.

13. Gardner DG. Peripheral ameloblastoma: a study of 21 cases, including 5 reported as basal cell carcinoma of the gingiva. Cancer 1977;39:1625-1633.

14. Baden E, Doyle JL, Petriella V. Malignant transformation of peripheral ameloblastoma. Oral Surg Oral Med Oral Pathol 1993;75:214-219.

15. Kishino M, Murakami S, Yuki M, et al. A immunohistochemical study of the peripheral ameloblastoma. Oral Dis 2007;13:575-580.

16. da Silveira EJ, Gordon-Nunez MA, Seabra FR, et al. Peripheral calcifying epithelial odontogenic tumor associated with generalized drug-induced gingival growth: a case report. J Oral Maxillofac Surg 2007;65:341-345.

17. de Oliveira MG, Chaves AC, Visioli F, et al. Peripheral clear cell variant of calcifying epithelial odontogenic tumor affecting 2 sites: report of a case. Oral Surg Oral Med Oral Pathol Oral Radiol Endod 2009;107:407-411.

18. Habibi A, Saghravanian N, Zare R, Jafarzadeh H. Clear cell variant of extraosseous calcifying epithelial odontogenic tumor: a case report. J Oral Sci 2009;51:485-488.

19. Abrahao AC, Camisasca DR, Bonelli BR, et al. Recurrent bilateral gingival peripheral calcifying epithelial odontogenic tumor (Pindborg tumor): a case report. Oral Surg Oral Med Oral Pathol Oral Radiol Endod 2009;108:e66-71.

20. Mesquita RA, Lotufo MA, Sugaya NN, De Araujo NS, De Araujo VC. Peripheral clear cell variant of calcifying epithelial odontogenic tumor: Report of a case and immunohistochemical investigation. Oral Surg Oral Med Oral Pathol Oral Radiol Endod 2003;95:198-204.

21. Buchner A, Merrell PW, Hansen LS, Leider AS. Peripheral (extraosseous) calcifying odontogenic cyst. A review of forty-five cases. Oral Surg Oral Med Oral Pathol 1991;72:65-70.

22. Iezzi G, Rubini C, Fioroni M, Piattelli A. Peripheral dentinogenic ghost cell tumor of the gingiva. J Periodontol 2007;78:1635-1638.

23. Seyedmajidi M, Feizabadi M. Peripheral calcifying odontogenic cyst. Arch Iran Med 2009;12:309-312.

24. Wong YK, Chiu SC, Pang SW, Cheng JC. Peripheral dentinogenic ghost cell tumour presenting as a gingival mass. Br J Oral Maxillofac Surg 2004;42:173-175.

25. Candido GA, Viana KA, Watanabe S, Vencio EF. Peripheral dentinogenic ghost cell tumor: a case report and review of the literature. Oral Surg Oral Med Oral Pathol Oral Radiol Endod 2009;108: e86-90.

26. Aytac-Yazicioglu D, Eren H, Görgün S. Peripheral odontogenic myxoma located on the maxillary gingiva: report of a case and review of the literature. Oral Maxillofac Surg 2008;12:167-171.

27. Chi AC, Owings JR Jr, Muller S. Peripheral odontogenic keratocyst: report of two cases and review of the literature. Oral Surg Oral Med Oral Pathol Oral Radiol Endod 2005;99:71-78.

28. Preston RD, Narayana N. Peripheral odontogenic keratocyst. J Periodontol 2005;76:2312-2315.

29. Faustino SE, Pereira MC, Rossetto AC, Oliveira DT. Recurrent peripheral odontogenic keratocyst: a case report. Dentomaxillofac Radiol 2008;37:412-414.

30. Ilief-Ala MA, Eisenberg E, Mathieu G. Peripheral complex odontoma in a pediatric dental patient: a case report. J Mass Dent Soc 2008;56:24-26.

31. Silva AR, Carlos-Bregni R, Vargas PA, de Almeida OP, Lopes MA. Peripheral developing odontoma in newborn. Report of two cases and literature review. Med Oral Patol Oral Cir Bucal 2009;14:e612-615.

32. Abughazaleh K, Andrus KM, Katsnelson A, White DK. Peripheral ameloblastic fibroma of the maxilla: report of a case and review of the literature. Oral Surg Oral Med Oral Pathol Oral Radiol Endod 2008;105:e46-48.

33. Buchner A, Sciubba JJ. Peripheral epithelial odontogenic tumors: a review. Oral Surg Oral Med Oral Pathol 1987;63:688-697.

34. Buchner A, Hansen LS. The histomorphologic spectrum of peripheral ossifying fibroma. Oral Surg Oral Med Oral Pathol 1987;63:452-461.

35. Cuisia ZE, Brannon RB. Peripheral ossifying fibroma—a clinical evaluation of 134 pediatric cases. Pediatr Dent 2001;23:245-248.

36. Kumar SK, Ram S, Jorgensen MG, Shuler CF, Sedghizadeh PP. Multicentric peripheral ossifying fibroma. J Oral Sci 2006;48:239-243.

37. Silva CO, Sallum AW, do Couto-Filho CE, Costa Pereira AA, Hanemann JA, Tatakis DN. Localized gingival enlargement associated with alveolar process expansion: peripheral ossifying fibroma coincident with central odontogenic fibroma. J Periodontol 2007;78:1354-1359.

38. Garcia de Marcos JA, Garcia de Marcos MJ, Arroyo Rodriguez SA, Chiarri Rodrigo JC, Poblet E. Peripheral ossifying fibroma: a clinical and immunohistochemical study of four cases. J Oral Sci 2010;52:95-99.

39. Katsikeris N, Kakarantza-Angelopoulou E, Angelopoulos AP. Peripheral giant cell granuloma. Clinicopathologic study of 224 new cases and review of 956 reported cases. Int J Oral Maxillofac Surg 1988;17:94-99.

40. Motamedi MH, Eshghyar N, Jafari SM, et al. Peripheral and central giant cell granulomas of the jaws: a demographic study. Oral Surg Oral Med Oral Pathol Oral Radiol Endod 2007;103: e39-43.

41. Ozden FO, Ozden B, Kurt M, Gunduz K, Gunhan O. Peripheral giant cell granuloma associated with dental implants: a rare case report. Int J Oral Maxillofac Implants 2009;24:1153-1156.

42. Friedrich RE, Eisenmann J, Roser K, Scheuer HA, Löning T. Expression of proteases in giant cell lesions of the jaws, tendon sheath and salivary glands. Anticancer Res 2010;30:1645-1652.

43. Epivatianos A, Antoniades D, Zaraboukas T, et al. Pyogenic granuloma of the oral cavity: comparative study of its clinicopathological and immunohistochemical features. Pathol Int 2005;55:391-397.

44. Cruz LE, Martos J. Granuloma gravidarum (pyogenic granuloma) treated with periodontal plastic surgery. Int J Gynaecol Obstet 2010;109:73-74.

45. das Chagas MS, Pinheiro Rdos S, Janini ME, Maia LC. Pyogenic granuloma: lobular capillary hemangioma in the upper lip of a 24-month-old child: case report. J Dent Child (Chic) 2009;76:237-240.

46. de Waal J, Dreyer WP. Oral medicine case book 22. Pyogenic granuloma. SADJ 2009;64:412-413.

47. Dojcinovic I, Richter M, Lombardi T. Occurrence of a pyogenic granuloma in relation to a dental implant. J Oral Maxillofac Surg 2010;68:1874-1876.

48. Wysocki GP, Brannon RB, Gardner DG, Sapp P. Histogenesis of the lateral periodontal cyst and the gingival cyst of the adult. Oral Surg Oral Med Oral Pathol 1980;50:327-334.

49. Nxumalo TN, Shear M. Gingival cyst in adults. J Oral Pathol Med 1992;21:309-313.

50. Bell RC, Chauvin PJ, Tyler MT. Gingival cyst of the adult: a review and a report of eight cases. J Can Dent Assoc 1997;63:533-535.

51. Breault LG, Billman MA, Lewis DM. Report of a gingival "surgical cyst" developing secondarily to a subepithelial connective tissue graft. J Periodontol 1997;68:392-395.

52. Buchner A, Hansen LS. The histomorphologic spectrum of the gingival cyst in the adult. Oral Surg Oral Med Oral Pathol 1979;48:532-539.

53. Cataldo E, Berkman MD. Cysts of the oral mucosa in newborns. Am J Dis Child 1968;116:44-48.

54. Ikemura K, Kakinoki Y, Nishio K, Suenaga Y. Cysts of the oral mucosa in newborns: a clinical observation. J UOEH 1983;5:163-168.

12 FIBRO-OSSEOUS LESIONS

Fibro-osseous lesions are diverse bone dysplasias and neoplasias that are characterized by the replacement of normal bone by fibrous connective tissue and dysplastic mineralization. In some cases, the radiographic and clinical features provide a definitive diagnosis because the histopathologic features are often identical. These lesions include varieties of fibrous dysplasia, cemento-osseous dysplasia, and central ossifying and cementifying fibromas.

FIBROUS DYSPLASIA

Definition. *Fibrous dysplasia* is a developmental fibro-osseous lesion that often results from an activating mutation in the gene that encodes the alpha subunit of stimulatory G protein (G[s] alpha) located at 20q13.2-13.3 (1). This mutation is not found in other fibro-osseous lesions such as cemento-osseous dysplasia and cemento-ossifying fibromas (2).

Clinical Features. Fibrous dysplasia has an equal sex predilection. Most cases are initially diagnosed in the second and third decades, with equal occurrence in both jaws (3). There may be significant expansion resulting in clinically evident malformations. In the maxilla and mandible, progressive malocclusion of the teeth can occur.

Monostotic fibrous dysplasia accounts for 80 to 85 percent of all cases and is limited to a single bone. Males and females are affected equally. Although lesions of the mandible are truly monostotic, maxillary lesions often spread to involve the zygoma, sphenoid, temporal or occipital bones. The term *craniofacial fibrous dysplasia* is often used to designate this distribution.

Polyostotic fibrous dysplasia is rare, and as the name implies, involves multiple bones. *Jaffe-Lichtenstein syndrome* consists of polyostotic fibrous dysplasia and café au lait pigmentations of the skin. *McCune-Albright syndrome* is polyostotic fibrous dysplasia associated with café au lait pigmentations and multiple endocrinopathies.

Radiographic Features. Radiographically, areas of bone involved with fibrous dysplasia are often described as showing a "ground glass" or homogeneous radiopaque appearance (fig. 12-1). The lesions are poorly defined and blend into the adjacent normal bone anatomy (4). Idiopathic bone cavity formation within fibrous dysplasia has been reported (5).

Microscopic Findings. Typically, there is a loose, cellular fibrous connective tissue stroma. Numerous small, irregular-shaped trabeculae of woven and lamellar bone are identified, often described metaphorically as "Chinese script" (fig. 12-2). The areas of mineralization are usually metaplastic, but small focal areas of osteoblastic rimming can be seen (fig. 12-3). Dysplastic bone fuses with normal bone at the margin of the lesion, a characteristic that distinguishes bone dysplasias from neoplasms such as cemento-ossifying fibroma. As lesions "mature" more lamellar trabeculae are seen.

Treatment and Prognosis. Therapeutic management is often dictated by the morbidity caused by progressive enlargements or because of cosmetic features. Recontouring of bone expansions is often delayed until after skeletal growth has ceased. Rare malignant changes have been reported in lesions of fibrous dysplasia, but most reports involve lesions inappropriately treated in the past with radiation.

CEMENTO-OSSIFYING FIBROMA

Definition. Although the microscopic features of all fibro-osseous lesions can be identical, the term *cemento-ossifying fibroma* is reserved for a true mesenchymal neoplasm with continuing growth potential that can lead to the significant displacement of teeth and cosmetic concerns.

Clinical Features. A literature review of 781 cases revealed a mean age for initial diagnosis of 31 years, with the greatest frequency in the fourth decade (6). Tumors occurred in females more often than males, and were three times more prevalent

151

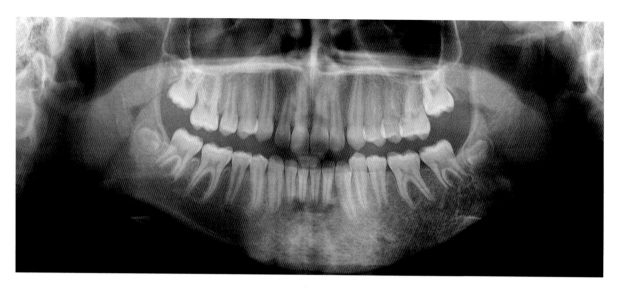

Figure 12-1

FIBROUS DYSPLASIA

A homogeneous radiolucency/radiopacity with diffuse borders extends from the right premolar region to the left third molar. There is loss of the inferior cortex of the mandible.

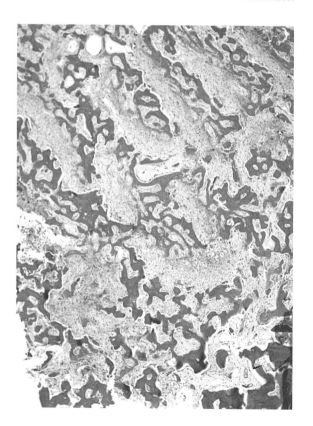 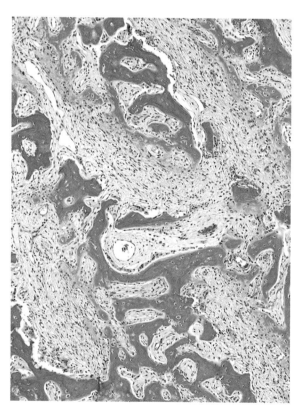

Figure 12-2

FIBROUS DYSPLASIA

Left: Irregular trabeculae of bone are in a loose fibrovascular connective tissue background.
Right: Irregular trabeculae of woven and lamellar bone are seen.

in the mandible than the maxilla. Two thirds were initially identified because of buccal cortical plate enlargement and the remainder were identified incidentally on radiographs made for other reasons. Most cases that involved the maxilla elevated the inferior border of the sinus.

Radiographic Features. Unlike dysplasias of bone, cemento-ossifying fibroma is a well-defined unilocular radiolucency with or without foci of homogeneous radiopaque areas (fig. 12-4). Tumors are entirely radiolucent or mostly radiopaque depending upon the amount of mineralized bone or cementum-like material contained within the tumor. Circumscription and delineation from surrounding normal bone distinguish this lesion as a true neoplasm rather than a dysplasia of bone.

Gross Findings. During surgical removal, these lesions usually shell out from the surrounding unaffected bone, resulting in gross specimens that exhibit a smooth periphery (fig. 12-5). This is in contrast to the bone dysplasias which are fused to surrounding normal bone and require sharp instrumentation for biopsy, resulting in a fragmented specimen.

Microscopic Findings. Microscopic examination reveals fibrous connective tissue with varying degrees of cellularity and mineralized product (fig. 12-6). The mineralizations often

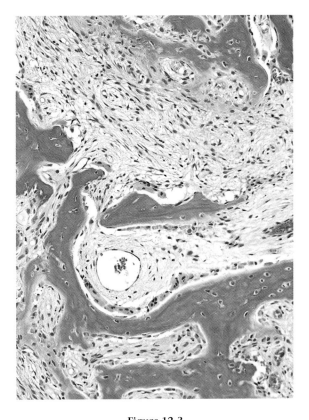

Figure 12-3

FIBROUS DYSPLASIA

Osteoblastic rimming and multinucleated osteoclasts border woven and lamellar bone trabeculae.

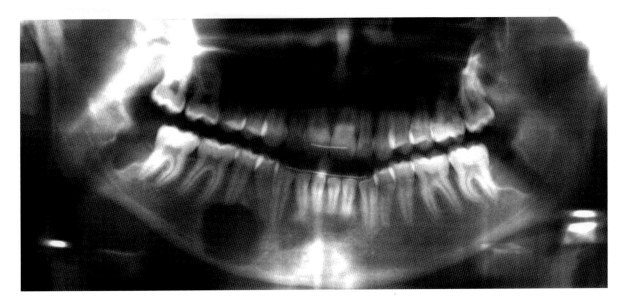

Figure 12-4

CEMENTO-OSSIFYING FIBROMA

A panoramic radiograph shows a well-demarcated radiolucency in the right mandibular premolar region.

Figure 12-5

CEMENTO-OSSIFYING FIBROMA

Grossly, these tumors shell-out from the surrounding normal bone.

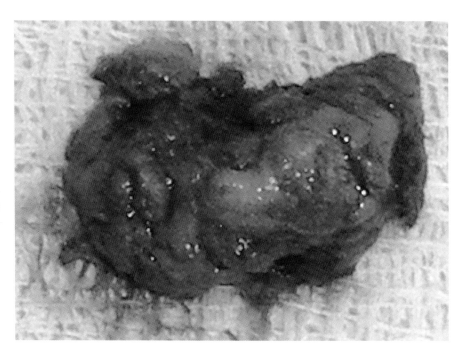

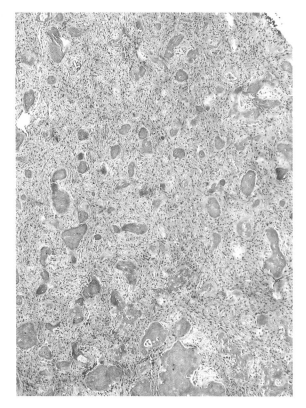 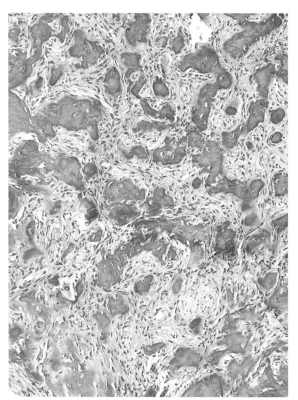

Figure 12-6

CEMENTO-OSSIFYING FIBROMA

Left: The cellular background of spindle cells has islands and trabeculae of woven and lamellar bone and acellular, basophilic cementum-like material.

Right: Islands and trabeculae of woven bone, lamellar bone, and cementum-like material are present.

are osteoid or woven bone spicules or poorly formed lamellar trabeculae. In some neoplasms, some of the mineralized product appears to be globules of acellular cementum. This diversity of mineralization patterns resembling bone or cementum suggests an odontogenic origin for some of these tumors, a feature seldom seen in fibrous dysplasia. Differentiating these neoplasms from variants of cemento-osseous dysplasias usually requires clinical and radiographic correlation.

Immunohistochemical Findings. *GNAS* mutations, which play a role in fibrous dysplasia, have not been identified in the pathogenesis of cemento-ossifying fibromas (2).

Treatment and Prognosis. Therapeutic management usually involves simple enucleation and curettage. Radiographic follow-up to assure complete resolution without recurrence is recommended.

One systematic review of the literature found follow-up for 218 cases and reported a recurrence rate of 12 percent (6). There is no evidence that cemento-ossifying fibromas undergo malignant change.

CEMENTO-OSSEOUS DYSPLASIA

Definition. *Cemento-osseous dysplasias* are a group of jaw bone abnormalities occurring in association with tooth-bearing sites. Although the exact tissue of origin is unknown, microscopic features have suggested that these lesions may originate from cells of the periodontal ligament. Based on radiographic presentation, they fall into three groups: focal, periapical, and florid (7–9). All three variants show identical microscopic features.

Focal cemento-osseous dysplasia accounts for approximately 90 percent of cases reported. These are single lesions occurring most often in the posterior mandible. They are identified most often in females between the third and sixth decades of life. The lesions are characteristically asymptomatic and often found during radiographic evaluation for other diseases.

Periapical cemento-osseous dysplasias are lesions that involve the periapical regions of permanent teeth, often in the mandibular anterior region. They can be single lesions, but often involve multiple apices of the incisors, canines, and premolars. They occur more often in females and blacks. Early developing lesions,

which are radiolucent, are frequently mistaken for periapical abscesses or cysts secondary to necrotic pulp disease of the teeth.

Florid cemento-osseous dysplasia describes multifocal lesions involving larger areas of the alveolar processes concurrently. This condition is seen most often in black females, middle aged or older. Radiographically, the lesions are often bilateral and often somewhat symmetrical in the anterior and posterior regions (8,10,11).

Clinical Features. Most lesions show little evidence of cortical plate expansion. This is an important factor which in many instances allows distinction of larger dysplasias from benign and malignant neoplasms and sclerosing inflammatory lesions of bone.

Radiographic Features. These lesions are completely radiolucent, mostly radiopaque, or any combination of the two (figs. 12-7–12-9). The appearance is a function of the degree of mineralization, which usually increases with the age of the lesion. The lesion borders may be diffuse or sharp, but there should be no peripheral cortication characteristic of a slowly expanding benign tumor or cyst. The lack of cortication distinguishes these dysplasias from neoplastic tumors, including cemento-ossifying fibromas, which are sharply demarcated from the surrounding bone by a thin corticated border (4). Cemento-osseous dysplasias have been reported in association with idiopathic bone cavities, which can be a confounding factor during radiographic evaluation (12).

Gross Findings. One feature that is characteristic of all variants of cemento-osseous dysplasia is fusion of the lesion to the surrounding bone. This feature requires sharp hand or rotary instruments to remove tissue for biopsy. As a result, most biopsy specimens consist of small, irregular bony fragments (fig. 12-10).

Microscopic Findings. All of the clinical variants demonstrate the same histopathologic features (figs. 12-10, 12-11). Early developing or immature lesions consist primarily of cellular fibrovascular connective tissue with numerous spindle-shaped fibroblasts, collagen, and small blood vessels. Small foci of mineralized tissue, resembling woven or lamellar bone or acellular cementum globules, is admixed within the soft tissue. As the lesions mature, there is a significant increase in the percentage of mineralized

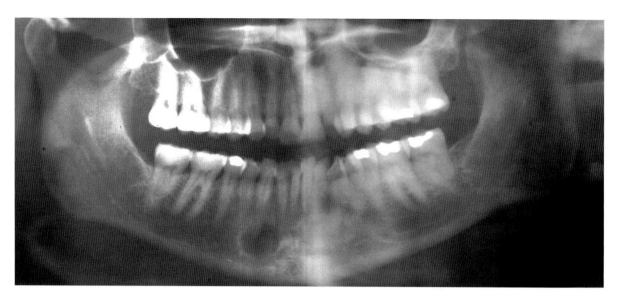

Figure 12-7

PERIAPICAL CEMENTO-OSSEOUS DYSPLASIA

An early lesion with minimal mineralization presents as a localized radiolucency involving the root of the mandibular right canine.

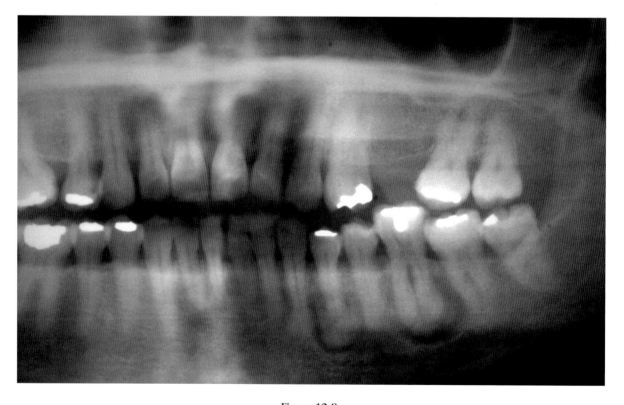

Figure 12-8

PERIAPICAL CEMENTO-OSSEOUS DYSPLASIA

Mature lesions of the left mandible present as radiolucencies with homogeneous central radiopacities associated with the roots of teeth.

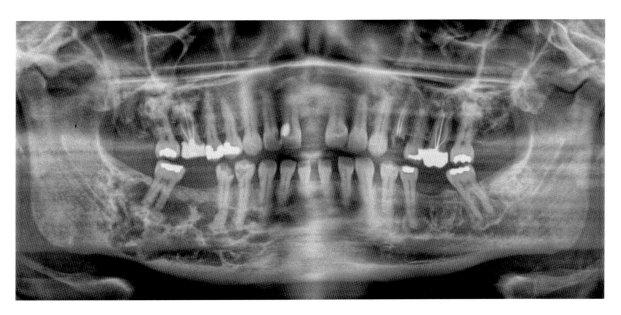

Figure 12-9

FLORID CEMENTO-OSSEOUS DYSPLASIA

Multiple radiopaque/radiolucent lesions involve the mandible and maxilla bilaterally.

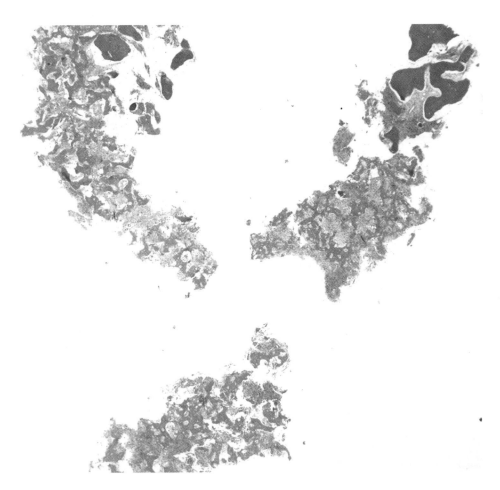

Figure 12-10

CEMENTO-OSSEOUS DYSPLASIA

Specimens are fragmented because dysplasias of bone are fused to the surrounding normal bone.

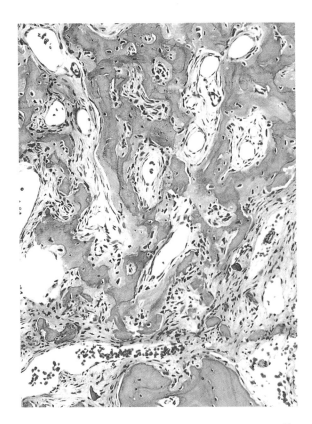 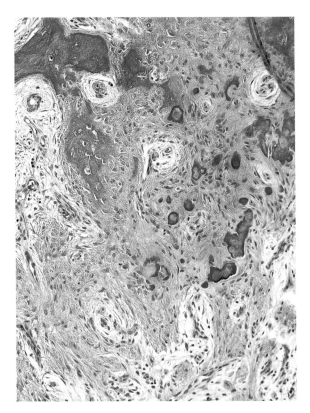

Figure 12-11

CEMENTO-OSSEOUS DYSPLASIA

Left: Irregular trabeculae and islands of woven and lamellar bone are noted in a background of fibrous connective tissue.

Right: Foci of eosinophilic, lamellar and woven bone are together with basophilic cementum-like material.

tissue. In mature lesions, islands of mineralization resembling bone or cementum are often fused, forming large sheets (fig. 12-12).

Immunohistochemical Findings. The *GNAS* mutations that play a role in fibrous dysplasia have not been identified in the pathogenesis of cemento-osseous dysplasia (2).

Treatment and Prognosis. As indicated above, a specific diagnosis usually depends on the correlation of radiographic and clinical features with the histopathology. In some instances, classic examples are diagnosed based on the clinical and radiographic features alone.

In cases where multiple lesions are identified, the biopsy of a single lesion is usually all that is necessary to provide a diagnosis. These lesions seldom expand and therefore cosmetic issues are not problematic.

In cases of florid cemento-osseous dysplasia, however, surgical procedures, including extraction of teeth in areas of mature dysplasias, may increase the risk of postoperative complications due to a decrease in bone vascularity (13). Additional long-term studies are needed to assess any possible issues related to the placement of osseous integrated implants within these lesions (11).

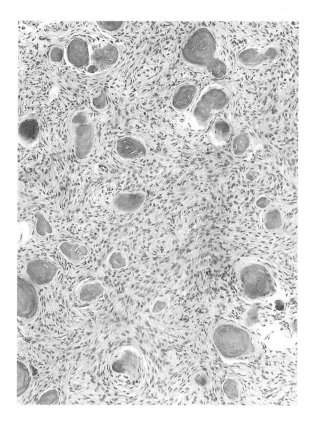 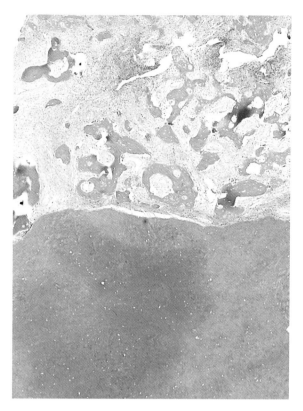

Figure 12-12

CEMENTO-OSSEOUS DYSPLASIA

Left: A background of spindle-shaped fibroblasts surrounds ovoid islands of basophilic cementum-like material.

Right: As these lesions undergo increased mineralization, sheets of woven and lamellar bone and acellular cementum-like material predominate.

REFERENCES

1. DiCaprio MR, Enneking WF. Fibrous dysplasia. Pathophysiology, evaluation, and treatment. J Bone Joint Surg Am 2005;87:1848-1864.

2. Patel MM, Wilkey JF, Abdelsayed R, D'Silva NJ, Malchoff C, Mallya SM. Analysis of GNAS mutations in cemento-ossifying fibromas and cemento-osseous dysplasias of the jaws. Oral Surg Oral Med Oral Pathol Oral Radiol Endod 2010;109:739-743.

3. Alsharif MJ, Sun ZJ, Chen XM, Wang SP, Zhao YF. Benign fibro-osseous lesions of the jaws: a study of 127 Chinese patients and review of the literature. Int J Surg Pathol 2009;17:122-134.

4. Bernaerts A, Vanhoenacker FM, Hintjens J, et al. Tumors and tumor-like lesions of the jaw mixed and radiopaque lesions. JBR-BTR 2006;89:91-99.

5. Ferretti C, Coleman H, Dent M, Altini M. Cystic degeneration in fibrous dysplasia of the jaws: a case report. Oral Surg Oral Med Oral Pathol Oral Radiol Endod 1999;88:337-342.

6. MacDonald-Jankowski DS. Ossifying fibroma: a systematic review. Dentomaxillofac Radiol 2009;38:495-513.

7. Regezi JA. Odontogenic cysts, odontogenic tumors, fibroosseous, and giant cell lesions of the jaws. Mod Pathol 2002;15:331-341.

8. MacDonald-Jankowski DS. Fibro-osseous lesions of the face and jaws. Clin Radiol 2004;59:11-25.

9. Mupparapu M, Singer SR, Milles M, Rinaggio J. Simultaneous presentation of focal cemento-osseous dysplasia and simple bone cyst of the mandible masquerading as a multilocular radiolucency. Dentomaxillofac Radiol 2005;34:39-43.

10. Goncalves M, Pispico R, Alves Fde A, Lugao CE, Goncalves A. Clinical, radiographic, biochemical and histological findings of florid cemento-osseous dysplasia and report of a case. Braz Dent J 2005;16:247-250.

11. Macdonald-Jankowski DS. Focal cemento-osseous dysplasia: a systematic review. Dentomaxillofac Radiol 2008;37:350-360.

12. Mahomed F, Altini M, Meer S, Coleman H. Cemento-osseous dysplasia with associated simple bone cysts. J Oral Maxillofac Surg 2005;63:1549-1554.

13. Bencharit S, Schardt-Sacco D, Zuniga JR, Minsley GE. Surgical and prosthodontic rehabilitation for a patient with aggressive florid cemento-osseous dysplasia: a clinical report. J Prosthet Dent 2003;90:220-224.

13 CARTILAGINOUS TUMORS

OSTEOCHONDROMA

Definition. *Osteochondroma* is a benign proliferation of bone with an intrinsic cartilaginous cap that extends from the surface of the bone. An alternative name is *osteocartilaginous exostosis*.

General Features. Likely not a true neoplasm, osteochondroma is nevertheless one of the most common benign tumors arising in enchondral bone of the skeleton. It is rarely found in the jaw, however. Karasu et al. (1) reported that less than 40 cases had been described as of 2005. The exact number of cases that exist in the literature is difficult to determine since differentiation from condylar hyperplasia can be difficult.

Since the condyle is predominantly cartilaginous in origin, the mandibular coronoid process and the mandibular condyle are the most frequently affected sites of osteochondroma in the jaws (2,3). The majority of extracondylar osteochondromas in this region occur on the coronoid process. Nevertheless, cases have been reported in the maxillary sinus, posterior maxilla, mandibular symphysis, parasymphyseal region, and zygomatic arch (3).

The etiology of osteochondroma is not known but some have hypothesized that trauma or inflammation plays a role. Some patients complain of pain in the region of the temporomandibular joint before there is evidence of a tumor, yet some authors dispute trauma or inflammation as being the only etiology for the development of osteochondromas in the jaw (3,4). Skeletal chondrosarcomas can develop in the cartilaginous cap of osteochondromas occurring elsewhere but this has not been reported in the jaw.

Clinical Features. Most patients are in their fourth to fifth decade at presentation and females are more commonly affected (5). Osteochondromas are generally slow-growing, progressive deformities likely to simulate unilateral condylar hyperplasia. Pain and dysfunction are common complaints. Patients may exhibit malocclusion, facial asymmetry, or prognathic deviation of the chin and cross-bite to the contralateral side (5). Some authors suggest that osteochondroma in the mandibular condyle arises consistently from the anteromedial surface at the site of the tendinous attachment (4). Yet, Vezeau et al. (3) noted that these tumors arise elsewhere on the condyle as well.

Long-term complications of untreated coronoid osteochondromas include pseudoarthrosis between the coronoid process and the zygomatic arch, also known as Jacob disease (6). Hearing loss has also been reported when extension of the osteochondroma results in obstruction of the external auditory canal (4). The clinical differential diagnosis of osteochondroma in the mandibular condyle should include other slow-growing masses such as giant cell tumor, condylar hyperplasia, fibro-osseous lesions, vascular malformation, and osteoma. Rarer reported condylar tumors include chondroblastoma, chondrosarcoma, osteoblastoma/osteoid osteoma, osteosarcoma, and metastatic tumors (3).

Radiographic Features. On radiographs, osteochondromas are exophytic and often dome shaped. As expected from the histologic features, these tumors are radio-opaque (7).

Microscopic Findings. Cartilage is evident on the surface of most osteochondromas (fig. 13-1). The cartilage is arranged in columns, simulating the epiphyseal plate (fig. 13-2). The cartilage can form a cap of 2 to 3 mm in thickness and may mineralize. Multinucleated cartilaginous cells are common and should not be considered a sign of malignancy (fig. 13-3); however, there may be no cartilage present or cartilage only covering part of the lesion. At the base of the lesion, cancellous bone, with both a woven and lamellar arrangement, may be present (fig. 13-4). The base and stalk contain bone marrow elements, fat, or both.

A pseudoarthrosis may be seen if the cartilaginous cap approaches other osseous structures,

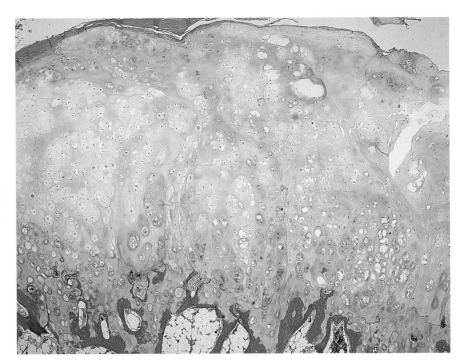

Figure 13-1

OSTEOCHONDROMA

This osteochondroma shows a zonal pattern with the ossified bone trabeculae directly associated with hyaline cartilage. The marrow spaces are filled with fat.

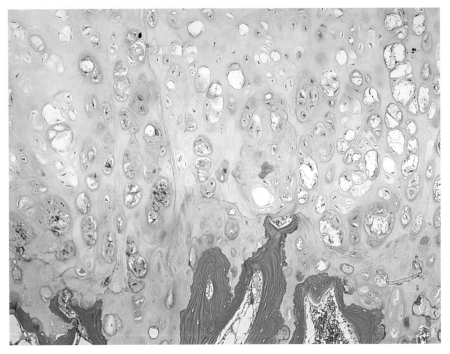

Figure 13-2

OSTEOCHONDROMA

Parallel arrays of chondrocytes extend directly toward the surface of the cartilage cap. There is marked variability in the size of the lacunae.

and in some cases a bursa is formed. It is thought that the cartilage cap proliferation ceases if the lesion stops growing (fig. 13-5).

Differential Diagnosis. The histologic and radiographic features usually allow for diagnosis. If only limited biopsy material is available, however, and no radiographs can be viewed, other cartilaginous tumors enter the differential diagnosis.

Treatment and Prognosis. Symptomatic osteochondromas are treated by resection. Incomplete excision has been reported to be associated with recurrence while completely excised lesions do not recur (5,8).

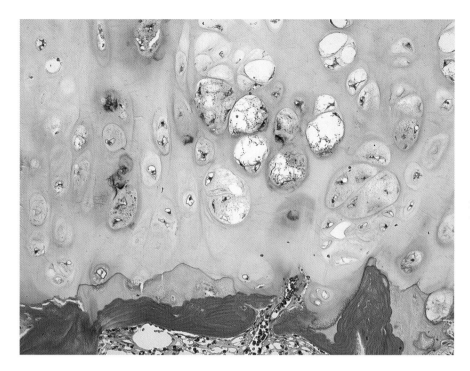

Figure 13-3

OSTEOCHONDROMA

Nuclear size is variable in the cartilaginous cells of osteochondroma.

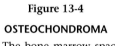

Figure 13-4

OSTEOCHONDROMA

The bone marrow spaces show only scant marrow elements in this osteochondroma.

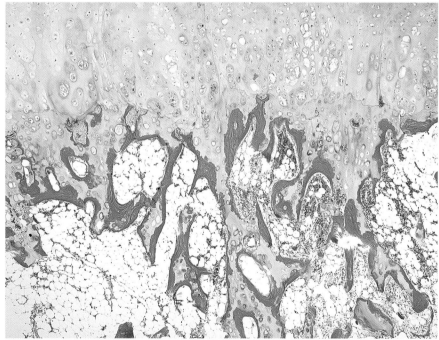

CHONDROBLASTOMA

Definition. *Chondroblastoma* is a benign tumor, usually occurring in the epiphyses of long bones, characterized by cartilaginous differentiation combined with mononuclear cells and giant cells.

General Features. Chondroblastomas are uncommon neoplasms of bone, accounting for only 1.4 percent of bone tumors in the Mayo Clinic files. These neoplasms usually occur at the ends of long bones but have been reported in the jaw (9–13). Bertoni et al. (9) described 30 cases that occurred in the facial bones and skull;

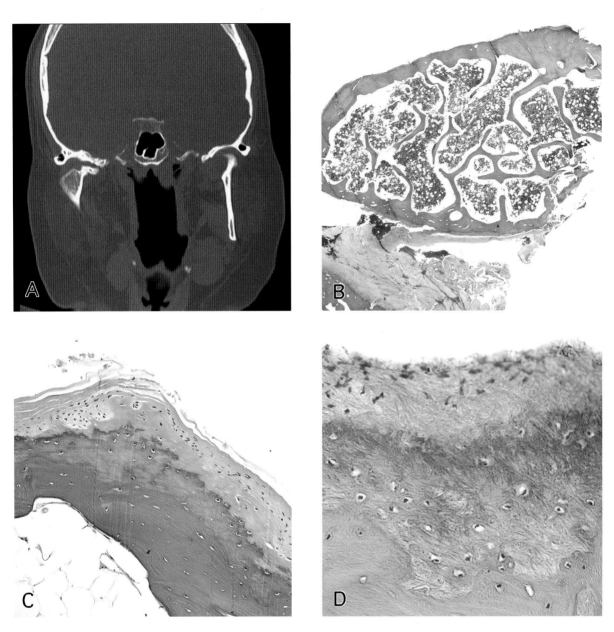

Figure 13-5

OSTEOCHONDROMA

A: Computerized tomography (CT) image of an osteochondroma extending from the medial surface of the right mandibular condyle. This forms a pseudoarthrosis with the base of the skull.

B: The base of the resected tumor in A is composed of a small stalk. The bone marrow spaces are filled with active elements of bone marrow formation. There is minimal cartilage present in the cap.

C: The cartilage cap of this osteochondroma shows minimal cartilage, suggesting that it has reduced proliferative capacity.

D: The fibrous tissue lying above the cartilage surface represents the fibrous portion of the pseudoarthrosis.

the temporal bone was the most common site in the skull, with the jaw accounting for 6 cases (all in the mandible).

Clinical Features. In the jaws, the mandible is nearly exclusively affected (9,10). Patients present with facial swelling, difficulty in opening the jaw, and pain. When considering chondroblastoma at all sites, approximately 75 percent of patients present in the second and third decades but the average age of patients with jaw tumors is often

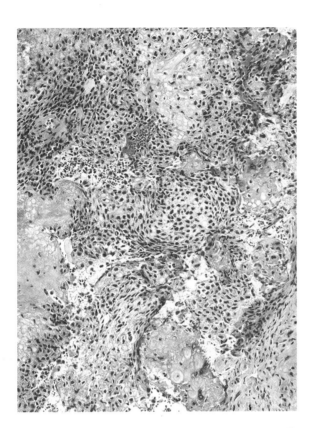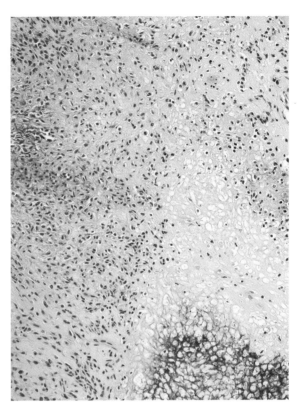

Figure 13-6

CHONDROBLASTOMA

Left: Chondroblastomas are composed of a variety of cell types including mononuclear cells with clear cytoplasm and admixed cartilage. The mononuclear cells are arranged in sheets as well as swirled nests. Hyaline cartilage is present in this image although the cartilaginous differentiation can also have a myxoid appearance.

Right: The cartilaginous differentiation in chondroblastoma can show myxochondroid differentiation as well as hyaline cartilage. Lace-like calcification surrounds individual cells.

in the third to fifth decade (9). Bertoni et al. (9) noted that in general, when chondroblastoma presents in a patient beyond the second or third decade, it is usually found in a location other than the long bones, such as the jaws.

Radiographic Features. In the long bones, chondroblastomas are sharply demarcated radiologically and appear as round or ovoid radiolucencies (10). The findings are similar in the mandible, although some authors have found lesions presenting as condylar enlargements with a sclerotic border. These radiographic findings are not specific for chondroblastoma and only suggest that the process is benign (10).

Microscopic Findings. The histologic appearance of chondroblastoma in the jaws is generally the same as in other sites. They are composed of mononuclear cells admixed with

pink- to blue-staining chondroid matrix, mineralization, and giant cells. In some tumors, the mineralization has a lace-like calcification that surrounds the mononuclear cells (figs. 13-6–13-8). Mitoses are usually found but are not atypical or numerous. Hemosiderin deposition is seen in most tumors. The cells, which are round to polygonal, have pale cytoplasm revealing a distinct, well-demarcated border (10). Their nuclei are ovoid and show a characteristic groove, giving a "coffee bean" appearance, or may show only a small nuclear membrane dent. Another characteristic finding is the presence of multinucleated giant cells. Chondroid differentiation is seen as either myxochondroid material or hyaline cartilage. Some investigators have reported seeing limited chondroid differentiation in some tumors, although this is not unusual

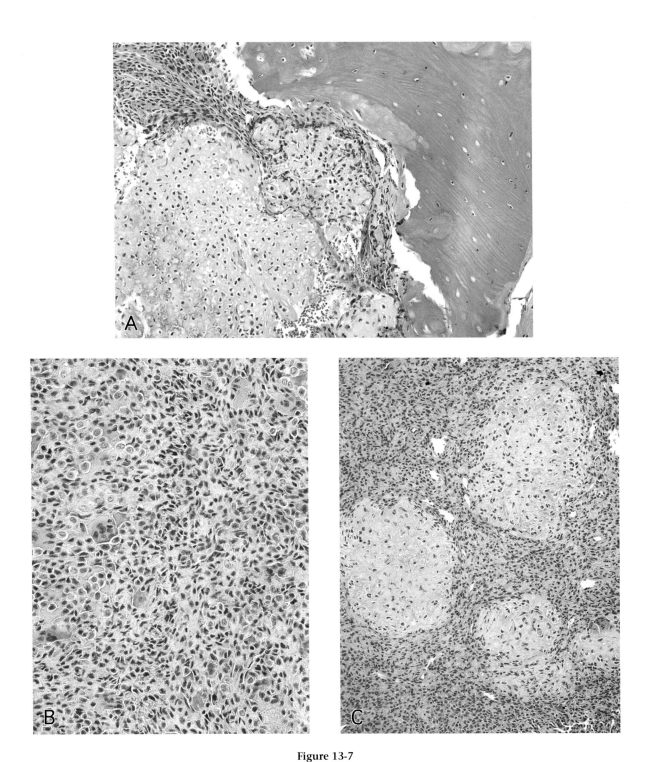

Figure 13-7

CHONDROBLASTOMA

A: A chondroblastoma with mononuclear cells and nodules of hyaline cartilage is abutting and eroding underlying bone.

B: This cellular focus in a chondroblastoma has no cartilaginous differentiation. The nuclei of the mononuclear cells are hyperchromatic and irregular in shape in the most crowded areas, but in the less densely packed areas, the cell nuclei are round. A tiny nucleolus is evident. Pale cytoplasm with well-defined cell borders is present. Scattered giant cells are present but are indistinct and appear to merge with the surrounding mononuclear cells.

C: Islands of hyaline cartilage are surrounded by a cellular proliferation.

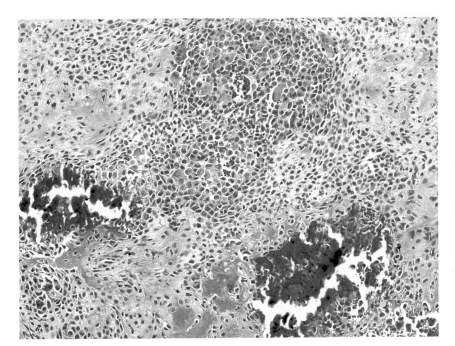

Figure 13-8

CHONDROBLASTOMA

There is pink staining of the chondroid matrix in this chondroblastoma in addition to the blue staining more often associated with hyaline cartilage. Islands of densely mineralized cartilage matrix stain a deep purple. The mononuclear cells show a variety of patterns, with some cells spread out with stroma between each cell and other areas where there is cellular crowding.

Figure 13-9

CHONDROBLASTOMA

The multinucleated giant cells in a background of mononucleated cells in this chondroblastoma give the appearance of giant cell tumor of bone as well as central giant cell tumor of the jaw.

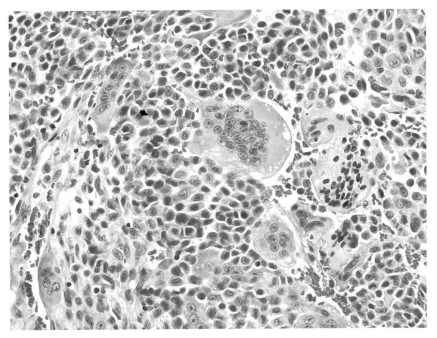

for chondroblastoma at any site (9). Aneurysmal bone cyst-like or central giant cell granuloma-like change may be frequent (figs. 13-9, 13-10). In the Bertoni et al. study of chondroblastoma of the bones of the skull and face (9), 22 of the 30 cases exhibited both of these features.

Immunohistochemical Findings. S-100 protein stains the nuclei of the mononuclear cells in chondroblastoma (11). The use of S-100 protein is usually not necessary to establish a diagnosis of chondroblastoma and the staining is not specific.

Cytologic Findings. The cytologic findings of chondroblastoma mirror the histologic findings but establishing the diagnosis is more challenging using only cytologic features. Smears of chondroblastoma show cellular aspirates with both mononuclear cells and osteoclast-like

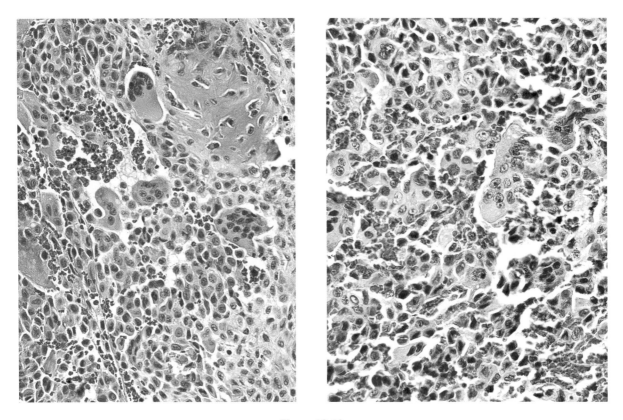

Figure 13-10

CHONDROBLASTOMA

Left: The combination of hemorrhage, giant cells, and mononuclear cells in this chondroblastoma resembles giant cell tumor of bone or solid areas of aneurysmal bone cyst. Pink staining cartilage is beginning to mineralize.

Right: Red blood cells are found between the mononuclear cells and giant cells of this chondroblastoma. The appearance is reminiscent of giant cell tumor of bone.

giant cells. Both these components occur in loose aggregates or singly (12). The cytoplasm of the mononuclear cells is distinct and well defined, and these cells contain folded nuclei. Chondroid matrix, sometimes with the characteristic lace-like calcification, is sometimes seen. Similar to the histologic findings, hemosiderin is commonly present and is often contained in the mononuclear cells.

Differential Diagnosis. Entities in the differential diagnosis of chondroblastoma include giant cell tumor and central giant cell reparative granuloma. The presence of cartilaginous differentiation separates these lesions but the chondroid differentiation can be sparse and thus must be sought for in any giant cell-containing lesion of the bone. Cytologic evaluation is hampered by sampling error in some cases, particularly when there is abundant giant cell

formation and the chondroid component is not sampled.

Treatment and Prognosis. Complete excision of chondroblastoma is the recommended therapy and results in a good outcome in most patients. Lesions treated only with curettage are more prone to recur (9).

CHONDROMYXOID FIBROMA

Definition. *Chondromyxoid fibroma* is a benign neoplasm characterized by a myxomatous stroma with spindled and stellate cells, all arranged in lobular formations. It may develop from cartilaginous remnants.

General Features. Few cases of chondromyxoid fibroma at any anatomic site have been documented in the literature. Those presenting in the jaw make up less than 5 percent of all chondromyxoid fibromas (14,15). The sites of

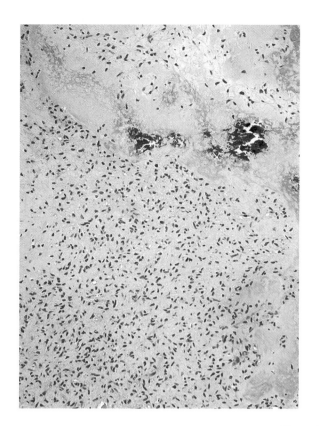
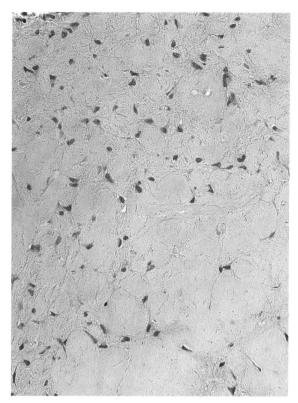

Figure 13-11

CHONDROMYXOID FIBROMA

Left: The pale-staining myxoid background is filled with small bland cells with indistinct cytoplasmic borders. The matrix has calcified in some areas. The central portion of this tumor is less cellular than the periphery.

Right: The hypocellular blue-staining myxoid background has scattered small, round to elongated, bland nuclei.

occurrence are compatible with an origin from developmental cartilaginous remnants (16–18). Most patients are in their third and fourth decades, and the mandible is more frequently affected than the maxilla. Swelling and pain are the presenting symptoms.

Radiographic Features. Radiographically, the tumor shows a distinct, punched-out radiolucent appearance with a thinned cortex but a sclerotic margin. Some lesions appear lobulated.

Microscopic Findings. The tumors are composed of varying amounts of chondroid, myxoid, and fibrous tissues, with the individual quantity of each of these components highly variable between tumors. This variability is important, since a limited biopsy may contain only one type of tissue and be difficult to interpret correctly. A low-power microscopic view of the tumor often shows a lobular arrangement and

a distinct peripheral concentration of cells (figs. 13-11, 13-12). This peripheral arrangement is heightened by the fact that the centers of the lobules are more hypocellular. Tumor calcification is present. The tumor cell cytoplasm is eosinophilic and the cells have both stellate and spindled morphology. The nuclei are variable in shape, and are spindled, round, or oval (fig. 13-13). Often, multinucleated giant cells are seen at the periphery of the lobules.

Differential Diagnosis. Myxomas or myxofibromas are the most likely jaw neoplasms to be confused with chondromyxoid fibroma (19), however, chondroblastoma and chondrosarcoma also should be considered. The lace-like calcification of chondroblastoma may be seen in chondromyxoid fibroma but the proliferating mononuclear cells with a grooved nucleus, present in chondroblastoma, as well as the frequent aneurysmal bone cyst-like changes

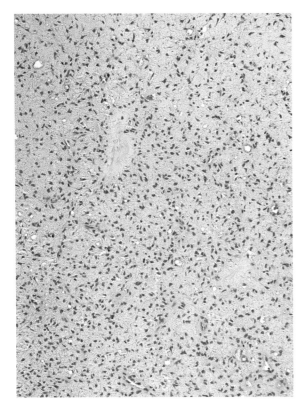

Figure 13-12

CHONDROMYXOID FIBROMA

Chondromyxoid fibromas can show moderate degrees of cellularity.

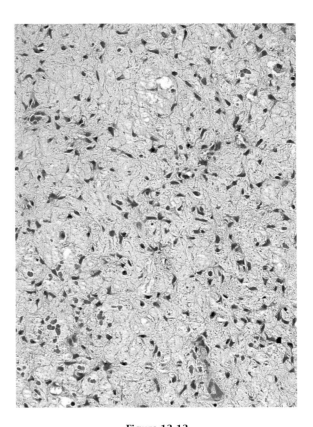

Figure 13-13

CHONDROMYXOID FIBROMA

Mild nuclear hyperchromasia is seen in this chondromyxoid fibroma. The nuclear shapes vary from round or oval to stellate and spindled.

and giant cell tumor-like areas, are not. Chondrosarcomas grow in a lobular pattern and may have myxoid changes but should exhibit more nuclear atypia (20).

Treatment and Prognosis. Thorough curettage of the lesion is considered adequate therapy.

CHONDROSARCOMA

Definition. *Chondrosarcoma* is a malignant neoplasm with cartilaginous differentiation. In the jaws particularly, many osteosarcomas produce cartilage, and therefore, any osteoid production by a mesenchymal lesion considered otherwise to have the features of chondrosarcoma should be designated as osteosarcoma.

General Features. Chondrosarcoma encompasses several types of malignant neoplasm that produce a cartilage matrix. The most common is *conventional chondrosarcoma*, representing nearly 90 percent of these lesions; other types,

such as *dedifferentiated, clear cell,* and *mesenchymal chondrosarcomas* make up the remainder. Chondrosarcoma of the jaws is rare but there is variability in the literature concerning its prevalence (21). Pindborg (22) found only one case of chondrosarcoma of the jaws in Denmark in the years 1943 to 1953. In a 50-year period in Japan, 35 cases involving the jaws and facial skeleton were found (23). Over half of these occurred in the maxilla and mandible, with the maxilla showing a slight predominance. In a period from 1960 to 1983, 1,302 jaw lesions, excluding cysts, were seen at a single institution in Nigeria; 14 (1.1 percent) of the lesions were chondrosarcomas (24). These 14 jaw chondrosarcomas occurred out of a total of 41 chondrosarcomas that were diagnosed in all bones in the same time period. This high percentage of chondrosarcoma of the jaw bones compared to chondrosarcoma of all sites is unusual.

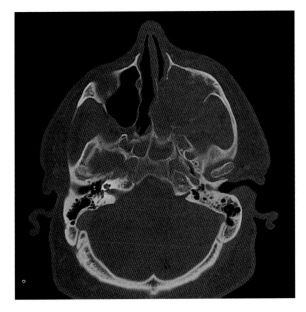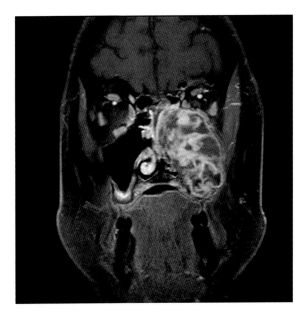

Figure 13-14

CHONDROSARCOMA

Left: This CT image reveals a large chondrosarcoma arising in the maxillary bone and destroying surrounding nasal structures.

Right: A magnetic resonance image (MRI) study of a recurrent chondrosarcoma that arose in the maxilla shows regions of cystic change that have occurred in this large tumor that invaded orbital structures.

Clinical Features. The maxilla is generally more commonly affected than the mandible. When the mandible is affected, the body and ramus are more likely involved (25). Chondrosarcoma also arises in the temporomandibular joint. The most common complaint at initial presentation is the presence of a mass. Pain is a less frequent to even rare presenting symptom (26–29).

Radiographic Features. Radiographically, chondrosarcoma presents as a poorly defined radiolucency that frequently contains areas of radiopacity scattered throughout. A widened periodontal membrane space can be seen on periapical dental radiographs when the teeth are involved (26,30). Computerized tomography (CT) is most useful to assess the tumor matrix and cortical involvement while magnetic resonance imaging (MRI) helps best characterize the extent of bone marrow and adjacent soft tissue extension (fig. 13-14).

Gross Findings. Typically, chondrosarcomas are lobulated, blue-gray translucent masses. Calcification is seen as white flecks.

Microscopic Findings. Chondrosarcomas are composed of atypical cartilaginous tissue arranged in lobules (figs. 13-15, 13-16). The cartilage matrix stains blue and contains lacunae that hold chondrocyte nuclei. Chondrosarcomas can also have myxoid foci that merge with cartilaginous tissue. In some instances, the myxoid areas have a liquefactive appearance, a finding suggested to be helpful in determining whether the lesion is indeed a malignant cartilaginous tumor (fig. 13-17) (31). A key finding in chondrosarcoma is the infiltrative nature of the lesion into the surrounding bone (fig. 13-18). As in many chondrosarcomas of long bones, the degree of atypia can be minimal (26). These tumors can be very difficult to separate from benign cartilaginous tumors, although some investigators are reluctant to accept a diagnosis of enchondroma in the jaw (32).

Histologic Types. Besides chondrosarcoma of usual type, variants include *clear cell* and *parosteal type* (31,33,34). *Mesenchymal chondrosarcoma* is discussed separately.

Most chondrosarcomas of the jaw are of low (grade 1) to intermediate (grade 2) grade. In the series by Saito et al. (35), no grade 3 chondrosarcomas of the maxilla or mandible were seen,

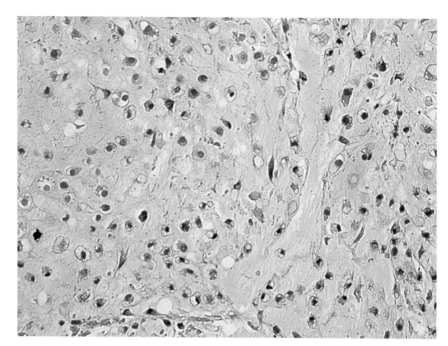

Figure 13-15

CHONDROSARCOMA

Top: There is distinct nuclear pleomorphism of the chondrocytes.

Bottom: The chondrocytes have lobular arrangements. At a low microscopic power, the disorganization and pleomorphism of the chondrocytes are evident.

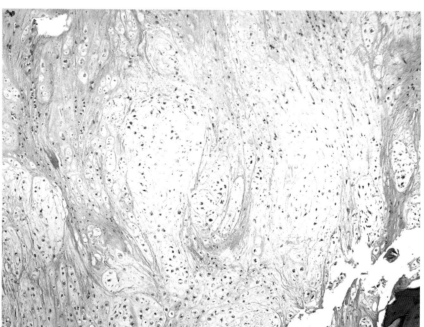

with the vast majority being grade 1 (26,35). High-grade tumors are unusual but can occur (figs. 13-19, 13-20).

Molecular and Cytogenetic Findings. A number of cell factors have been implicated in chondrosarcomas including hypoxia-inducible factor, cyclooxygenase 2 (COX2), insulin-like growth factor, matrix metalloproteinase, and parathyroid hormone-like hormone (36,37). In addition, similar to enchondromas, constitutive hedgehog signaling is present in chondrosarcomas and AKT, an important kinase for cell survival, is highly active in these neoplasms (36,37).

Numerous genetic abnormalities exist in chondrosarcoma (38). Using an array-based comparative genomic hybridization technique, Hallor et al. (39) found that most of 67 chondrosarcomas had genomic imbalances. No copy

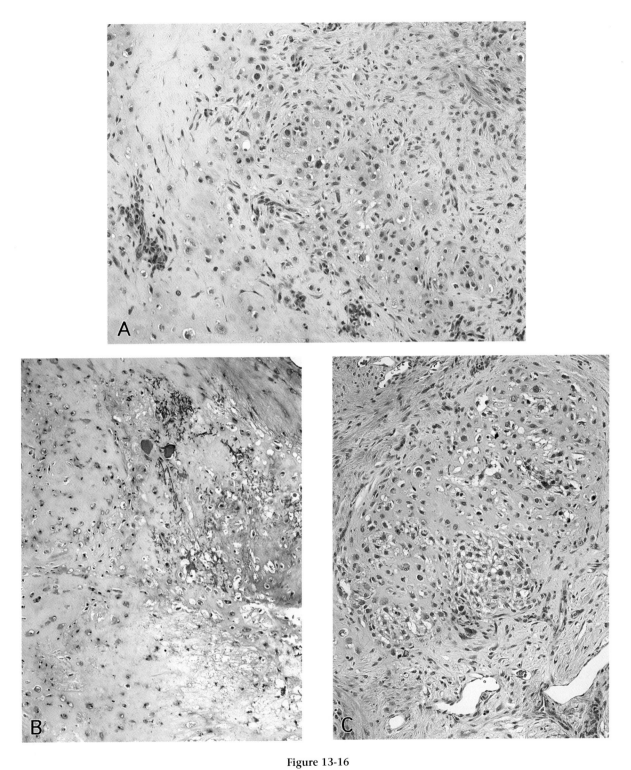

Figure 13-16

CHONDROSARCOMA

A: Significant nuclear atypia is present in this chondrosarcoma.

B: Light mineralization of the atypical cartilage cells can be found in chondrosarcomas.

C: Chondrosarcoma often retains a lobular growth pattern even when it extends into the surrounding soft tissues, as in this case.

Figure 13-17

CHONDROSARCOMA

Liquefactive change is a very useful diagnostic change in atypical cartilage tumors, pointing to a diagnosis of chondrosarcoma.

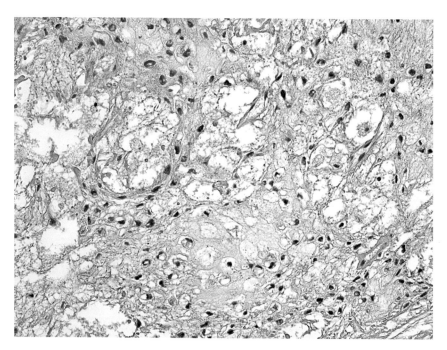

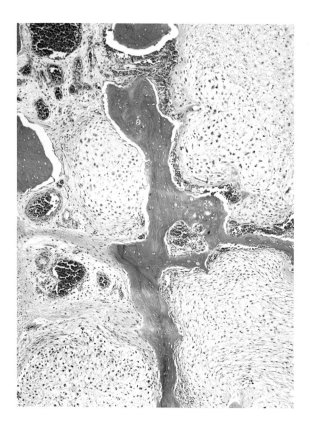

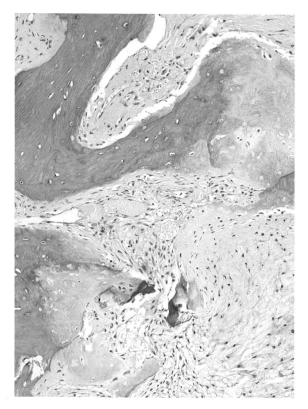

Figure 13-18

CHONDROSARCOMA

Left: The tumor is infiltrating underlying normal bone.
Right: Infiltration of surrounding bone is a useful diagnostic feature in chondrosarcoma.

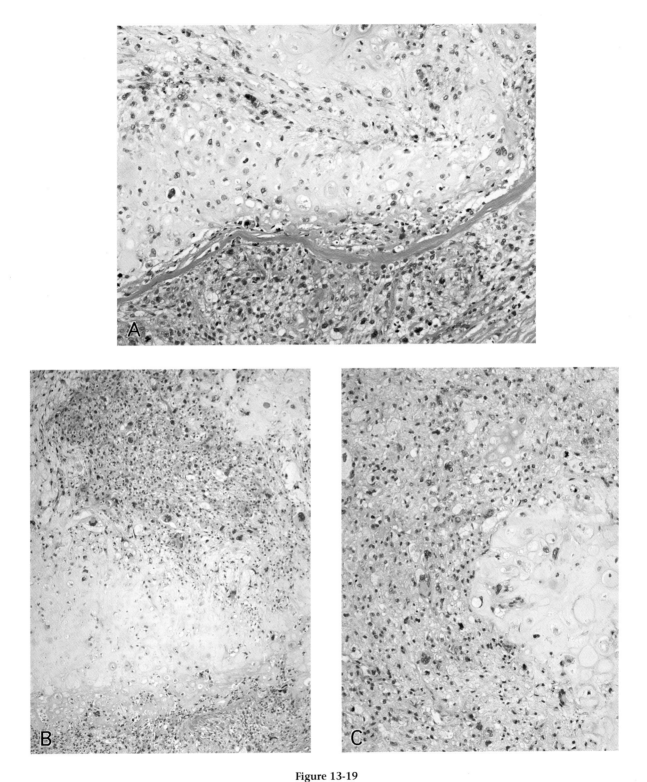

Figure 13-19

CHONDROSARCOMA

A: Low- and high-grade differentiation is present in this tumor.
B: A combination of low- and high-grade differentiation is illustrated. Markedly atypical, large chondrocytic nuclei are seen.
C: High-grade chondrosarcoma.

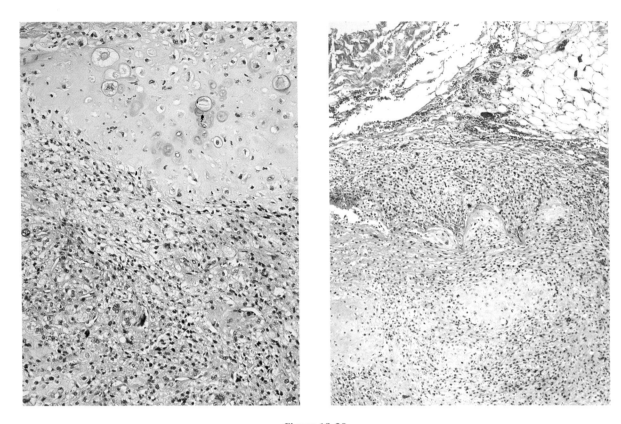

Figure 13-20

CHONDROSARCOMA

Left: High-grade chondrosarcoma is associated with a low-grade component.
Right: Chondrosarcoma extends into surrounding adipose soft tissue.

number imbalance, however, was related to metastatic potential or tumor associated death. In a study of 59 cases by Mandahl et al. (40), genomic imbalances were found in at least 10 cases and numerous chromosomal losses in at least 10 or more of the cases: 1p36, 1p13-p22, 4, 5q13-q31, 6q22-qter, 7p13-pter, 9p22-pter, 10p, 10q24-qter, 11p13-pter, 11q25, 12q15-qter, 13q21-qter, 14q24-qter, 18p, 18q22-qter, 19, 20pter-q11, 21q, and 22q13. In this study, loss of 13q was an independent prognostic factor for metastasis, regardless of tumor grade or size. Sjogren et al. (41) found that unbalanced rearrangement was common in their study of chondrosarcoma, with recurrent breakpoints noted at Xq21, 6p10, 9p13, 20p11, and 22q11-12.

Differential Diagnosis. The most important entity in the differential diagnosis of chondrosarcoma in the jaws is osteosarcoma. Osteosarcomas of the jaws show extensive cartilaginous differentiation. Only a small focus of osteoid is

sufficient for a diagnosis of osteosarcoma in the setting of an atypical chondroid jaw neoplasm. For this reason, it is critical to examine all of the material submitted as a biopsy or resection in a cartilaginous tumor of the jaws.

Edentulous patients can develop osteocartilaginous metaplasia of the alveolar ridge which can mimic neoplasm (32). On occasion, this metaplastic mass contains atypical cartilage that mimics chondrosarcoma.

Grade 1 chondrosarcomas may be difficult to separate from benign cartilaginous tumors and the evaluation of the radiographic and clinical features of the lesion's invasiveness and destructive nature is very important. The degree of cellularity in grade 1 tumors is often not marked, nor is there marked nuclear atypia. Grade 2 tumors have larger nuclei that are also much more hyperchromatic.

Some investigators consider all purely cartilaginous neoplasms of the jaws as likely malignant, thus questioning the acceptance of diagnosis of enchondroma in the jaws. Caution should be exercised with attention always given to the clinical and radiographic findings.

Myxomas of the jaws can potentially simulate the myxoid degenerative material seen within chondrosarcomas but they do not contain cartilaginous foci. Chondromyxoid fibroma and chondroblastoma, discussed elsewhere in this chapter, have additional distinct histologic features and are not composed of pure cartilage. Mesenchymal chondrosarcomas have cartilaginous differentiation but also exhibit a small, hyperchromatic cell population (42).

Treatment and Prognosis. Because of the rarity of chondrosarcoma of the jaws, there are no evidence-based treatment protocols (23). Many of the current treatment strategies are based on chondrosarcoma outside of the head and neck region or other types of sarcomas. Chondrosarcoma is treated primarily with wide en-bloc resection, ideally with 2- to 3-cm margins (43). Of all adjuvant therapies, radiotherapy is given postoperatively most frequently, often when margins are positive (21,43–45).

Chondrosarcoma of the jaws is a locally destructive process and metastases are rare (35). In the Mayo Clinic series (35), which had a nearly 10-year follow-up, the overall actuarial survival rates at 5, 10, and 15 years were 68 percent, 54 percent, and 44 percent, respectively. In general, the larger size of the lesion and the more central (near the maxillary sinus or mandibular ramus) rather than peripheral (alveolar ridge, mandibular body) location correlate with a poorer outcome. Prado et al. (46), in a study of 16 head and neck chondrosarcomas, most of which were in the maxilla and mandible, showed an overall survival rate of 56 percent for 5 years; larger tumors conferred a worse prognosis. Gadwal et al. (47) suggested that chondrosarcomas occurring in the pediatric population may have a relatively good prognosis.

MESENCHYMAL CHONDROSARCOMA

Definition. *Mesenchymal chondrosarcoma* is a rare malignant tumor that has a biphasic growth pattern of a poorly differentiated cellular component juxtaposed to cartilaginous foci. It occurs in both bone and soft tissues.

General Features. These are rare neoplasms. Unni et al. (48) noted that the Mayo Clinic

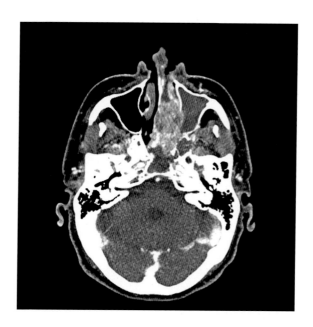

Figure 13-21

MESENCHYMAL CHONDROSARCOMA

Positron emission tomography (PET) CT image of a mesenchymal chondrosarcoma that arises in the maxilla and fills the maxillary antrum, destroying the nasal structures. It extends to the base of the skull.

recorded 32 cases out of a total of 1,023 conventional chondrosarcomas. In their series, one third of the tumors occurred in the soft tissues. While these neoplasms are rare, accounting for less than 2 percent of all chondrosarcomas, the jaw is one of the most common sites for mesenchymal chondrosarcoma, comprising slightly over 20 percent of the cases in some series (49–52).

Clinical Features. Mesenchymal chondrosarcoma presents more in younger patients than conventional chondrosarcoma, although there can be a wide age range. In a study of 19 patients by Vencio et al. (53), 16 were less than 30 years of age. Conventional chondrosarcoma more frequently affects the maxilla but mesenchymal chondrosarcoma more commonly affects the mandible (49).

Radiographic Features. Mesenchymal chondrosarcomas have the same radiographic features as conventional chondrosarcomas, presenting as a lytic tumor along with stippled calcification (54). They can attain large size while giving few symptoms (fig. 13-21).

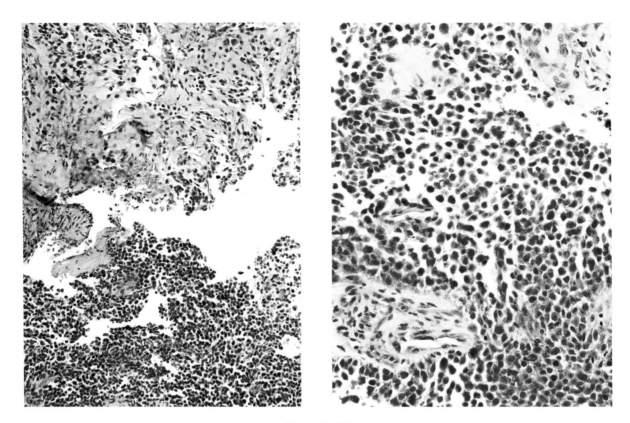

Figure 13-22

MESENCHYMAL CHONDROSARCOMA

Left: Mesenchymal chondrosarcoma with an area of small, hyperchromatic cells with no stroma as well as an area of myxoid stroma.

Right: A nearly solid population of tumor cells with minimal stroma is seen in this mesenchymal chondrosarcoma. The tumor cells are round to oval and markedly hyperchromatic.

Microscopic Findings. Mesenchymal chondrosarcoma is composed of a population of small, hyperchromatic, atypical cells as well as cartilage-producing cells. One of the most striking histologic aspects of the tumor is that the two cell types, noncartilaginous and cartilaginous, are abruptly separated in the tumor (fig. 13-22). The amount of each of these elements is variable between tumors. The small cells have dark, round nuclei and in many, but not all tumors, are classically arranged in a hemangiopericytoma-like pattern with irregular slit-like to antler-shaped vessels. In other areas this population of cells forms irregular sheets or a spindle arrangement with a dense fibrous stroma (fig. 13-23). The cartilage is variable in cellularity and its matrix varies from mottled blue-pink to pink.

Molecular and Cytogenetic Findings. Cytogenetic abnormalities have been described in mesenchymal chondrosarcomas but there are no consistent or characteristic karyotypic changes exhibited by these neoplasms (55,56). Wehrli et al. (57) found that Sox9, a master regulator of cartilage differentiation, was expressed in mesenchymal chondrosarcoma, but not in other small round cell tumors. In a study by Fanburg-Smith et al. (58), the authors found that the expression of Sox9 could be used, along with expression of osteocalcin, in the immunohistologic separation of mesenchymal chondrosarcoma from small cell osteosarcoma. Their findings of rare nuclear beta-catenin expression at the interface between hyaline cartilage and small round cells suggest involvement by the APC/Wnt pathway during endochondral ossification in the morphologically benign hyaline cartilage component of mesenchymal chondrosarcoma.

Differential Diagnosis. The most likely tumors in the differential diagnosis are neoplasms with a growth pattern similar to

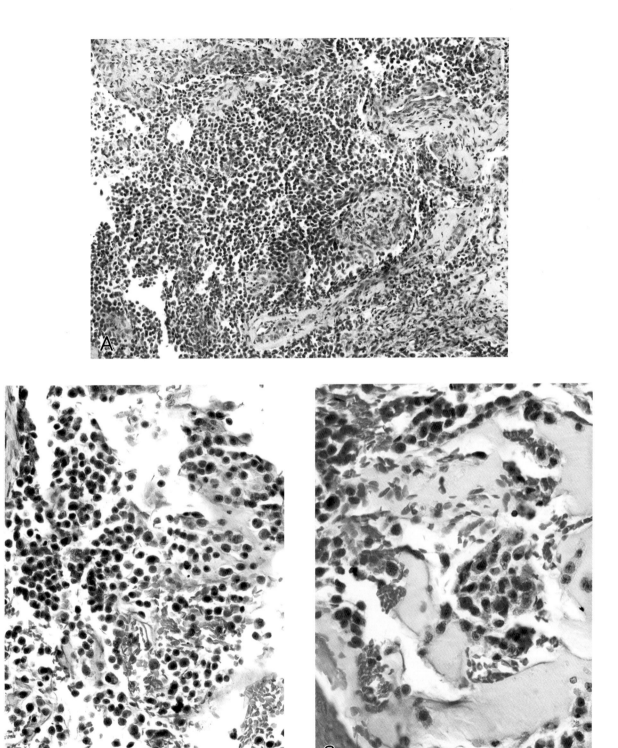

Figure 13-23

MESENCHYMAL CHONDROSARCOMA

A: A fibrous stroma with larger vessels, some with thick walls, is seen in this mesenchymal chondrosarcoma.

B: The cells of mesenchymal chondrosarcoma have minimal amounts of poorly demarcated, eosinophilic cytoplasm.

C: The tumor cells are embedded in a myxoid stroma.

hemangiopericytoma. This includes hemangiopericytoma as well as other tumors that could demonstrate such a pattern, such as monophasic synovial sarcoma.

Spread and Metastases. If mesenchymal chondrosarcoma metastasizes, it does so to the lungs primarily.

Treatment and Prognosis. Mesenchymal chondrosarcoma is treated by surgical ablation (59). There are too few cases, particularly in the jaw, to determine whether specific adjuvant therapies are of value. Some patients have had long follow-up periods with no recurrence while others have quickly succumbed to the disease (50). In a study by Vencio et al. (53), the 5-year and 10-year survival rates for tumors in the jaw were 82 and 56 percent, respectively. These survival rates are superior to those of this neoplasm occurring at other sites.

REFERENCES

Osteochondroma

1. Karasu HA, Ortakoglu K, Okcu KM, Gunhan O. Osteochondroma of the mandibular condyle: report of a case and review of the literature. Mil Med 2005;170:797-801.
2. Loftus MJ, Bennett JA, Fantasia JE. Osteochondroma of the mandibular condyles. Report of three cases and review of the literature. Oral Surg Oral Med Oral Pathol 1986;61:221-226.
3. Vezeau PJ, Fridrich KL, Vincent, SD. Osteochondroma of the mandibular condyle: literature review and report of two atypical cases. J Oral Maxillofac Surg 1995;53:954-963.
4. Seki H, Fukuda M, Takahashi T, Iino M. Condylar osteochondroma with complete hearing loss: report of a case. J Oral Maxillofac Surg 2003;61:131-133.
5. Peroz I, Scholman HJ, Hell B. Osteochondroma of the mandibular condyle: a case report. Int J Oral Maxillofac Surg 2002;31:455-456.
6. Escuder i de la Torre O, Vert Klok E, Mari i Roig A, Mommaerts MY, Pericot i Ayats J. Jacob's disease: Report of two cases and review of the literature. J Craniomaxillofac Surg 2001;29:372-376.
7. Zhang J, Wang H, Li X, et al. Osteochondromas of the mandibular condyle: Variance in radiographic appearance on panoramic radiographs. Dentomaxillofac Radiol 2008;37:154-160.
8. Ward BB, Pires CA, Feinberg SE. Osteochondromas of the mandible: case reports and rationale for treatment. J Oral Maxillofac Surg 2005;63:1039-1044.

Chondroblastoma

9. Bertoni F, Unni KK, Beabout JW, Harner SG, Dahlin DC. Chondroblastoma of the skull and facial bones. Am J Clin Pathol 1987;88:1-9.
10. Kondoh T, Hamada Y, Kamei K, Seto K. Chondroblastoma of the mandibular condyle: report of a case. J Oral Maxillofac Surg 2002;60:198-203.
11. Unni KK, Inwards CY, Kindblom LG, Wold, LE. Tumors of the bones and joints. AFIP Atlas of Tumor Pathology, 4th Series, Fascicle 2. Washington, DC: American Registry of Pathology; 2005:61-67.
12. Cabrera RA, Almeida M, Mendonca ME, Frable WJ. Diagnostic pitfalls in fine-needle aspiration cytology of temporomandibular chondroblastoma: report of two cases. Diagn CytoPathol 2006;34:424-429.
13. Payne M, Yusuf H. Benign chondroblastoma involving the mandibular condyle. Br J Oral Maxillofac Surg 1987;25:250-255.

Chondromyxoid Fibroma

14. Batsakis JG, Raymond AK. Chondromyxoid fibroma. Ann Otol Rhinol Laryngol 1989;98(Pt 1):571-572.
15. Lingen MW, Solt DB, Polverini PJ. Unusual presentation of a chondromyxoid fibroma of the mandible. Report of a case and review of the literature. Oral Surg Oral Med Oral Pathol 1993;75:615-621.
16. Damm DD, White DK, Geissler RH,Jr, Drummond JF, Gonty AA. Chondromyxoid fibroma of the maxilla. Electron microscopic findings and review of the literature. Oral Surg Oral Med Oral Pathol 1985;59:176-183.

17. Hammad HM, Hammond HL, Kurago ZB, Frank JA. Chondromyxoid fibroma of the jaws. Case report and review of the literature. Oral Surg Oral Med Oral Pathol Oral Radiol Endod 1998;85:293-300.

18. Muller S. Unusual presentation of a chondromyxoid fibroma of the mandible. Oral Surg Oral Med Oral Pathol 1993;76:552.

19. Thompson SH, Weathers DR, Vatral JJ. Chondromyxoid fibroma of the jaws. Head Neck Surg 1982;4:330-334.

20. Unni KK, Inwards CY, Kindblom LG, Wold, LE Tumors of the bones and joints. Atlas of Tumor Pathology, 4th Series, Fascicle 2. Washington, DC: American Registry of Pathology; 2005:67-73.

Chondrosarcoma

21. Koch BB, Karnell LH, Hoffman HT, et al. National cancer database report on chondrosarcoma of the head and neck. Head Neck 2000;22:408-425.

22. Pindborg JJ. The incidence rate of jaw sarcomas in Denmark, 1943 to 1953. Oral Surg Oral Med Oral Pathol 1961;14:276-279.

23. Sato K, Nukaga H, Horikoshi T. Chondrosarcoma of the jaws and facial skeleton: a review of the Japanese literature. J Oral Surg 1977;35:892-897.

24. Ajagbe HA, Daramola JO, Junaid TA. Chondrosarcoma of the jaw: review of fourteen cases. J Oral Maxillofac Surg 1985;43:763-766.

25. Happonen RP, Heikinheimo K, Aitasalo K, Ekfors TO, Calonius PE. Chondrosarcoma of the jaws. Review of the literature and report of two cases. Proc Finn Dent Soc 1985;81:135-141.

26. Garrington GE, Collett WK. Chondrosarcoma. II. Chondrosarcoma of the jaws: analysis of 37 cases. J Oral Pathol 1988;17:12-20.

27. Merrill RG, Yih WY, Shamloo J. Synovial chondrosarcoma of the temporomandibular joint: a case report. J Oral Maxillofac Surg 1997;55:1312-1316.

28. Oliveira RC, Marques KDS, Mendonca AR, Mendonca EF, Silva MRB, Batista AC, et al. Chondrosarcoma of the temporomandibular joint: a case report in a child. J Orofac Pain 2009;23:275-281.

29. Sesenna E, Tullio A, Ferrari S. Chondrosarcoma of the temporomandibular joint: a case report and review of the literature. J Oral Maxillofac Surg 1997;55:1348-1352.

30. Hackney FL, Aragon SB, Aufdemorte TB, Holt GR, Van Sickels JE. Chondrosarcoma of the jaws: Clinical findings, histopathology, and treatment. Oral Surg Oral Med Oral Pathol 1991;71:139-143.

31. Unni KK, Inwards CY, Kindblom LG, Wold, LE Tumors of the bones and joints. Atlas of Tumor Pathology, 4th Series, Fascicle 2. Washington, DC: American Registry of Pathology 2005:73-86.

32. Daley TD, Damm DD, Wysocki GP, Weir JC. Atypical cartilage in reactive osteocartilagenous metaplasia of the traumatized edentulous mandibular ridge. Oral Surg Oral Med Oral Pathol Oral Radiol Endod 1997;83:26-29.

33. Bernasconi G, Preda L, Padula E, Baciliero U, Sammarchi L, Bellomi M. Parosteal chondrosarcoma, a very rare condition of the mandibular condyle. Clin Imaging 2004;28:64-68.

34. Slootweg PJ. Clear-cell chondrosarcoma of the maxilla: report of a case. Oral Surg Oral Med Oral Pathol 1980;50:233-237.

35. Saito K, Unni KK, Wollan PC, Lund BA. Chondrosarcoma of the jaw and facial bones. Cancer 1995;76:1550-1558.

36. Bovee JV, Hogendoorn PC. Molecular pathology of sarcomas: concepts and clinical implications. Virchows Arch 2010;456:193-199.

37. Bovee JV, Hogendoorn PC, Wunder JS, Alman BA. Cartilage tumours and bone development: Molecular pathology and possible therapeutic targets. Nat Rev Cancer 2010;10:481-488.

38. Bell WC, Klein MJ, Pitt MJ, Siegal GP. Molecular pathology of chondroid neoplasms: part 2, malignant lesions. Skeletal Radiol 2006;35:887-894.

39. Hallor KH, Staaf J, Bovee JV, et al. Genomic profiling of chondrosarcoma: chromosomal patterns in central and peripheral tumors. Clin Cancer Res 2009;15:2685-2694.

40. Mandahl N, Gustafson P, Mertens F, et al. Cytogenetic aberrations and their prognostic impact in chondrosarcoma. Genes Chromosomes Cancer 2002;33:188-200.

41. Sjögren H, Orndal C, Tingby O, Meis-Kindblom JM, Kindblom LG, Stenman G. Cytogenetic and spectral karyotype analyses of benign and malignant cartilage tumours. Int J Oncol 2004;24:1385-1391.

42. Pellitteri PK, Ferlito A, Fagan JJ, Suarez C, Devaney KO, Rinaldo A. Mesenchymal chondrosarcoma of the head and neck. Oral Oncol 2007;43:970-975.

43. Carlson ER, Panella T, Holmes JD. Sarcoma of mandible. J Oral Maxillofac Surg 2004;62:81-87.

44. Mohammadinezhad C. Chondrosarcoma of the jaw. J Craniofac Surg 2009;20:2097-2100.

45. Sammartino G, Marenzi G, Howard CM, et al. Chondrosarcoma of the jaw: a closer look at its management. J Oral Maxillofac Surg 2008;66:2349-2355.

46. Prado FO, Nishimoto IN, Perez DE, Kowalski LP, Lopes MA. Head and neck chondrosarcoma: Analysis of 16 cases. Br J Oral Maxillofac Surg 2009;47:555-557.

47. Gadwal SR, Fanburg-Smith JC, Gannon FH, Thompson LD. Primary chondrosarcoma of the head and neck in pediatric patients: a clinicopathologic study of 14 cases with a review of the literature. Cancer 2000;88:2181-2188.

Mesenchymal chondrosarcoma

48. Unni KK, Inwards CY, Kindblom LG, Wold, LE Tumors of the bones and joints. AFIP Atlas of Tumor Pathology, 4th Series, Fascicle 2. Washington, DC: American Registry of Pathology 2005:99-104.
49. Nakashima Y, Unni KK, Shives TC, Swee RG, Dahlin DC. Mesenchymal chondrosarcoma of bone and soft tissue. A review of 111 cases. Cancer 1986;57:2444-453.
50. Angiero F, Vinci R, Sidoni A, Stefani M. Mesenchymal chondrosarcoma of the left coronoid process: Report of a unique case with clinical, histopathologic, and immunohistochemical findings, and a review of the literature. Quintessence Int 2007;38:349-355.
51. Takahashi K, Sato K, Kanazawa H, Wang XL, Kimura T. Mesenchymal chondrosarcoma of the jaw—report of a case and review of 41 cases in the literature. Head Neck 1993;15:459-464.
52. Tien N, Chaisuparat R, Fernandes R, et al. Mesenchymal chondrosarcoma of the maxilla: case report and literature review. J Oral Maxillofac Surg 2007;65:1260-1266.
53. Vencio EF, Reeve CM, Unni KK, Nascimento AG. Mesenchymal chondrosarcoma of the jaw bones: Clinicopathologic study of 19 cases. Cancer 1998;82:2350-2355.
54. Chidambaram A, Sanville P. Mesenchymal chondrosarcoma of the maxilla. J Laryngol Otol 2000;114:536-539.
55. Bell WC, Klein MJ, Pitt MJ, Siegal GP. Molecular pathology of chondroid neoplasms: part 2, malignant lesions. Skeletal Radiol 2006;35:887-894.
56. Li S, Siegal GP. Small cell tumors of bone. Adv Anat Pathol 2010;17:1-11.
57. Wehrli BM, Huang W, De Crombrugghe B, Ayala AG, Czerniak B. Sox9, a master regulator of chondrogenesis, distinguishes mesenchymal chondrosarcoma from other small blue round cell tumors. Hum Pathol 2003;34:263-269.
58. Fanburg-Smith JC, Auerbach A, Marwaha JS, Wang Z, Rushing EJ. Reappraisal of mesenchymal chondrosarcoma: novel morphologic observations of the hyaline cartilage and endochondral ossification and beta-catenin, Sox9, and osteocalcin immunostaining of 22 cases. Hum Pathol 2010;41:653-662.
59. Pellitteri PK, Ferlito A, Fagan JJ, Suarez C, Devaney KO, Rinaldo A. Mesenchymal chondrosarcoma of the head and neck. Oral Oncol 2007;43:970-975.

14 OSSEOUS LESIONS

GIANT CELL LESIONS

Central jaw lesions that are characterized by multinucleated osteoclast-like giant cells include central giant cell granuloma; brown tumors of primary, secondary, and tertiary hyperparathyroidism; and cherubism. Other lesions, including tooth-related inflammatory conditions and a variety of cysts and tumors, have foci of foreign body-type giant cells, often with cholesterol clefts or areas of foreign material. The lesions described below all have giant cells as a component of the primary tumor or systemic condition.

Central Giant Cell Granuloma

Definition. *Central giant cell granuloma* is widely considered to be a reactive condition but is included here because of its neoplastic behavior. The term giant cell granuloma was coined by Jaffe in 1953 (1). Cells of the jawbones, the periodontal ligament, or the dental follicle, originating from the neural crest, may be involved in the pathogenesis of these tumors.

General Features. In the absence of additional clinical or radiographic information, many pathologists prefer to use the term central giant cell lesion because the radiographic and clinical features of giant cell granulomas are indistinguishable from brown tumors of hyperparathyroidism and cherubism. Most, but not all information suggests that giant cell granulomas of the jaws should be distinguished from giant cell tumors in long bones, which are more aggressive, occur in older populations, and have higher rates of recurrence and malignant change. Furthermore, giant cell tumors of bone appear to develop only in cartilaginous and not membranous bones.

In a retrospective evaluation of 93 cases of maxillofacial central giant cell granulomas and giant cell tumors of the axial/appendicular skeleton, however, Resnick et al. (2) identified more similarities than differences and suggested that they

are similar if not the same disease. The sample included 45 jaw lesions and 48 extragnathic tumors. Controlling for location and clinical behavior, the authors suggested that any behavioral differences could be explained by the earlier diagnosis and treatment of maxillofacial giant cell lesions because of facial exposure and dental screening examinations including radiographs.

Some cases of central giant cell granuloma occur in association with *Noonan syndrome* and *neurofibromatosis type 1* (NF1) (3,4). A case of bilateral central giant cell granulomas in the mandible of a 12-year-old girl, with no evidence of systemic disease, cherubism, Noonan syndrome, or NF1 has been reported (5). A syndrome linked to the *HRPT2* gene includes hyperparathyroidism with associated giant cell lesions of bone and multiple ossifying fibromas (6).

As indicated above, brown tumor of primary, secondary, or tertiary hyperparathyroidism must be included in the differential diagnosis of central bony lesions with giant cells. Primary hyperparathyroidism is characteristically the result of uncontrolled production of parathyroid hormone (PTH) brought on by a functional parathyroid adenoma, or occasionally, parathyroid hyperplasia. Most patients with primary hyperparathyroidism are older than 50 years. Woman are affected more often than men. The classic triad of signs and symptoms are characterized as stones, bones, and groans: the term stones is the increased prevalence of nephroliths resulting from elevated serum calcium levels, bones is the osseous changes often seen in conjunction with hyperparathyroidism described below, and groans refers to the tendency for patients to develop duodenal ulcers.

Secondary hyperparathyroidism is almost always the result of chronic low levels of serum calcium associated with renal disease. Tertiary hyperparathyroidism is a less common condition seen in patients treated for secondary hyperparathyroidism after a successful kidney

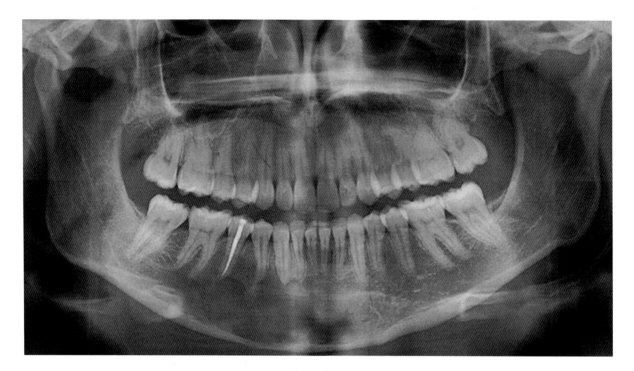

Figure 14-1

CENTRAL GIANT CELL GRANULOMA

A panoramic radiograph shows a well-defined, multilocular radiolucency of the right body of the mandible.

transplant. Patients with this rare condition may continue to develop giant cell lesions of the jaw (7).

Clinical Features. Central giant cell granulomas occur in a wide age range, from 2 to 80 years of age, although the majority occur in individuals under 20 years. There is a slight female predominance and most lesions are identified in the anterior mandible (8,9). Central giant cell granulomas involving the condylar head have been reported (10,11).

Auclair et al. (12) evaluated a series of giant cell tumors of long bones and giant cell granulomas of the jaw and found that there was a female predilection for both lesions and that both tumors were often first diagnosed in the third decade. In their analysis of 22 cases, 14 involved women and 8 men of an age range of 7 to 81 years. Sixteen were located in the mandible and 6 in the maxilla. Painless swelling was the most common clinical feature in 18 of the cases. In an analysis of 80 cases by Kaffe et al. (13), 50 percent of tumors were located in the molar, ramus, and tuberosity, and not in the deciduous teeth-bearing area.

Based on a series of studies, giant cell lesions are divided into two categories. Nonaggressive lesions constitute most tumors that are asymptomatic, slowly growing, and show no tooth root resorption or cortical perforation. Aggressive lesions are characterized by pain or paresthesia, root resorption, cortical perforation, and a higher recurrence rate following curettage (2,9,14).

Radiographic Features. Radiographically, central giant cell granulomas appear similar to other benign odontogenic neoplasms and cysts. The tumors present as an asymptomatic radiolucency with corticated borders that characteristically displace teeth and other anatomic structures (fig. 14-1). Tooth root resorption and cortical perforation, as noted above, are seen in aggressive lesions. The lesions may be unilocular or multilocular based primarily on size. In an analysis of 80 cases, slightly more than 50 percent were multilocular and the correlation between the lesion's size and its locularity was statistically significant, with larger lesions assuming a multilocular appearance (13). Only 6 percent of the lesions crossed the midline of the

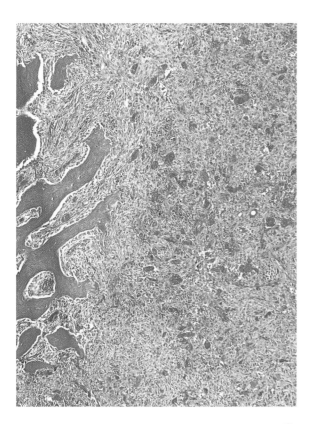 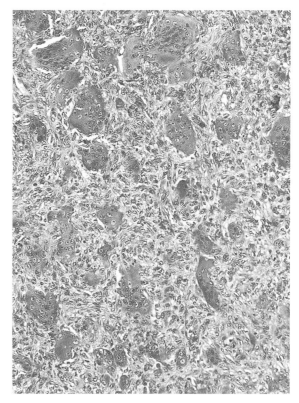

Figure 14-2

CENTRAL GIANT CELL GRANULOMA

Left: At medium power, trabeculae of bone are seen adjacent to vascular connective tissue with numerous giant cells.
Right: At higher power, numerous thin-walled vascular channels are noted within the fibrovascular stroma, along with numerous multinucleated giant cells.

jaw, a feature that was considered in the past as typical for central giant cell granulomas. In an analysis of 22 cases, 13 lesions were entirely radiolucent, 15 were unilocular, and 14 showed well-defined but not sclerotic margins (10). Computerized tomographic (CT) images in 5 patients clearly showed bony trabeculae within the lesions.

Both primary and secondary hyperparathyroidism can cause radiographic changes throughout the skeleton. In the jaws there is often a loss of distinct trabeculae, and the overall appearance of the bone becomes more homogeneous. The lamina dura surrounding the roots of teeth becomes less evident and in some cases the cortical plates, even at the inferior border of the mandible, appear thinned and less prominent. The term "ground glass" is often used to describe the appearance of bone in advanced cases of hyperparathyroidism.

Gross Findings. Central giant cell lesions grossly appear as hemorrhagic, amorphous soft tissue fragments. Following demineralization, focal hard tissue nodules are identified as irregular islands and trabeculae of woven and lamellar bone.

Microscopic Findings. There is a background of spindle-shaped mesenchymal cells with numerous multinucleated giant cells, thin-walled vascular channels, hemorrhage, and hemosiderin (fig. 14-2). It has been proposed that the spindle cells are of monocyte/microphage linage which differentiate into the osteoclastic giant cells. The giant cells occur in small groups or are distributed throughout the lesion. Most giant cells are round or ovoid, and contain as many as 20 nuclei. Some studies have found that the giant cells of the jaw lesions contain significantly fewer nuclei than the giant cells of long bone lesions; there is some overlap in most lesions (12,15).

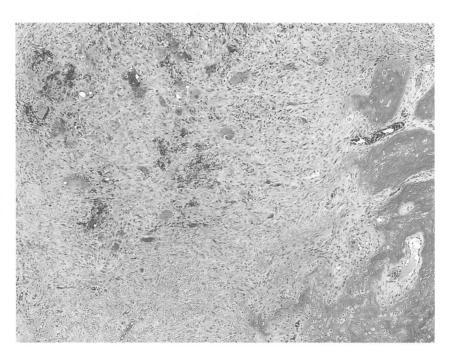

Figure 14-3

COLLISION TUMOR

This hybrid tumor consists of a central ossifying fibroma on the right and a central giant cell granuloma on the left.

Osteoid, woven, and lamellar bone complete with osteoplastic rimming may be focally identified. Giant cell granulomas and central ossifying fibroma collision tumors have been described (fig. 14-3) (16–18).

The brown tumor of hyperparathyroidism is microscopically identical to central giant cell granulomas. Both tumors show a background of spindle cells with extensive hemorrhage and numerous multinucleated giant cells. Areas of osteoid woven and lamellar bone with osteoblastic rimming are identified.

In primary hyperparathyroidism, elevated PTH levels and serum calcium above 10.5 mg/dL are characteristic. The serum phosphate level is often below 2.5 mg/dL. Alkaline phosphatase is elevated in some cases with extensive bone disease.

Secondary hyperparathyroidism, the mechanisms of which are complex and not completely understood, is the result of long-standing hypocalcemia. In most cases it is associated with chronic renal disease. The loss of normal renal function causes a decrease in phosphate excretion and the resultant hyperphosphatemia decreases serum calcium levels. In addition, the loss of renal parenchyma results in less synthesis of vitamin D to an active form, causing less absorption of calcium. Further, the sensitivity of osteoblasts to PTH is decreased if there is vitamin D deficiency.

Immunohistochemical Findings. Some studies have suggested that aggressive and nonaggressive variants of giant cell granuloma can be separated based on the argyrophilic nucleolar organizer regions (AgNOR) staining of mononuclear cells (19). However, in a recent evaluation of AgNOR as a marker of proliferation in 21 cases of central giant cell granulomas, 8 cases of aneurysmal bone cyst, 6 cases of cherubism, and 6 cases of brown tumor of hyperparathyroidism, no significant differences were identified (20).

The lineage of the mononuclear and multinuclear cells has been controversial. Special stains have previously shown the giant cells to be osteoclasts, and alkaline phosphatase–containing osteoblasts also account for the formation of bone. O'Malley et al. (21), however, when comparing aggressive and nonaggressive central giant cell granulomas using antibodies to CD34, CD68, factor XIIIa, alpha-smooth muscle actin, prolyl 4-hydroxylase, Ki-67, and p53 protein, concluded that central giant cell granulomas are primarily fibroblastic and myofibroblastic tumors in which macrophages appear to play a secondary role. The tumor cells showed no differentiation toward endothelial cells or macrophage-related dendrocytes (factor XIIIa), and the cellular phenotypes and numbers of cells in the cell cycle were similar in both aggressive and nonaggressive tumors.

Using staining techniques for CD68 and tartrate-resistant acid phosphatase (TRAP) proteins in 20 giant cell lesions, a more recent study showed that 99 percent of multinucleated giant cells were positive for TRAP antibody and about 90 percent were positive for CD68 (22). In the mononuclear cells, 14 percent of cases stained for TRAP antibody and 8 percent for CD68. This reinforces the evidence that the multinucleated giant cells are osteoclasts, and at least some of the mononuclear cells are of macrophage/monocyte lineage.

Additional studies have suggested that the development of giant cell lesions of the jaw as well as cherubism is possibly mediated by overexpression of nuclear factor of activated T-cell (NFATc1) proteins in the nucleus of the multinucleated cells (23). MSX1 protein, a classic transcription regulator that promotes cell proliferation and inhibits cell differentiation, has been shown to be present in the multinucleated giant cells and mononucleated stromal cells of central giant cell granulomas (24).

PTH-related peptide and PTH receptor type 1 are expressed by multinucleated giant cells and stromal cells with vesicular nuclei, whereas these proteins are expressed to a lesser extent in multinucleated giant cells and stromal cells with pyknotic nuclei (24). In an evaluation of CD34 as a molecular marker for predicting the clinical behavior of giant cell tumors, staining density levels of more than 2.5 percent were associated with aggressive clinical behavior (25).

Treatment and Prognosis. Central giant cell lesions are characteristically treated with simple curettage. Following the treatment of 29 cases (28 with curettage and 1 with en bloc resection), 5 cases recurred (26). All recurrent cases had cortical perforation at the time of initial treatment. Recurrent lesions seem to occur more often in younger patients (12). The distribution of the giant cells and the frequency of osteoid within the lesions also indicate an increased possibility of recurrence (9).

Recent reports have suggested that some central giant cell granulomas may be treated nonsurgically with injections of corticosteroids, calcitonin, interferon, and monoclonal antibodies to vascular endothelial growth factor, while some require more aggressive surgery including resection (14,27–30). In a series of 21 cases treated with intralesional injection of 20 mg/mL of triamcinolone hexacetonide diluted in an anesthetic solution of 2 percent lidocaine/epinephrine 1:200,000 in the proportion 1:1, dosed as 1.0 mL of the solution for every 1 cm^3 of radiographic area of the lesion, totaling 6 biweekly applications, two patients showed a negative response to the treatment and underwent surgical resection, 4 showed a moderate response, and 15 showed a good response (31). Eight of the 19 who had a moderate to good response to the injections underwent subsequent osteoplasty to reestablish bony contours for aesthetic purposes. In these 8 cases, microscopic examination of the post-treatment tissue revealed only mature or dysplastic bone with rare multinucleated giant cells. In contrast, in a systematic review of previous randomized controlled trials from 1950 to 2009 regarding surgical and nonsurgical treatment, no good evidence was identified to support nonsurgical treatment (32). Distraction osteogenesis following bone graft placement has been utilized for reconstruction following surgical removal (33).

Cherubism

Definition. *Cherubism* was first described by Jones in 1933 (34) as an autosomal-dominant familial condition with variable penetrance (35). Lesions usually manifest in early childhood between ages 1 and 4 years. The characteristic giant cell lesions usually involve the maxillary and mandibular posterior regions bilaterally. The term cherubism is the result of bilateral maxillary lesions resulting in a resemblance to the cherubs seen in Renaissance art (36).

General Features. Cherubism is related to an exon 9-*SH3BP2* mutation that has not been identified in central giant cell granulomas (37–39). An additional missence mutation has been identified in exon 4 (40). Studies in mice have shown that *SH3BP2* regulates bone homeostasis not only through osteoclast-specific effects, but also through effects on osteoblast differentiation and function (41,42).

Some cases of cherubism are associated with *Noonan syndrome* (43,44). The association of cherubism with gingival fibromatosis, epilepsy, mental retardation, stunted growth, and hypertrichosis is referred as *Ramon syndrome* (45).

Radiographic Features. Radiographs characteristically show unilocular or multilocular well-corticated radiolucencies involving the maxilla

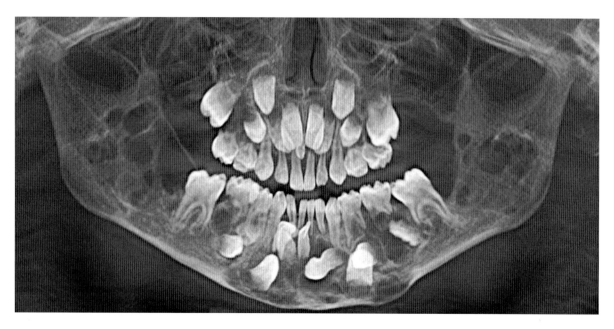

Figure 14-4

CHERUBISM

A cone beam computerized tomography (CT) panoramic reconstruction shows multiloculated radiolucencies bilaterally involving the mandible and maxilla.

and mandible bilaterally (fig. 14-4). The term soap-bubble has been used to describe the multilocular radiolucencies. Because these tumors occur in young children, multiple unerupted teeth at various levels of formation often appear to be floating within these radiolucencies.

Microscopic Findings. The lesions of cherubism are microscopically indistinguishable from central giant cell granulomas. A fibrovascular stroma with numerous mononuclear spindle cells, osteoclast-like multinucleated giant cells, hemorrhage, and osteoid and woven bone is seen (fig. 14-5). Giant cells are often located in small groups. Biopsies from older patients usually show bone with more fibrosis and fewer giant cells.

Immunohistochemical Findings. The development of giant cell lesions of the jaw, including cherubism, is possibly mediated by the overexpression of nuclear factor of activated T-cell (NFAT) protein in multinucleated cells (23). The spindle-shaped stromal cells express a ligand for the receptor activator of nuclear factor kappaB (RANKL), which may have a role in the differentiation of osteoclast precursor cells to multinucleated giant cells in cherubism (46).

Treatment and Prognosis. Therapy is often aimed at maintaining function and cosmetics. Intervention at an early, appropriate time is necessary to prevent long-term functional and aesthetic issues (47,48). Some reports advocate a two-stage surgical approach involving curettage and recontouring the maxillary lesions in stage one, and subsequent curettage and recontouring of the mandibular lesions several months later (49). Anti-tumor necrosis factor (TNF) therapy and the use of calcitonin are nonsurgical options in some cases (39,50).

ANEURYSMAL BONE CYST

Definition. *Aneurysmal bone cyst* is a proliferative blood-filled lesion occurring in bone. It can be associated with other lesions of bone, in which case it is deemed secondary. It is uncommon in the jaw.

General Features. The etiology of aneurysmal bone cyst has long remained unclear but recent strong evidence shows that it may represent a neoplasm rather than a reactive process in lesions that are primary rather than secondary (51,52). First described by Jaffe and Lichtenstein in 1942 as a solitary unicameral bone cyst, it

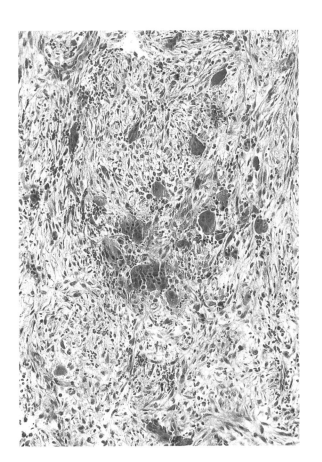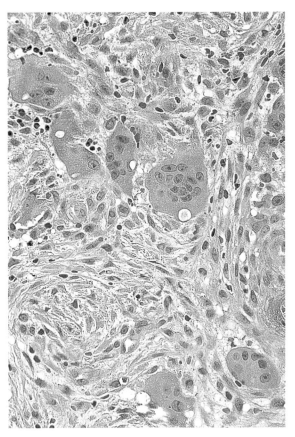

Figure 14-5

CHERUBISM

Left: Fibrovascular connective tissue with numerous multinucleated giant cells is seen.
Right: At high power, a fibrovascular connective tissue background surrounds multinucleated giant cells.

was further defined by both authors and became known as *Jaffe-Lichtenstein disease* (53,54). Both authors subsequently described the lesion as aneurysmal bone cyst, a term that is descriptive but apt. The lesion is predominantly cystic but because it is blood-filled and has a pushing border, and aneurysmal is a reasonable adjective (55,56). A curious aspect of this tumor is that it can be associated with a wide variety of non-neoplastic and neoplastic bony lesions such as giant cell tumor, chondroblastoma, solitary or unicameral bone cyst, or more rarely, osteosarcoma, nonosteogenic fibroma, osteoblastoma, hemangioendothelioma, hemangioma, and fracture site (57).

Clinical Features. Aneurysmal bone cyst occurs primarily in patients in the first and second decades of life. Pain and rapid swelling are the most common complaints (58). There is a pre-

dilection for the mandible over the maxilla by a 2 to 1 or 3 to 1 margin (59,60). The temporomandibular joint is also affected (61).

Radiographic Features. Radiographically, there is usually a lytic lesion, sometimes with ill-defined borders. In some patients the lesion is mixed lucent and solid, and rarely radiopaque (62,63). The border of the lesion may extend through the cortex of the bone into the soft tissues. Imaging techniques such a CT sometimes demonstrate fluid levels (64,65).

Gross Findings. Aneurysmal bone cyst can be unilocular or multilocular. On occasion it is resected intact but usually the specimen is obtained by biopsy and curettage (fig. 14-6). Since the lesion is predominantly cystic, what was a large lesion clinically and radiographically, is reduced to small hemorrhagic soft tissue fragments when received by the pathologist.

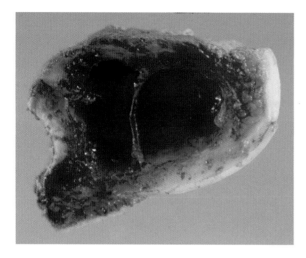

Figure 14-6

ANEURYSMAL BONE CYST

Above: This aneurysmal bone cyst was resected and reveals only several large cysts in the bone.

Right: Numerous small cysts with scarring and fibrosis are seen.

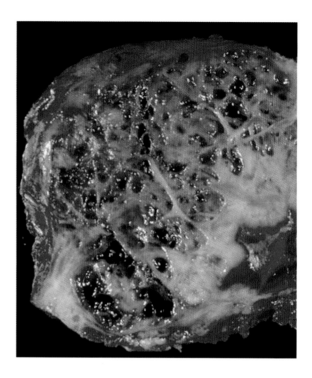

Microscopic Findings. The low-power magnification shows irregular cysts filled with fresh or degenerated blood or are empty (fig. 14-7). The walls of the cysts contain a significant amount of mineralization, osteoid, or bone (fig. 14-8). The osseous proliferations are lined at their periphery by osteoblasts. The lining of the cyst is thin and intervening septa are primarily composed of fibrous tissue with variable cellularity (fig. 14-9). The septa also contain multinucleated giant cells and hemosiderin deposition, the latter associated with the abundant blood and fibrin present (figs. 14-10, 4-11). The spindled cells are arranged in a loose pattern, in distinction to the more packed arrangement in a giant cell tumor, a lesion that is often in the histologic differential diagnosis (fig. 14-12). A common finding is the presence of mitotic figures. These can be numerous but are not atypical. As aneurysmal bone cysts can form in response to other bone lesions, there can be an admixture of the inciting lesion as well as the aneurysmal bone cyst (fig. 14-13).

There may be no cystic component, and such cases are termed *solid pattern* or *solid variant* (66,67). These tumors still have a loosely arranged stroma with spindle cells. Osteoid production is common in the intervening areas of the spindled cells.

Molecular Findings. Recent evidence has shown clonal chromosome band 17p13 translocations that put the *USP6* oncogene under the control of the regulatory promoter, *CDH11*. Rearrangements of *USP6* or *CDH11* are found in a high percentage of aneurysmal bone cysts. It appears that the molecular abnormalities are localized to the spindle cells of the tumor, which are likely progenitors of osteoblasts. The rearrangements do not appear to correlate to clinical or pathologic findings, such as recurrence. These rearrangements have not been found in secondary aneurysmal bone cysts (52). Ye et al. (51) have further elucidated how this translocation, which results in a *TRE17/USP6* translocation, is potentially involved in aneurysmal bone cyst. *TRE17* encodes a ubiquitin-specific protease (USP) and is implicated in the regulation of matrix metalloproteinases (MMPs), the latter of which can effect osteolysis and bone matrix remodeling.

Differential Diagnosis. Because of its spindled and hemorrhagic microscopic appearance, aneurysmal bone cyst can be confused with a number of other lesions of bone. The tumor cells of giant cell tumor are packed together and are more oval than the spindled-shaped cells in aneurysmal bone cyst. Solid variants of aneurysmal bone cyst can cause some difficulties, however. The overall looseness of

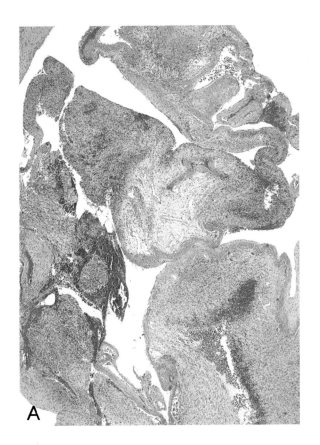

Figure 14-7

ANEURYSMAL BONE CYST

A: A mixture of solid and cystic areas is present.

B: Aneurysmal bone cysts can be predominantly cystic.

C: The cyst lining is composed of organizing blood, which will form into fibrous tissue.

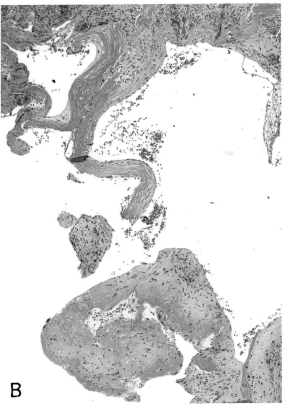

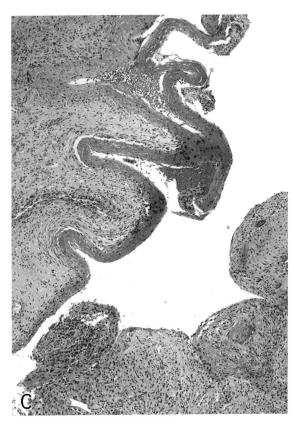

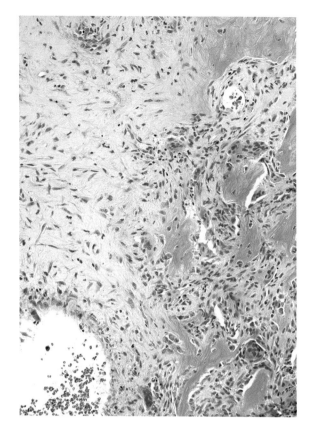

Figure 14-8

ANEURYSMAL BONE CYST

Osteoid production is present in this lesion.

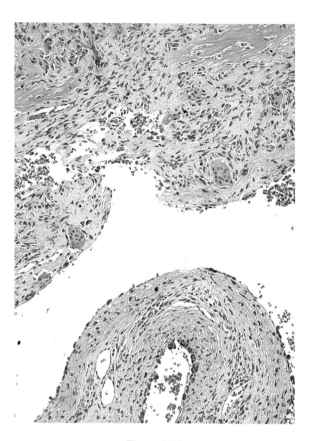

Figure 14-9

ANEURYSMAL BONE CYST

A thin lining is present on the wall of a septum.

Figure 14-10

ANEURYSMAL BONE CYST

Giant cells can be seen in this aneurysmal bone cyst. The degree of cellularity is variable in this tumor.

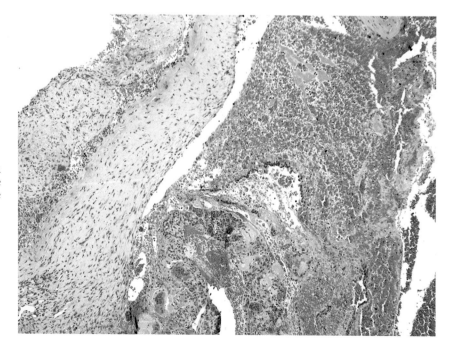

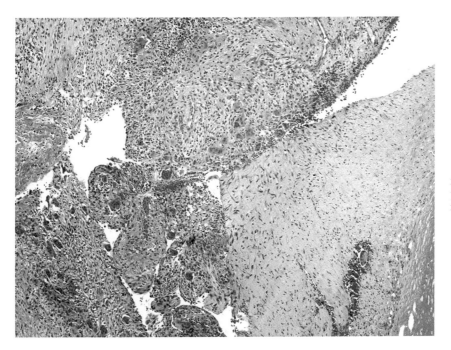

Figure 14-11

ANEURYSMAL BONE CYST

Giant cells are admixed in moderately cellular areas juxtaposed to hypocellular fibrous areas.

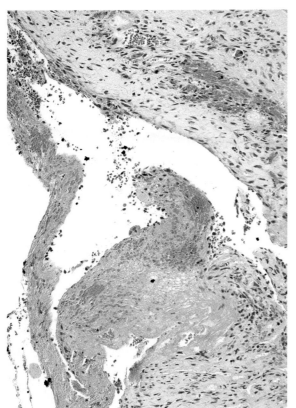
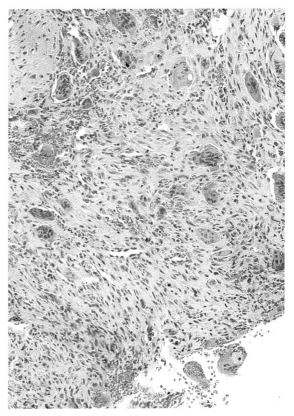

Figure 14-12

ANEURYSMAL BONE CYST

Left: Fibrin is attached focally to the wall of the cyst.
Right: Numerous giant cells are seen in a fibrovascular stroma.

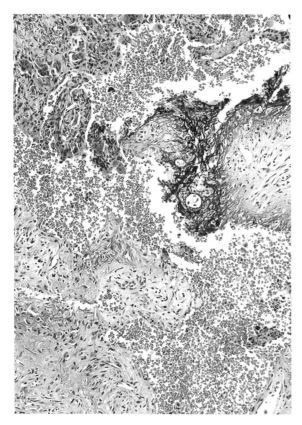

Figure 14-13

ANEURYSMAL BONE CYST

Aneurysmal bone cyst formation accompanies this chondroblastoma.

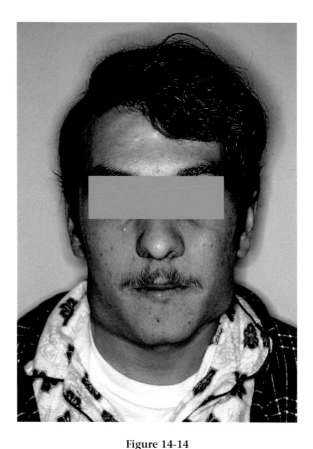

Figure 14-14

OSTEOMAS OF MANDIBLE IN GARDNER SYNDROME

Deformity of both sides of the mandible is produced by multiple mandibular osteomas.

the cells in aneurysmal bone cyst helps in the differentiation. Telangiectatic osteosarcoma is also composed of blood-filled spaces and can appear similar at low-power magnification but closer examination reveals that the cells within the walls of the cysts are very atypical.

Treatment and Prognosis. Curettage is the usual treatment. Some authors have noted significant recurrence rates (58,56,60). Incomplete removal usually results in cure but has also been associated with recurrence or persistence in large lesions (68). Recurrence of the lesion after thorough curettage or enucleation should suggest consideration of other processes.

OSTEOMA

Definition. *Osteomas* are tumorous growths composed of mature cancellous bone, but whether they represent a true identifiable entity is debated by some.

General Features. In the most recent Atlas of Tumor Pathology Fascicle, Tumors of the Bones and Joints (69), osteoma is not mentioned in the classification of bone tumors. The problem with defining osteoma as an entity is that reactive processes of bone can histologically mimic exactly the findings of osteoma. Most tumors reported to be osteomas are in the craniofacial region and involve the sinuses. They rarely involve the jawbones. They are often associated with Gardner syndrome (70–73). This syndrome, also known as familial adenomatous polyposis syndrome, shows a constellation of findings including colon polyps that develop adenocarcinomas, odontomas, fibromatosis, and epidermal inclusion cysts. The colon polyps in these patients develop at a young age and subsequent adenocarcinomas of the colon can be seen in third decade (figs. 14-14–14-16).

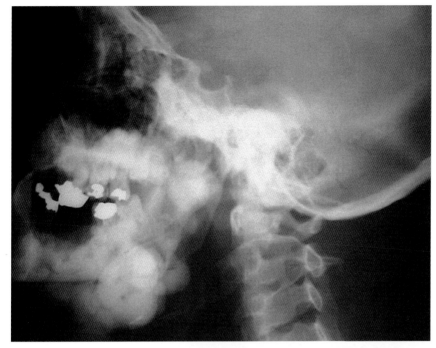

Figure 14-15

OSTEOMAS OF MANDIBLE IN GARDNER SYNDROME

Dense, sclerotic, circumscribed masses are present within the body of the mandible.

Figure 14-16

MULTIPLE ADENOMATOUS POLYPS IN GARDNER SYNDROME

The mucosa is studded with adenomatous polyps.

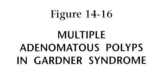

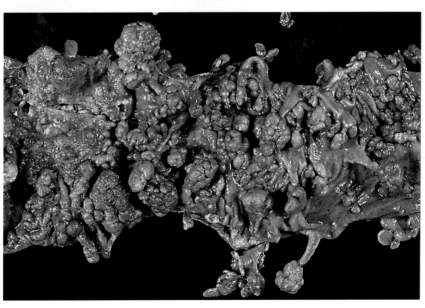

Clinical Features. Osteomas are classified as *peripheral, central,* or *extraosseous* (74,75). It is thought that the peripheral osteoma arises from the periosteum while the central osteoma from the endosteum. Extraosseous osteomas usually arise in muscle. Most osteomas of the jaws are peripheral, with only rare central osteomas reported (76,77). When involving the bones of the jaws, osteomas mostly occur on the lingual surface of the mandible and occasionally the maxilla, although no specific area of the jaws is immune. The radiographic features of osteomas are not specific but show the lesion to be densely sclerotic with distinct circumscription.

Microscopic Findings. Osteomas are composed of mature bone, usually of cancellous type (fig. 14-17). There is no specific histology, however, that defines osteoma and thus the clinical and radiographic findings are of importance.

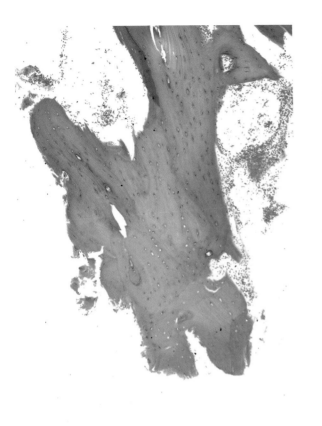 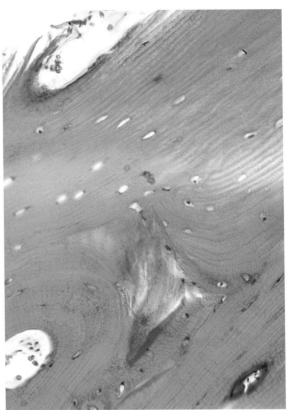

Figure 14-17

OSTEOMA

Left: Mature cancellous bone is evident in this osteoma. The histologic findings are not specific and appear identical to those of mature bone.

Right: Osteocytes are seen within the matrix of an osteoma. This osseous material was removed from a patient with Gardner syndrome.

Differential Diagnosis. Osteoma requires diagnosis by the clinical findings and radiographic images. Osteomas must be differentiated from tori by the clinical findings since the histologic features are identical.

While peripheral osteomas are easy to diagnose when radiographic images are correlated, central osteomas are more difficult to classify. The differential diagnosis includes central ossifying fibroma, condensing osteitis, idiopathic osteosclerosis, osteoblastoma, cementoblastoma, complex odontoma, and bone islands (77). Histologic separation of osteoma from some of these lesions can be nearly impossible. The bone formation of osteoma is mature and does not have the features of well-differentiated surface osteosarcoma.

Treatment and Prognosis. Treatment is required when the bony growth interferes with normal functions or is aesthetically disfiguring (78). Conservative procedures are used when possible. Osteomas do not recur. Those associated with Gardner syndrome, however, may continue to appear.

OSTEOBLASTOMA/OSTEOID OSTEOMA

Definition. *Osteoblastoma* is a benign bone-forming neoplasm. *Osteoid osteoma* is identical to osteoblastoma, and the two are separated on the basis of overall size as well as the presence of a nidus in osteoid osteoma. Osteoid osteomas are less than 1 cm in diameter; osteoblastomas are greater than 2 cm. For tumors between the sizes of 1 and 2 cm, the diagnosis is relegated to pathologic and radiographic interpretation.

General Features. Osteoblastoma occurring in the jaws is a rare tumor and its exact incidence

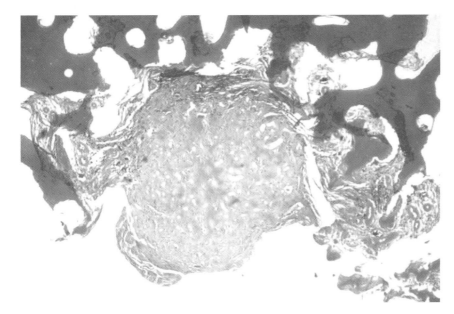

Figure 14-18

OSTEOID OSTEOMA

Low-power view shows a dense nidus.

is difficult to determine. Some authorities have included cementoblastoma with their cases of osteoblastoma, since the histologic features are identical (79). Further clouding the issue of separation from cementoblastoma is that some suggest that osteoblastomas occurring in the jaws have a tendency to be attached to a tooth root, a conclusion not shared by all (80,81). Osteoblastomas are more frequently reported than osteoid osteomas in the jaws.

Clinical Features. Patients with osteoblastomas or osteoid osteomas have complaints of painful swelling (82,83). Most patients present in the first, second, and third decades of life and the mandible is more often involved than the maxilla (83,84). When in the mandible, the body of mandible is more often affected but any site in this bone is possible. Osteoid osteomas characteristically cause pain that is worse at night and is alleviated immediately after oral consumption of nonsteroidal anti-inflammatory medication.

Radiographic Features. On radiographs, osteoid osteoma is distinguished most usually by having a distinct central nidus of proliferation with surrounding reactive and sclerotic bone. On panoramic radiographs, a circular radiopacity is seen and CT shows a rounded sclerotic lesion. Uptake of tracer material occurs in the area corresponding to active growth (85).

The radiographic appearance of osteoblastoma is that of a sharply demarcated mass. The tumors are predominantly sclerotic but can appear lytic or have a mixed radiolucent/radiopaque appearance.

Microscopic Findings. Osteoid osteoma is histologically similar to osteoblastoma but classically presents with a central nidus of very dense bone which is surrounded by bone spicules in a cellular stroma (fig. 14-18). Osteoblastomas are composed of woven bone spicules that are separated by a cellular spindled stroma (fig. 14-19). The stroma is well vascularized and the bone spicules are rimmed by osteoblasts. In addition, numerous multinucleated osteoclasts are present, both attached to the osseous spicules and within the intervening stroma (fig. 14-20). An important finding is the lack of atypical cells in the stroma. Osteoblastoma can exhibit large dense areas of mineralized material identical to that of cementoblastoma (fig. 14-21). Although osteoblastomas may be very cellular, there is no atypia as seen in osteosarcoma (fig. 14-22).

A variant of osteoblastoma has been described, the so-called *aggressive osteoblastoma* although not all authorities agree on its existence (86,87). These tumors have a higher recurrence rate (50 percent) than usual osteoblastoma (fig. 14-23). The key findings in aggressive osteoblastoma are larger epithelioid osteoblasts and sheet-like

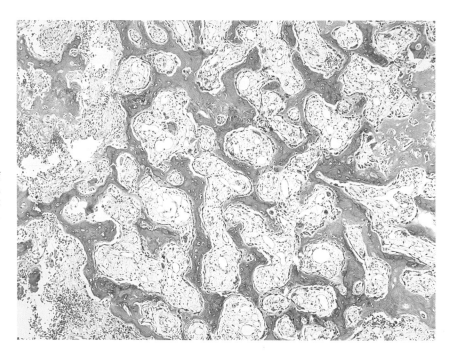

Figure 14-19

OSTEOBLASTOMA

A criss-crossed network of osseous trabeculae is seen. A loose myxoid stroma is present between the osseous trabeculae.

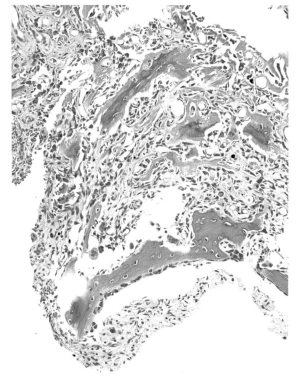

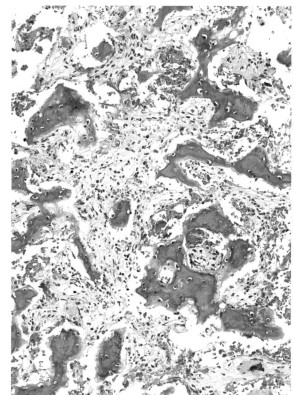

Figure 14-20

OSTEOID OSTEOMA

Left: Some of the osseous trabeculae are rimmed by a single layer of osteoblasts. The intervening loose stroma is moderately cellular but no atypical stromal cells are seen.

Right: A loose myxoid stroma separates the osseous trabeculae. There is minimal osteoblastic rimming.

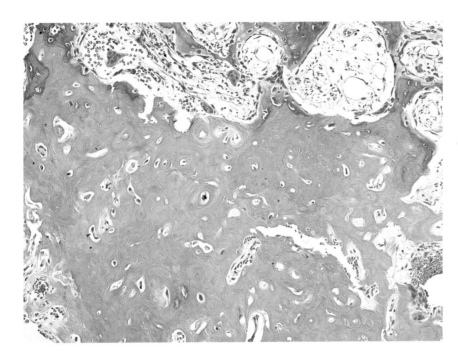

Figure 14-21

OSTEOBLASTOMA

A densely mineralized area is seen in an osteoblastoma. There is marked similarity to the dense mineralized matrix seen in cementoblastoma (see figs. 7-16, 7-17).

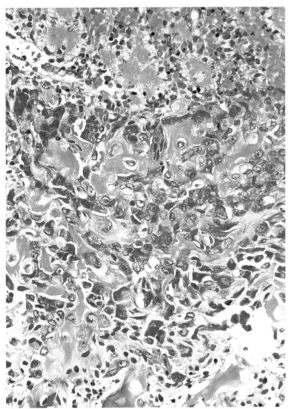
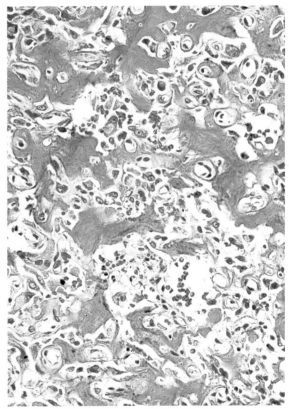

Figure 14-22

OSTEOBLASTOMA

Left: Numerous osteoblasts with osteoid production are present.
Right: A cellular osteoblastoma reveals osteoid production. The stroma shows no atypical cells.

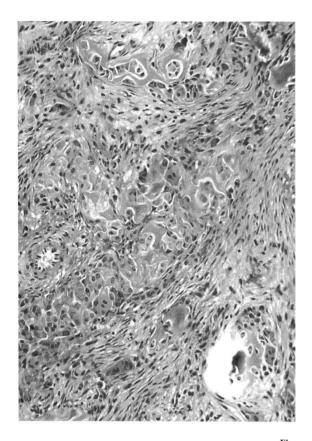 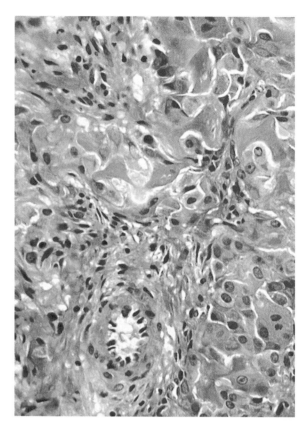

Figure 14-23

AGGRESSIVE OSTEOBLASTOMA

Left: The osteoid trabeculae have a delicate, ribbon-like quality and the osteoblasts are large with epithelioid characteristics. These areas fulfill the histologic criteria for aggressive osteoblastoma.

Right: Higher magnification demonstrates the presence of large epithelioid-type osteoblasts with prominent eosinophilic nucleoli surrounding delicate spicules of woven bone. This lesion recurred twice following local resection.

osteoid. While mitoses can be seen, they are not atypical. The osteoid trabeculae were reported to be increased in size when compared to those of osteoblastoma of usual type. One of the tumors in the series of gnathic osteoblastomas of Rawal et al. (88) had histologic features compatible with aggressive osteoblastoma but the lesion did not exhibit an aggressive clinical course. Rare cases of osteoblastoma developing into osteosarcoma have been reported (89).

Differential Diagnosis. The entities in the histologic differential diagnosis of osteoid osteoma and osteoblastoma are osteosarcoma, ossifying fibroma, and cementoblastoma (90). On small biopsies, the histologic separation of osteoblastoma and osteosarcoma can be difficult. Osteosarcomas have an irregular margin seen both radiographically as well as histologically. Unni et al. (79) stressed the importance of seeing the margins of osteosarcoma infiltrate into the surrounding normal bone. These authors also pointed out that the stroma of osteoblastoma that intervenes between the osseous trabeculae is loose rather than filled with atypical osteoblasts and that the trabeculae are rimmed by a single layer of osteoblasts and not the multiple layers more characteristic of osteosarcoma.

Treatment and Prognosis. Complete surgical curettage is the treatment of choice (88). Osteoblastomas have an approximate recurrence rate of 10 percent, although it is not clear whether this recurrence rate is due to incomplete excision. Some authors suggest that complete excision results in few recurrences (79).

OSTEOSARCOMA

Definition. *Osteosarcoma* is a malignant neoplasm producing either osteoid, bone, or both. Affecting the mandible as well as the maxilla, it usually presents in older patients. Although histologically similar to osteosarcoma in the long bones, it differs clinically from those tumors in that it often has an earlier diagnosis, a higher median survival rate, a lower incidence of distant metastasis, and a higher incidence of local recurrence (90).

General Features. Osteosarcoma is the most common primary malignant bone tumor, accounting for 40 to 60 percent of all primary malignancies of bone. About 6 to 10 percent of osteosarcomas occur in the head and neck, primarily in the mandible and maxilla (91–95). Most studies show that more cases arise in the mandible than the maxilla (95–100). The average age of patients presenting with osteosarcoma of the jaws ranges from the 30s to early 40s, which is much older than that of patients with osteosarcoma of the long bones. The gender distribution generally shows a near equal balance, although some studies show a slight female predominance while others a slight male predominance.

The incidence of osteosarcoma of the jaws varies. In the Netherlands, it is estimated to be at least 0.14 per 1,000,000 population (101). In Japan, 114 cases of osteosarcoma of the maxillofacial region were reported during a 60-year period (99). Ajagbe et al. (102) reviewed the osteogenic jaw sarcomas in Nigeria from 1960 to 1984. In this 24-year period, 21 osteosarcomas of the jaws were seen out of 1,375 jaw lesions, excluding cysts. During this period, 107 total osteosarcomas (including jaw lesions) were seen. Rarely, osteosarcoma can metastasize to the jaws (103–105).

Although most osteosarcomas are sporadic in nature, a number of diseases, syndromes, and even iatrogenic conditions are associated with osteosarcoma. Paget disease is associated with the development of osteosarcoma although the jaw is not a common site (106,107). In a Mayo Clinic series (98), 4.3 percent of osteosarcomas associated with Paget disease were in the jaw, with 1.4 percent in the maxilla and 2.9 percent in the mandible. Other syndromes and diseases associated with the development of osteosarcoma include fibrous dysplasia, hereditary retinoblastoma,

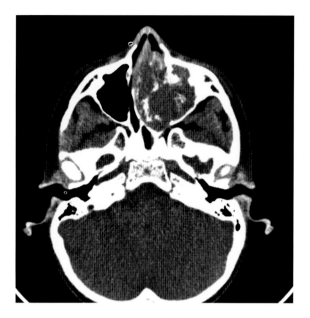

Figure 14-24

OSTEOSARCOMA

CT image of a large chondroblastic osteosarcoma arising in the maxilla. There is destruction of the underlying maxillary space and extension into the nasal cavity. Heterogeneous densities represent mineralization of some of the matrix.

Ollier disease, Blum syndrome, Werner syndrome, Li-Fraumeni syndrome, and Rothmund-Thomson syndrome (98,108). Dental implants have been associated with osteosarcoma. Postradiation osteosarcomas have been reported (110,111,119). Radiation-induced osteosarcomas are aggressive and often elude early detection and timely intervention, rapidly leading to early death (112).

Clinical and Radiographic Features. The most common presenting features of osteosarcoma in the jaws are swelling, pain, ulceration, loosened teeth, and numb chin (100). The radiologic diagnosis of osteosarcoma of the jaws can be difficult because of its variable appearance. Areas of radiopacity are mixed with areas of radiolucency (113). CT is particularly useful in the diagnosis and surgical management of the disease (fig. 14-24) (114). The radiographic differentiation of osteogenic sarcoma, osteomyelitis, and fibrous dysplasia of the jaw may be difficult. Some of the radiologic features of osteosarcoma include widening of the mandibular canal, widening of the periodontal ligament space, permeative lesion borders, stippled appearance of the bone, destruction of cortical outlines, and perpendicular spiculations representing periosteal new bone formation (115–117). In postradiation osteosarcomas, the radiographic abnormalities occur in portions of bones at the borders of the radiation field (118,119).

Gross Findings. The gross appearance of osteosarcoma is variable but most have a fleshy appearance and texture admixed with varying degrees of mineralization and chondroid areas.

Microscopic Findings. The histologic type of osteosarcoma dictates many of the microscopic findings (Table 14-1). The overlying principal in the diagnosis is the finding of osteoid production by a sarcomatous stroma (fig. 14-25). The intervening stromal cells are atypical, a finding of practical use in the separation from benign entities that also produce osteoid (fig. 14-26). Osteosarcomas that are not of low grade are usually not difficult to discern as malignant since they produce osteoid and have a stroma characterized by highly atypical cells. It is important to emphasize that only a small amount of osteoid production by the tumor is required to qualify it as osteosarcoma.

Table 14-1
HISTOLOGIC TYPES OF OSTEOSARCOMA
Osteoblastic
Chondroblastic
Low-grade fibroblastic
High-grade fibroblastic
Small cell
Telangiectatic

Surface osteosarcomas
    Parosteal
    Periosteal
    High-grade surface

Well-differentiated central Epithelioid Low-grade intraosseous

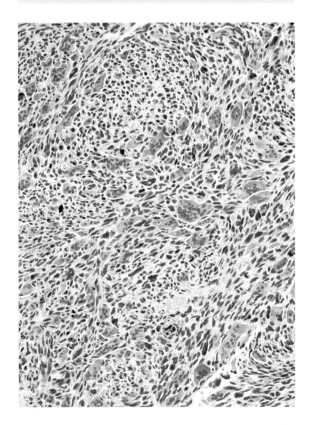 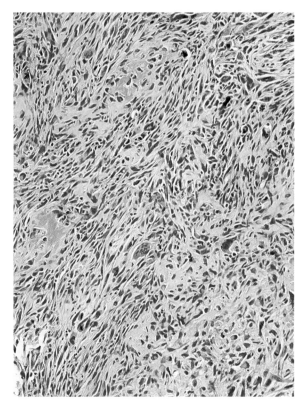

Figure 14-25

OSTEOSARCOMA

Left: This high-grade osteosarcoma cannot be diagnosed by this image alone because of the lack of demonstrable osteoid.
Right: The same tumor shows osteoid production.

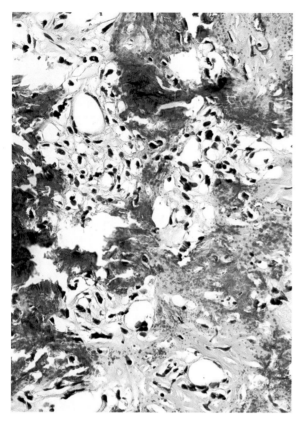

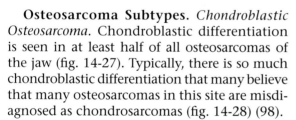

Figure 14-26

OSTEOSARCOMA

Atypical stromal cells are present.

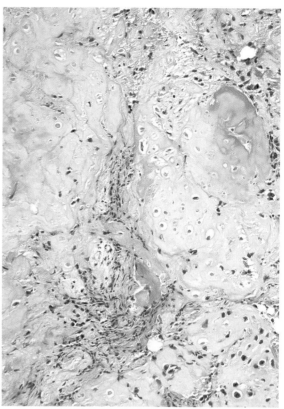

Figure 14-27

CHONDROBLASTIC OSTEOSARCOMA

Abundant cartilage is present with disorganized and atypical nuclei. A small focus of eosinophilic osteoid is seen.

Osteosarcoma Subtypes. *Chondroblastic Osteosarcoma.* Chondroblastic differentiation is seen in at least half of all osteosarcomas of the jaw (fig. 14-27). Typically, there is so much chondroblastic differentiation that many believe that many osteosarcomas in this site are misdiagnosed as chondrosarcomas (fig. 14-28) (98).

Osteoblastic Osteosarcoma. Osteoblastic osteosarcoma is characterized by predominant osteoid formation by malignant stromal cells (figs. 14-29–14-31). While in the Mayo Clinic experience (98), osteoblastic osteosarcoma is the most common subtype, chondroblastic osteosarcoma is the predominant subtype of the jaw in most other series.

Surface Osteosarcoma. Surface osteosarcoma variants grow on the surface of the bone. These include *parosteal osteosarcoma, periosteal osteosarcoma,* and *high-grade surface osteosarcoma* (120–123).

Parosteal osteosarcoma of the head and neck region is a rare, low-grade variant of osteosarcoma, but has the potential to recur after simple local excision (121,122,124). Radiographically, this tumor is a densely mineralized mass adherent to the surface of the bone. While all surface osteosarcomas are rare, parosteal osteosarcoma is the most common of the three subtypes. Microscopically, the surface of parosteal sarcoma has a cartilaginous cap simulating an osteochondroma. The tumors generally have mature-appearing bony trabeculae with intervening bland spindle cells, although in some cases the stroma is more cellular with mild to moderate atypia (figs. 14-30, 14-31).

Periosteal osteosarcoma of the jaw is rare with very few cases reported (123,125,126). Periosteal osteosarcomas can show extensive chondroid differentiation and significant nuclear atypia.

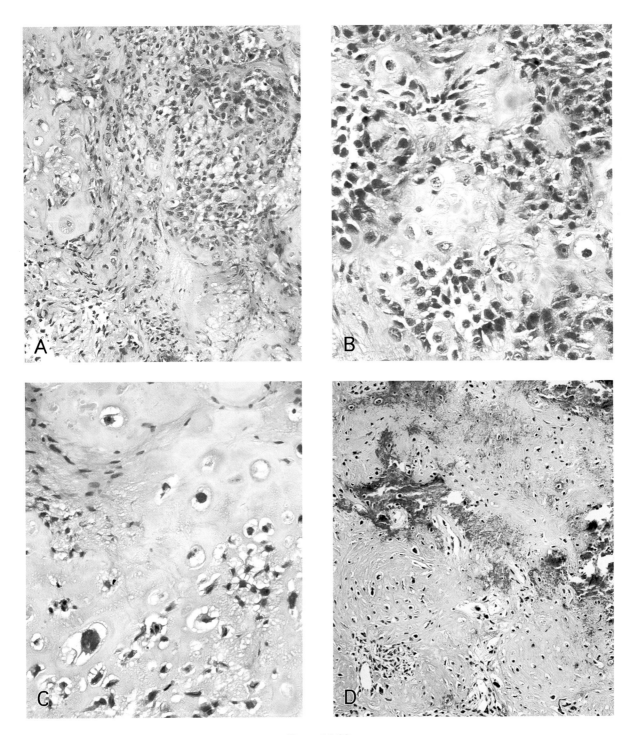

Figure 14-28

CHONDROBLASTIC OSTEOSARCOMA

A: Chondroblastic osteosarcoma shows extensive cartilaginous differentiation with minimal to no osteoid in much of the tumor.

B: Chondroblastic osteosarcoma mimics high-grade chondrosarcoma.

C: Marked nuclear atypia and cells with cartilaginous differentiation.

D: This chondroblastic osteosarcoma (seen also in fig. 14-24) exhibits an area with minimal cartilaginous differentiation but with prominent osseous differentiation. Sampling of these tumors is critical to find diagnostic foci.

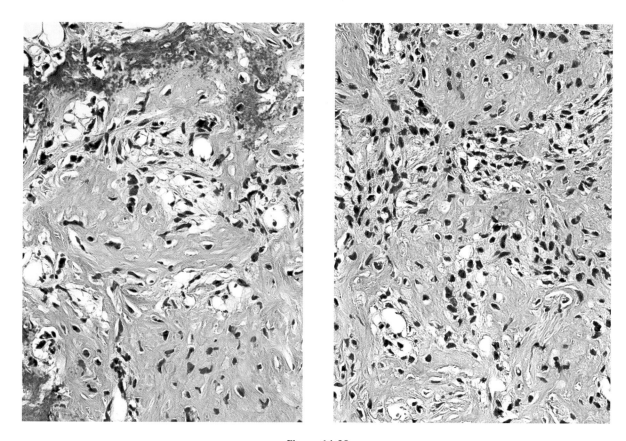

Figure 14-29

OSTEOBLASTIC OSTEOSARCOMA

Left: Osteoblastic osteosarcoma shows abundant eosinophilic osteoid. Flocculent mineralization is often seen.

Right: The osteoid in this osteoblastic osteosarcoma is arranged in a nodular pattern. The nuclei are densely hyperchromatic and irregular.

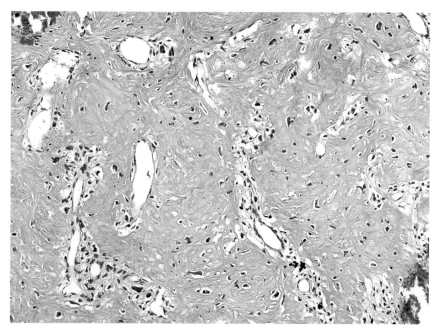

Figure 14-30

OSTEOBLASTIC OSTEOSARCOMA

At first look, this osteoblastic osteosarcoma has a rather banal appearance. The abundant osteoid matrix and scattered hyperchromatic nuclei, however, are those of osteosarcoma.

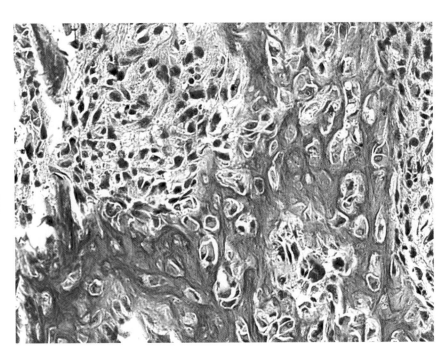

Figure 14-31

OSTEOBLASTIC OSTEOSARCOMA

Malignant stromal cells are seen with abundant osteoid production.

Telangiectatic Osteosarcoma. The telangiectatic variant of osteosarcoma is also rare in the jaw. It is characterized by vascular lakes filled with blood. The surrounding tissue is composed of osteoid-producing osteoblasts. Aneurysmal bone cyst should not be diagnosed for what is a telangiectatic osteosarcoma (127).

Epithelioid Osteosarcoma. This is a rare subtype of osteosarcoma with aggressive behavior. Histologic and ultrastructural examinations show a high-grade neoplasm consisting of sheets of epithelioid cells with focal osteoid formation (128).

Low-Grade Intraosseous Osteosarcoma. These neoplasms resemble benign proliferations except that they include cortical bone destruction, soft tissue infiltration, irregular bone production with foci of abundant osteoid, and mild cellular atypia. In some cases, incomplete excision has been associated with transformation to high-grade osteosarcoma (125,126,129,130).

Histologic Grading. Osteosarcomas of the jaws are usually of lower histologic grade than osteosarcomas occurring elsewhere. Nevertheless, any grade of osteosarcoma is possible in this location. Grading is categorized as grades 1, 2, or 3 on an increasing scale, with grade 3 having the least or poorest differentiation. Some grading schemes utilize a 1 to 4 scheme.

Immunohistochemical Findings. Immunohistochemistry is generally of limited value in the diagnosis of osteosarcoma. Some potential traps in immunohistochemical studies of osteosarcoma exist as some tumors express keratins in some but not all studies (131,132). Jaw osteosarcomas express p53 but the expression is not always linked to biologic behavior. In one study, p53 expression was linked to chondroblastic differentiation and aneuploidy (133). In an immunohistochemical study of 25 head and neck osteosarcomas, 52 percent of the tumors were positive for p53, 24 percent for murine double minute (MDM)2, 84 percent for cyclin-dependent kinase (CDK)4, 92 percent for proliferating cell nuclear antigen (PCNA), and 88 percent for Ki-67 (134).

Cytologic Findings. The cytologic features seen on fine needle aspiration of osteosarcoma depend on the subtype of osteosarcoma. The chondroblastic subtype has lacunar cells that can be either mononuclear or binucleate. These tumors also show a myxoid to chondroid background, often best appreciated with Giemsa-based stains (135). The osteoblastic subtype often shows distinctly pleomorphic nuclei and atypical mitoses. The latter is useful in helping establish a diagnosis of malignancy. The cell shape varies from round to oval and may have an appearance similar to osteoblasts, with an eccentric nucleus and a perinuclear hof (135).

Cytogenetic Findings. Genetic analyses have revealed numerous regions of chromosomal losses, rearrangements, and amplifications. While no specific pattern can be assigned to osteosarcoma, certain chromosomes and chromosomal regions are often affected more commonly. These include gain on chromosome 1, and losses involving chromosomes 9, 10, 13, and 17 (136). Common chromosomal rearrangements have been found in 1p11–13, 1q10–12, 1q11,1q21–22, 4q27–33, 6p23–25, 7p13–22, 7q11–36, 11p10–5, 11p14–15, 12p13, 14p11–13, 15p11–13, 17p12–13, 19q13, and 22q11–13 (136,137).

Molecular Findings. Gene expression profiling has been investigated in osteosarcomas but at this point, there are no specific molecular markers that can identify osteosarcoma on a consistent or clinically applicable basis (138–142). Certain molecular markers, however, shed light on tumorigenesis.

The *RB1* tumor suppressor gene is one of the most widely recognized genes having a role in the development of osteosarcoma. Located at chromosome 13q14, the loss of this tumor suppressor gene accounts for the common occurrence of osteosarcoma in patients with retinoblastoma and is also found in sporadic osteosarcoma (137).

The *p53* gene is also commonly involved in osteosarcoma, in either sporadic cases or those associated with defined syndromes or diseases. *p53* abnormalities are common in many sporadic osteosarcomas and consist of inactivation of function by either allele loss, gene rearrangement, or point mutations. In the Li-Fraumeni syndrome, where osteosarcoma is the second most common malignancy with an incidence of approximately 10 percent, germline mutations of *p53* are observed (137). In sporadic tumors, the frequency of *p53* mutations is associated with the degree of differentiation, with 40 to 50 percent of high-grade tumors having mutations while low-grade tumors are associated with nearly no mutations (137).

The REC-Q helicases, which are DNA unwinding proteins, are associated with mutations in rare syndromes such as Bloom syndrome, Werner syndrome, and Rothmund-Thomson syndrome, all of which are associated with osteosarcoma (94,137).

Differential Diagnosis. Fibrous dysplasia of bone is a condition in which both fibrous and osseous tissues replace the underlying cancellous bone, and this benign process must be differentiated from low-grade osteosarcoma (143). One key differentiating feature of fibrous dysplasia is that it does not invade the surrounding bone marrow space or existing bone trabeculae (98). Osteosarcoma also invades soft tissues, a finding not seen in fibrous dysplasia. Although fibrous dysplasia can produce trabeculae similar to those of low-grade osteosarcoma, foam cells, common in fibrous dysplasia, are not present in osteosarcoma. Osteosarcoma can arise in fibrous dysplasia; when this rare occurrence does happen, the tumor is usually is of high grade (144). Parosteal osteosarcomas are extremely rare in the jaws. While the histologic features of parosteal osteosarcoma, particularly on a limited biopsy, may resemble the osseous proliferation in fibrous dysplasia, the clinical and radiographic findings of the two lesions are not similar.

In fine needle aspirations, the cytologic differential diagnosis always includes reactive osteoblasts that can mimic malignant osteoblasts; however, the chromatin pattern is not clumped and is more regular in reactive osteoblasts (135). The clinical and radiographic findings are of great importance in their separation.

Spread and Metastases. Osteosarcoma of the jaws is usually a locally aggressive disease but distant metastasis has been reported in up to 21 percent of patients (101).

Treatment and Prognosis. The treatment of osteosarcoma of the jaws is based on surgical therapy as the cornerstone with the goal of complete excision (98). The resection margins should be as wide as possible, with some authors suggesting a 1-cm margin as minimum, although in the craniofacial region attaining wide margins is more difficult than in long bones (90). Some investigators suggest that radiotherapy and chemotherapy should be considered in those cases where there are inadequate resection margins or distant spread (90).

In a study of osteosarcomas involving the jaws as well as extragnathic sites in the head and neck, Jasnau et al. (145) found that multidisciplinary treatment resulted in long-term survival in well over two thirds of affected patients. Extragnathic sites and failure to achieve and maintain local surgical control emerged as strong negative prognostic factors. Smeele et al. (146) in their study of craniofacial osteosarcomas also found that chemotherapy improved overall and disease-free survival.

For Van Es et al. (101) the overall 10-year survival rate was 59 percent. Distant metastasis occurred in 21 percent and local recurrences in 31 percent of the cases. Survival was significantly better for patients with small tumors and after radical surgery. Long-term survival after treatment was good if complete surgical excision was achieved.

The rarity of osteosarcoma of the jaws precludes large studies for the evaluation of chemotherapy or radiotherapy, as is the case for osteosarcoma of the long bones. Nevertheless, some patients have shown some benefit with chemotherapy (147). Using a small patient sample size, Theil et al. (148) concluded that radical resection of the tumor combined with high-dose chemotherapy, according to standard protocols, is the most effective treatment for craniofacial osteosarcomas. Chemotherapy given preoperatively must be assessed as to its effectiveness after the surgical resection. This requires examining the entire resected specimen and estimating the degree of tumor necrosis. This is best accomplished with tumor mapping of the resected bony specimen using published protocols (149). Tumors with less than 95 percent tumor necrosis are considered as nonresponders and patients are then given additional chemotherapy.

Guadagnolo et al. (150) investigated patient survival after receiving surgery alone versus surgery and radiotherapy. Some patients received chemotherapy in addition. The addition of radiotherapy improved overall survival and local control compared to surgery alone or surgery plus chemotherapy for patients with positive or uncertain resection margins. In a small series of patients, Nissanka (151) found that chemotherapeutic adjuvants in addition to surgery appeared to be more successful than radiotherapeutic adjuvants in addition to surgery.

Patient prognosis depends on the tumor grade and tumor size on presentation, as well as the completeness of initial surgery as monitored by resection margins (152). Fernandes et al. (91) reported that 12 of 14 patients with osteosarcoma of the jaws survived long term.

REFERENCES

Giant Cell Lesions

1. Jaffe HL. Giant-cell reparative granuloma, traumatic bone cyst, and fibrous (fibro-osseous) dysplasia of the jawbones. Oral Surg Oral Med Oral Pathol 1953;6:159-175.
2. Resnick CM, Margolis J, Susarla SM, et al. Maxillofacial and axial/appendicular giant cell lesions: unique tumors or variants of the same disease?—A comparison of phenotypic, clinical, and radiographic characteristics. J Oral Maxillofac Surg 2010;68:130-137.
3. Beneteau C, Cave H, Moncla A, et al. SOS1 and PTPN11 mutations in five cases of Noonan syndrome with multiple giant cell lesions. Eur J Hum Genet 2009;17:1216-1221.
4. Chrcanovic BR, Gomez RS, Freire-Maia B. Neurofibromatosis type 1 associated with bilateral central giant cell granuloma of the mandible. J Craniomaxillofac Surg 2011;39:538-543.
5. Orhan E, Erol S, Deren O, Sevin A, Ekici O, Erdogan B. Idiopathic bilateral central giant cell reparative granuloma of jaws: a case report and literature review. Int J Pediatr Otorhinolaryngol 2010;74:547-552.
6. Jackson CE, Norum RA, Boyd SB, et al. Hereditary hyperparathyroidism and multiple ossifying jaw fibromas: a clinically and genetically distinct syndrome. Surgery 1990;108:1006-12; discussion 1012-3.

7. Magalhaes DP, Osterne RL, Alves AP, Santos PS, Lima RB, Sousa FB. Multiple brown tumours of tertiary hyperparathyroidism in a renal transplant recipient: a case report. Med Oral Patol Oral Cir Bucal 2009;15:e10-13.

8. Waldron CA, Shafer WG. The central giant cell reparative granuloma of the jaws. An analysis of 38 cases. Am J Clin Pathol 1966;45:437-447.

9. Whitaker SB, Waldron CA. Central giant cell lesions of the jaws. A clinical, radiologic, and histopathologic study. Oral Surg Oral Med Oral Pathol 1993;75:199-208.

10. Sun ZJ, Cai Y, Zwahlen RA, Zheng YF, Wang SP, Zhao YF. Central giant cell granuloma of the jaws: clinical and radiological evaluation of 22 cases. Skeletal Radiol 2009;38:903-909.

11. Jadu FM, Pharoah MJ, Lee L, Baker GI, Allidina A. Central giant cell granuloma of the mandibular condyle: a case report and review of the literature. Dentomaxillofac Radiol 2011;40:60-64.

12. Auclair PL, Cuenin P, Kratochvil FJ, Slater LJ, Ellis GL. A clinical and histomorphologic comparison of the central giant cell granuloma and the giant cell tumor. Oral Surg Oral Med Oral Pathol 1988;66:197-208.

13. Kaffe I, Ardekian L, Taicher S, Littner MM, Buchner A. Radiologic features of central giant cell granuloma of the jaws. Oral Surg Oral Med Oral Pathol Oral Radiol Endod 1996;81:720-726.

14. Rovelo MO, Kim R, Mascarenhas L, Hammoudeh J, Urata MM. Recurrent and refractory giant cell tumor of the jaw. J Craniofac Surg 2009;20:2245-2248.

15. Abrams B, Shear M. A histological comparison of the giant cells in the central giant cell granuloma of the jaws and the giant cell tumor of long bone. J Oral Pathol 1974;3:217-223.

16. de Lima Mde D, de Aquino Xavier FC, Vanti LA, de Lima PS, de Sousa SC. Hybrid central giant cell granuloma and central odontogenic fibroma-like lesion of the mandible. Otolaryngol Head Neck Surg 2008;139:867-868.

17. Tosios KI, Gopalakrishnan R, Koutlas IG. So-called hybrid central odontogenic fibroma/central giant cell lesion of the jaws. A report on seven additional cases, including an example in a patient with cherubism, and hypotheses on the pathogenesis. Head Neck Pathol 2008;2:333-338.

18. Younis RH, Scheper MA, Lindquist CC, Levy B. Hybrid central odontogenic fibroma with giant cell granuloma-like component: case report and review of literature. Head Neck Pathol 2008;2:222-226.

19. Whitaker SB, Vigneswaran N, Budnick SD, Waldron CA. Giant cell lesions of the jaws: evaluation of nucleolar organizer regions in lesions of varying behavior. J Oral Pathol Med 1993;22:402-405.

20. Sadri D, Hejazi M, Jahanbani J, Forouzandeh A. Quantitative analysis of argyrophilic nuclear organizer regions in giant cell lesions of jaws. J Oral Pathol Med 2010;39:431-434.

21. O'Malley M, Pogrel MA, Stewart JC, Silva RG, Regezi JA. Central giant cell granulomas of the jaws: phenotype and proliferation-associated markers. J Oral Pathol Med 1997;26:159-163.

22. Torabinia N, Razavi SM, Shokrolahi Z. A comparative immunohistochemical evaluation of CD68 and TRAP protein expression in central and peripheral giant cell granulomas of the jaws. J Oral Pathol Med 2010;40:334-337.

23. Amaral FR, Brito JA, Perdigao PF, et al. NFATc1 and TNFalpha expression in giant cell lesions of the jaws. J Oral Pathol Med 2010;39:269-274.

24. Houpis CH, Tosios KI, Papavasileiou D, et al. Parathyroid hormone-related peptide (PTHrP), parathyroid hormone/parathyroid hormone-related peptide receptor 1 (PTHR1), and MSX1 protein are expressed in central and peripheral giant cell granulomas of the jaws. Oral Surg Oral Med Oral Pathol Oral Radiol Endod 2010;109:415-424.

25. Susarla SM, August M, Dewsnup N, Faquin WC, Kaban LB, Dodson TB. CD34 staining density predicts giant cell tumor clinical behavior. J Oral Maxillofac Surg 2009;67:951-956.

26. Minic A, Stajcic Z. Prognostic significance of cortical perforation in the recurrence of central giant cell granulomas of the jaws. J Craniomaxillofac Surg 1996;24:104-108.

27. Shirani G, Abbasi AJ, Mohebbi SZ, Shirinbak I. Management of a locally invasive central giant cell granuloma (CGCG) of mandible: report of an extraordinary large case. J Craniomaxillofac Surg 2011;39:530-533.

28. Romero M, Romance A, Garcia-Recuero I, Fernandez A. Orthopedic and orthodontic treatment in central giant cell granuloma treated with calcitonin. Cleft Palate Craniofac J 2011;48:519-525.

29. Allon DM, Anavi Y, Calderon S. Central giant cell lesion of the jaw: nonsurgical treatment with calcitonin nasal spray. Oral Surg Oral Med Oral Pathol Oral Radiol Endod 2009;107:811-818.

30. Tosco P, Tanteri G, Iaquinta C, et al. Surgical treatment and reconstruction for central giant cell granuloma of the jaws: a review of 18 cases. J Craniomaxillofac Surg 2009;37:380-387.

31. Nogueira RL, Teixeira RC, Cavalcante RB, Ribeiro RA, Rabenhosrt SH. Intralesional injection of triamcinolone hexacetonide as an alternative treatment for central giant-cell granuloma in 21 cases. Int J Oral Maxillofac Surg 2010;39:1204-1210.

32. Suarez-Roa Mde L, Reveiz L, Ruiz-Godoy Rivera LM, et al. Interventions for central giant cell granuloma (CGCG) of the jaws. Cochrane Database Syst Rev. 2009;(4):CD007404.

33. de Moraes M, Sato FR, Germano AR, Bastos PL. Distraction osteogenesis of iliac bone graft as a reconstruction after central giant cell granuloma curettage. Implant Dent 2009;18:126-131.

Cherubism

34. Jones WA. Familial multilocular cystic disease of the jaws. Am J Cancer 1933;17:946-950.

35. Jones WA. Further observations regarding familial multilocular cystic disease of the jaws. Br J Radiol 1938;11:227-241.

36. Peters WJ. Cherubism: a study of twenty cases from one family. Oral Surg Oral Med Oral Pathol 1979;47:307-311.

37. Lietman SA, Prescott NL, Hicks DG, Westra WH, Levine MA. SH3BP2 is rarely mutated in exon 9 in giant cell lesions outside cherubism. Clin Orthop Relat Res 2007;459:22-27.

38. Idowu BD, Thomas G, Frow R, Diss TC, Flanagan AM. Mutations in SH3BP2, the cherubism gene, were not detected in central or peripheral giant cell tumours of the jaw. Br J Oral Maxillofac Surg 2008;46:229-230.

39. Brix M, Peters H, Lebeau J. [Cherubism.] Rev Stomatol Chir Maxillofac 2009;110:293-298. [French]

40. Carvalho VM, Perdigao PF, Amaral FR, de Souza PE, De Marco L, Gomez RS. Novel mutations in the SH3BP2 gene associated with sporadic central giant cell lesions and cherubism. Oral Dis 2009;15:106-110.

41. Mukherjee PM, Wang CJ, Chen IP, et al. Cherubism gene Sh3bp2 is important for optimal bone formation, osteoblast differentiation, and function. Am J Orthod Dentofacial Orthop 2010;138:140-141.

42. Wang CJ, Chen IP, Koczon-Jaremko B, et al. Pro-416Arg cherubism mutation in Sh3bp2 knock-in mice affects osteoblasts and alters bone mineral and matrix properties. Bone 2010;46:1306-1315.

43. Dunlap C, Neville B, Vickers RA, O'Neil D, Barker B. The Noonan syndrome/cherubism association. Oral Surg Oral Med Oral Pathol 1989;67:698-705.

44. Betts NJ, Stewart JC, Fonseca RJ, Scott RF. Multiple central giant cell lesions with a Noonan-like phenotype. Oral Surg Oral Med Oral Pathol 1993;76:601-607.

45. Suhanya J, Aggarwal C, Mohideen K, Jayachandran S, Ponniah I. Cherubism combined with epilepsy, mental retardation and gingival fibromatosis (Ramon syndrome): a case report. Head Neck Pathol 2010;4:126-131.

46. Lee JY, Jung YS, Kim SA, Lee SH, Ahn SG, Yoon JH. Investigation of the SH3BP2 gene mutation in cherubism. Acta Med Okayama 2008;62:209-212.

47. Mortellaro C, Bello L, Lucchina AG, Pucci A. Diagnosis and treatment of familial cherubism characterized by early onset and rapid development. J Craniofac Surg 2009;20:116-120.

48. Pontes FS, Ferreira AC, Kato AM, et al. Aggressive case of cherubism: 17-year follow-up. Int J Pediatr Otorhinolaryngol 2007;71:831-835.

49. Raposo-Amaral CE, de Campos Guidi M, Warren SM, et al. Two-stage surgical treatment of severe cherubism. Ann Plast Surg 2007;58:645-651.

50. de Lange J, van den Akker HP, Scholtemeijer M. Cherubism treated with calcitonin: report of a case. J Oral Maxillofac Surg 2007;65:1665-1667.

Aneurysmal Bone Cyst

51. Ye Y, Pringle LM, Lau AW, et al. TRE17/USP6 oncogene translocated in aneurysmal bone cyst induces matrix metalloproteinase production via activation of NF-kappaB. Oncogene 2010;29:3619-3629.

52. Oliveira AM, Perez-Atayde AR, Inwards CY, et al. USP6 and CDH11 oncogenes identify the neoplastic cell in primary aneurysmal bone cysts and are absent in so-called secondary aneurysmal bone cysts. Am J Pathol 2004;165:1773-1780.

53. Jaffe HL, Lichtenstein L. Solitary unicameral bone cyst: with emphasis on the roentgen picture, the pathologic appearance and the pathogenesis. Arch Surg 1942;44:1004-1025.

54. Lichtenstein L. Aneurysmal bone cyst: observations on fifty cases. J Bone Joint Surg 1957;39A:873-882.

55. Sun ZJ, Sun HL, Yang RL, Zwahlen RA, Zhao YF. Aneurysmal bone cysts of the jaws. Int J Surg Pathol 2009;17:311-322.

56. Toljanic JA, Lechewski E, Huvos AG, Strong EW, Schweiger JW. Aneurysmal bone cysts of the jaws: a case study and review of the literature. Oral Surg Oral Med Oral Pathol 1987;64:72-77.

57. Levy WM, Miller AS, Bonakdarpour A, Aegerter E. Aneurysmal bone cyst secondary to other osseous lesions. report of 57 cases. Am J Clin Pathol 1975;63:1-8.

58. Motamedi MH, Navi F, Eshkevari PS, et al. Variable presentations of aneurysmal bone cysts of the jaws: 51 cases treated during a 30-year period. J Oral Maxillofac Surg 2008;66:2098-2103.

59. Kershisnik M, Batsakis JG. Aneurysmal bone cysts of the jaws. Ann Otol Rhinol Laryngol 1994;103:164-165.

60. Matt BH. Aneurysmal bone cyst of the maxilla: case report and review of the literature. Int J Pediatr Otorhinolaryngol. 1993;25:217-226.

61. Warner BF, Luna MA, Robert Newland T. Temporomandibular joint neoplasms and pseudotumors. Adv Anat Pathol 2000;7:365-381.

62. Kaffe I, Naor H, Calderon S, Buchner A. Radiological and clinical features of aneurysmal bone cyst of the jaws. Dentomaxillofac Radiol 1999;28:167-172.

63. Vergel De Dios AM, Bond JR, Shives TC, McLeod RA, Unni KK. Aneurysmal bone cyst. A clinicopathologic study of 238 cases. Cancer 1992;69:2921-2931.

64. Hudson TM. Fluid levels in aneurysmal bone cysts: a CT feature. AJR Am J Roentgenol 1984;142:1001-1004.

65. Hudson TM, Hamlin DJ, Fitzsimmons JR. Magnetic resonance imaging of fluid levels in an aneurysmal bone cyst and in anticoagulated human blood. Skeletal Radiol 1985;13:267-270.

66. Bertoni F, Bacchini P, Capanna R, et al. Solid variant of aneurysmal bone cyst. Cancer 1993;71:729-734.

67. Perrotti V, Rubini C, Fioroni M, Piattelli A. Solid aneurysmal bone cyst of the mandible. Int J Pediatr Otorhinolaryngol 2004;68:1339-1344.

68. Ettl T, Stander K, Schwarz S, Reichert TE, Driemel O. Recurrent aneurysmal bone cyst of the mandibular condyle with soft tissue extension. Int J Oral Maxillofac Surg 2009;38:699-703.

Osteoma

69. Unni KK, Inwards CY, Kindblom LG, Wold LE. Tumors of the bones and joints. AFIP Atlas of Tumor Pathology, 4th Series, Fascicle 2. Washington, DC: American Registry of Pathology; 2005.

70. Kubo K, Miyatani H, Takenoshita Y, et al. Widespread radiopacity of jaw bones in familial adenomatosis coli. J Craniomaxillofac Surg 1989;17:350-353.

71. Lee BD, Lee W, Oh SH, Min SK, Kim EC. A case report of Gardner syndrome with hereditary widespread osteomatous jaw lesions. Oral Surg Oral Med Oral Pathol Oral Radiol Endod 2009;107:e68-72.

72. Sayan NB, Ucok C, Karasu HA, Gunhan O. Peripheral osteoma of the oral and maxillofacial region: A study of 35 new cases. J Oral Maxillofac Surg 2002;60:1299-1301.

73. Woldenberg Y, Nash M, Bodner L. Peripheral osteoma of the maxillofacial region. Diagnosis and management: a study of 14 cases. Med Oral Patol Oral Cir Bucal 2005;10(Suppl 2):E139-142.

74. Iatrou IA, Leventis MD, Dais PE, Tosios KI. Peripheral osteoma of the maxillary alveolar process. J Craniofac Surg 2007;18:1169-1173.

75. Johann AC, de Freitas JB, de Aguiar MC, de Araujo NS, Mesquita RA. Peripheral osteoma of the mandible: case report and review of the literature. J Craniomaxillofac Surg 2005;33:276-281.

76. Kamel SG, Kau CH, Wong ME, Kennedy JW, English JD. The role of cone beam CT in the evaluation and management of a family with Gardner's syndrome. J Craniomaxillofac Surg 2009;37:461-468.

77. Kaplan I, Nicolaou Z, Hatuel D, Calderon S. Solitary central osteoma of the jaws: a diagnostic dilemma. Oral Surg Oral Med Oral Pathol Oral Radiol Endod 2008;106:e22-29.

78. Chen CT, Adriane K. Endoscopic resection of a mandibular body and condylar osteoma. Minim Invasive Ther Allied Technol 2008;17:323-325.

Osteoblastoma/Osteoid Osteoma

79. Unni KK, Inwards CY, Kindblom LG, Wold LE. Tumors of the bones and joints. AFIP Atlas of Tumor Pathology, 4th Series, Fascicle 2. Washington, DC: American Registry of Pathology; 2005:119-134.

80. Slootweg PJ. Cementoblastoma and osteoblastoma: a comparison of histologic features. J Oral Pathol Med 1992;21:385-389.

81. van der Waal I, Greebe RB, Elias EA. Benign osteoblastoma or osteoid osteoma of the maxilla. Report of a case. Int J Oral Surg 1983;12:355-358.

82. Capodiferro S, Maiorano E, Giardina C, Lacaita MG, Lo Muzio L, Favia G. Osteoblastoma of the mandible: clinicopathologic study of four cases and literature review. Head Neck 2005;27:616-621.

83. Jones AC, Prihoda TJ, Kacher JE, Odingo NA, Freedman PD. Osteoblastoma of the maxilla and mandible: a report of 24 cases, review of the literature, and discussion of its relationship to osteoid osteoma of the jaws. Oral Surg Oral Med Oral Pathol Oral Radiol Endod 2006;102:639-650.

84. el-Mofty S, Refai H. Benign osteoblastoma of the maxilla. J Oral Maxillofac Surg 1989;47:60-64.

85. Ida M, Kurabayashi T, Takahashi Y, Takaqi M, Sasaki T. Osteoid osteoma in the mandible. Dentomaxillofac Radiol 2002;31:385-387.

86. Dorfman HD, Weiss SW. Borderline osteoblastic tumors: problems in the differential diagnosis of aggressive osteoblastoma and low-grade osteosarcoma. Semin Diagn Pathol 1984;1:215-234.

87. Ohkubo T, Hernandez JC, Ooya K, Krutchkoff DJ. "Aggressive" osteoblastoma of the maxilla. Oral Surg Oral Med Oral Pathol 1989;68:69-73.

88. Rawal YB, Angiero F, Allen CM, Kalmar JR, Sedghizadeh PP, Steinhilber AM. Gnathic osteoblastoma: Clinicopathologic review of seven cases with long-term follow-up. Oral Oncol 2006;42:123-130.

89. Wozniak AW, Nowaczyk MT, Osmola K, Golusinski W. Malignant transformation of an osteoblastoma of the mandible: case report and review of the literature. Eur Arch Otorhinolaryngol 2010;267:845-849.

Osteosarcoma

90. Ketabchi A, Kalavrezos N, Newman L. Sarcomas of the head and neck: a 10-year retrospective of 25 patients to evaluate treatment modalities, function and survival. Br J Oral Maxillofac Surg 2010;49:116-120.

91. Fernandes R, Nikitakis NG, Pazoki A, Ord RA. Osteogenic sarcoma of the jaw: a 10-year experience. J Oral Maxillofac Surg 2007;65:1286-1291.

92. Azizi T, Motamedi MH, Jafari SM. Gnathic osteosarcomas: a 10-year multi-center demographic study. Indian J Cancer 2009;46:231-233.

93. Chindia ML. Osteosarcoma of the jaw bones. Oral Oncol 2001;37:545-547.

94. Ottaviani G, Jaffe N. The epidemiology of osteosarcoma. Cancer Treat Res 2010;152:3-13.

95. Chidzonga MM, Mahomva L. Sarcomas of the oral and maxillofacial region: A review of 88 cases in Zimbabwe. Br J Oral Maxillofac Surg 2007;45:317-318.

96. Batsakis JG. Osteogenic and chondrogenic sarcomas of the jaws. Ann Otol Rhinol Laryngol 1987;96:474-475.

97. Delgado R, Maafs E, Alfeiran A, et al. Osteosarcoma of the jaw. Head Neck 1994;16:246-252.

98. Unni KK, Inwards CY, Kindblom LG, Wold LE. Tumors of the bones and joints. AFIP Atlas of Tumor Pathology, 4th Series, Fascicle 2. Washington, DC: American Registry of Pathology; 2005:149-150.

99. Tanzawa H, Uchiyama S, Sato K. Statistical observation of osteosarcoma of the maxillofacial region in Japan. Analysis of 114 Japanese cases reported between 1930 and 1989. Oral Surg Oral Med Oral Pathol 1991;72:444-448.

100. Clark JL, Unni KK, Dahlin DC, Devine KD. Osteosarcoma of the jaw. Cancer 1983;51:2311-2316.

101. van Es RJ, Keus RB, van der Waal I, Koole R, Vermey A. Osteosarcoma of the jaw bones. Long-term follow up of 48 cases. Int J Oral Maxillofac Surg 1997;26:191-197.

102. Ajagbe HA, Junaid TA, Daramola JO. Osteogenic sarcoma of the jaw in an African community: report of twenty-one cases. J Oral Maxillofac Surg 1986;44:104-106.

103. Singh HB, Singh H, Chakraborty M. Metastatic osteosarcoma of the maxilla. J Laryngol Otol 1978;92:619-622.

104. Dayal PK, Patil S, Suvarna P, Srinivasan SV. Maxillary metastasis of osteosarcoma. Indian J Dent Res 1997;8:86-89.

105. Nakamura T, Ishimaru J, Mizui T, et al. Osteosarcoma metastatic to the mandible: A case report. Oral Surg Oral Med Oral Pathol Oral Radiol Endod 2001;91:452-454.

106. Vincent SD, Lilly GE, Ruskin JD. Recurrent enlargement of the left maxillary alveolus. J Oral Maxillofac Surg 1993;51:671-675.

107. Cheng YS, Wright JM, Walstad WR, Finn MD. Osteosarcoma arising in Paget's disease of the mandible. Oral Oncol 2002;38:785-792.

108. Larizza L, Roversi G, Volpi L. Rothmund-Thomson syndrome. Orphanet J Rare Dis 201029;5:2.

109. McGuff HS, Heim-Hall J, Holsinger FC, Jones AA, O'Dell DS, Hafemeister AC. Maxillary osteosarcoma associated with a dental implant: report of a case and review of the literature regarding implant-related sarcomas. J Am Dent Assoc 2008;139:1052-1059.

110. Kasthoori JJ, Wastie ML. Radiation-induced osteosarcoma of the maxilla. Singapore Med J 2006;47:907-909.

111. Prakash O, Varghese BT, Mathews A, Nayak N, Ramchandran K, Pandey M. Radiation induced osteogenic sarcoma of the maxilla. World J Surg Oncol 2005;3:49.

112. Chabchoub I, Gharbi O, Remadi S, et al. Postirradiation osteosarcoma of the maxilla: a case report and current review of literature. J Oncol 2009;2009:876138.

113. Bennett JH, Thomas G, Evans AW, Speight PM. Osteosarcoma of the jaws: a 30-year retrospective review. Oral Surg Oral Med Oral Pathol Oral Radiol Endod 2000;90:323-332.

114. Bianchi SD, Boccardi A. Radiological aspects of osteosarcoma of the jaws. Dentomaxillofac Radiol 1999;28:42-47.

115. Petrikowski CG, Pharoah MJ, Lee L, Grace MG. Radiographic differentiation of osteogenic sarcoma, osteomyelitis, and fibrous dysplasia of the jaws. Oral Surg Oral Med Oral Pathol Oral Radiol Endod 1995;80:744-750.

116. Slootweg PJ, Muller H. Osteosarcoma of the jaw bones. Analysis of 18 cases. J Maxillofac Surg 1985;13:158-166.

117. Yagan R, Radivoyevitch M, Bellon EM. Involvement of the mandibular canal: early sign of osteogenic sarcoma of the mandible. Oral Surg Oral Med Oral Pathol 1985;60:56-60.

118. Lee YY, Van Tassel P, Nauert C, Raymond AK, Edeiken J. Craniofacial osteosarcomas: plain film, CT, and MR findings in 46 cases. AJR Am J Roentgenol 1988;150:1397-1402.

119. Shao Z, He Y, Wang L, Hu H, Shi H. Computed tomography findings in radiation-induced osteosarcoma of the jaws. Oral Surg Oral Med Oral Pathol Oral Radiol Endod 2010;109:e88-94.

120. Isokane M, Sumida T, Okuhira T, Shintani S, Hamakawa H. Surface osteosarcoma: 2 case reports. Am J Otolaryngol 2006;27:349-352.

121. Hewitt KM, Ellis G, Wiggins R, Bentz BG. Parosteal osteosarcoma: case report and review of the literature. Head Neck 2008;30:122-126.

122. Bianchi SD, Boccardi A, Pomatto E, Valente G. Parosteal osteosarcoma of the maxilla. Dentomaxillofac Radiol 1997;26:312-314.

123. Piattelli A, Favia GF. Periosteal osteosarcoma of the jaws: report of 2 cases. J Periodontol 2000;71:325-329.

124. Newland JR, Ayala AG. Parosteal osteosarcoma of the maxilla. Oral Surg Oral Med Oral Pathol 1977;43:727-734.

125. Raubenheimer EJ, Noffke CE. Low-grade intraosseous osteosarcoma of the jaws. Oral Surg Oral Med Oral Pathol Oral Radiol Endod 1998;86:82-85.

126. Ruiz-Godoy RL, Meneses-Garcia A, Mosqueda-Taylor A, De la Garza-Salazar J. Well-differentiated intraosseous osteosarcoma of the jaws: experience of two cases from the Instituto Nacional de Cancerologia, Mexico. Oral Oncol 1999;35:530-533.

127. Chan CW, Kung TM, Ma L. Telangiectatic osteosarcoma of the mandible. Cancer 1986;58:2110-2115.

128. Cozza R, Devito R, De Ioris MA, et al. Epithelioid osteosarcoma of the jaw. Pediatr Blood Cancer 2009;52:877-879.

129. Diniz AF, Filho JA, Alencar Rde C, et al. Low-grade central osteosarcoma of the mandible: a case study report. Oral Surg Oral Med Oral Pathol Oral Radiol Endod 2007;103:246-252.

130. Zhao W, Cure J, Castro CY. Low-grade osteosarcoma of the jaw. Ann Diagn Pathol 2002;6:373-377.

131. Regezi JA, Zarbo RJ, McClatchey KD, Courtney RM, Crissman JD. Osteosarcomas and chondrosarcomas of the jaws: immunohistochemical correlations. Oral Surg Oral Med Oral Pathol 1987;64:302-307.

132. Kim J, Ellis GL, Mounsdon TA. Usefulness of antikeratin immunoreactivity in osteosarcomas of the jaw. Oral Surg Oral Med Oral Pathol 1991;72:213-217.

133. Oliveira P, Nogueira M, Pinto A, Almeida MO. Analysis of p53 expression in osteosarcoma of the jaw: correlation with clinicopathologic and DNA ploidy findings. Hum Pathol 1997;28:1361-1365.

134. Junior AT, de Abreu Alves F, Pinto CA, Carvalho AL, Kowalski LP, Lopes MA. Clinicopathological and immunohistochemical analysis of twenty-five head and neck osteosarcomas. Oral Oncol 2003;39:521-530.

135. Akerman M, Domanski HA, Jonsson K. Cytological features of bone tumours in FNA smears I: osteogenic tumours. Monogr Clin Cytol 2010;19:18-30.

136. Bridge JA, Nelson M, McComb E, et al. Cytogenetic findings in 73 osteosarcoma specimens and a review of the literature. Cancer Genet Cytogenet 1997;95:74-87.

137. Kansara M, Thomas DM. Molecular pathogenesis of osteosarcoma. DNA Cell Biol 2007;26:1-18.

138. Baird K, Davis S, Antonescu CR, et al. Gene expression profiling of human sarcomas: insights into sarcoma biology. Cancer Res 2005;65:9226-9235.

139. Leonard P, Sharp T, Henderson S, et al. Gene expression array profile of human osteosarcoma. Br J Cancer 2003;89:2284-2288.

140. Sadikovic B, Yoshimoto M, Al-Romaih K, Maire G, Zielenska M, Squire JA. In vitro analysis of integrated global high-resolution DNA methylation profiling with genomic imbalance and gene expression in osteosarcoma. PLoS One 2008;3:e2834.

141. Sadikovic B, Yoshimoto M, Chilton-MacNeill S, Thorner P, Squire JA, Zielenska M. Identification of interactive networks of gene expression associated with osteosarcoma oncogenesis by integrated molecular profiling. Hum Mol Genet 2009;18:1962-1975.

142. Davicioni E, Wai DH, Anderson MJ. Diagnostic and prognostic sarcoma signatures. Mol Diagn Ther 2008;12:359-374.

143. Yamashiro M, Komori A. Osteosarcoma mimicking fibrous dysplasia of the jaw. Int J Oral Maxillofac Surg 1987;16:112-115.

144. Present D, Bertoni F, Enneking WF. Osteosarcoma of the mandible arising in fibrous dysplasia. A case report. Clin Orthop Relat Res 1986;(204):238-244.

145. Jasnau S, Meyer U, Potratz J, et al. Craniofacial osteosarcoma experience of the cooperative German-Austrian-Swiss osteosarcoma study group. Oral Oncol 2008;44:286-294.

146. Smeele LE, Kostense PJ, van der Waal I, Snow GB. Effect of chemotherapy on survival of craniofacial osteosarcoma: a systematic review of 201 patients. J Clin Oncol 1997;15:363-367.

147. Oda D, Bavisotto LM, Schmidt RA, et al. Head and neck osteosarcoma at the University of Washington. Head Neck 1997;19:513-523.

148. Thiele OC, Freier K, Bacon C, Egerer G, Hofele CM. Interdisciplinary combined treatment of craniofacial osteosarcoma with neoadjuvant and adjuvant chemotherapy and excision of the tumour: a retrospective study. Br J Oral Maxillofac Surg 2008;46:533-536.

149 Abdul-Karim FW, Bauer TW, Kilpatrick SE, Raymond KA, Siegal GP, Association of Directors of Anatomic and Surgical Pathology. Recommendations for the reporting of bone tumors. Association of Directors of Anatomic and Surgical Pathology. Hum Pathol 2004;35:1173-1178.

150. Guadagnolo BA, Zagars GK, Raymond AK, Benjamin RS, Sturgis EM. Osteosarcoma of the jaw/ craniofacial region: outcomes after multimodality treatment. Cancer 2009;115:3262-3270.

151. Nissanka EH, Amaratunge EA, Tilakaratne WM. Clinicopathological analysis of osteosarcoma of jaw bones. Oral Dis 2007;13:82-87.

152. Lewis M, Perl A, Som PM, Urken ML, Brandwein MS. Osteogenic sarcoma of the jaw. A clinicopathologic review of 12 patients. Arch Otolaryngol Head Neck Surg 1997;123:169-174.

15 FIBROUS LESIONS

CONGENITAL FIBROMATOSIS (MYOFIBROMATOSIS)

Definition. *Congenital fibromatosis* is a proliferative process in which there is a neoplastic proliferation characterized by cells with a spindled appearance, best categorized as myofibroblasts. Usually this process is a solitary proliferation but multiple sites can be affected, and rarely, there is visceral involvement. Synonyms include *infantile myofibromatosis, myofibroma* (for a single lesion), or *myofibromatosis* (when multiple lesions exist).

General Features. Congenital fibromatosis is the most common fibroblastic-myofibroblastic tumor in children and adolescents (1). Most patients are infants, under the age of 2 years. Nevertheless, congenital fibromatosis can occur in older children and adolescents as well as adults, prompting some authorities to prefer the term myofibroma or myofibromatosis. The tumors are well recognized for their ability to spontaneously regress (2–4). The process manifests as solitary, multicentric, or generalized (5). The head and neck region is the most common site of occurrence and, in children, the mandible is the most frequently affected site. Mandibular involvement in adults is unusual (2,3,6).

Clinical Features. The lesions can present as an asymptomatic jaw expansion (7). Those in tooth-bearing areas can result in tooth mobility or tooth displacement.

Radiographic Features. On plain radiographic films, congenital fibromatosis appears most often as a unilocular radiolucency but a few are multilocular (4). When unilocular and in association with a tooth, the radiographic features mimic those of an odontogenic cyst (3,8). Shibuya et al. (9) reported an increased uptake on positron emission spectroscopy (PET) in a myofibroma in a 12-year-old. The lesions can attain a large size and push surrounding structures. The assessment of many of these lesions is often best appreciated on computerized tomography (CT) or magnetic resonance images (MRI) (figs. 15-1, 15-2).

Microscopic Findings. Histologically, congenital fibromatosis has several interesting features. Unni et al. (10) emphasize the distinctly nodular appearance and note, overall, that the lesion is hypocellular (fig. 15-3). Nuclear atypia is not present. Others have described a zoning arrangement with the peripheral portions of the tumor having a spindle cell morphology while the center has cells that are smaller with pale round nuclei. The spindled tumor cells have tapered nuclei and pale pink cytoplasm.

Immunohistochemical Findings. Immunohistochemical studies are positive for vimentin and alpha-smooth muscle actin. Sugatani et al. (2) found no tumors positive for desmin, S-100 protein, neuron-specific enolase, or myoglobin.

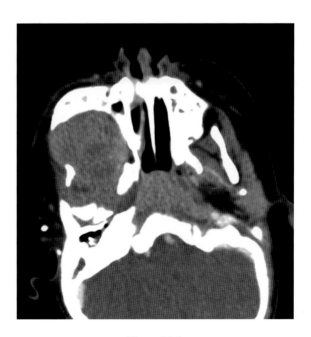

Figure 15-1

CONGENITAL FIBROMATOSIS

Computerized tomography (CT) image of maxillary involvement by congenital fibromatosis.

215

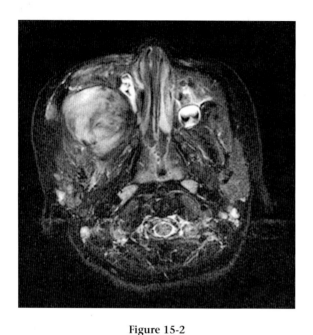

Figure 15-2

CONGENITAL FIBROMATOSIS

Magnetic resonance imaging (MRI) reveals the pushing, rounded border of congenital fibromatosis.

Genetic Findings. Some controversy exists about the inheritance of this disease. A recent paper by Zand et al. (11) suggests that in familial cases, an autosomal dominant rather than an autosomal recessive process occurs.

Differential Diagnosis. The differential diagnosis includes a sarcoma with spindle cells such as leiomyosarcoma. Most leiomyosarcomas have significant nuclear atypia and lack the zoning pattern of congenital fibromatosis. Juvenile fibromatosis, an aggressive lesion, should be eliminated (12). Infantile fibrosarcoma is much more cellular (5).

Treatment and Prognosis. Unless the tumor causes loss of function, no specific treatment is necessary and many lesions resolve with no surgical intervention. Infants with visceral involvement have a poor clinical outlook.

DESMOPLASTIC FIBROMA

Definition. *Desmoplastic fibroma* is a histologically benign but locally aggressive intraosseous tumor with a high likelihood of local

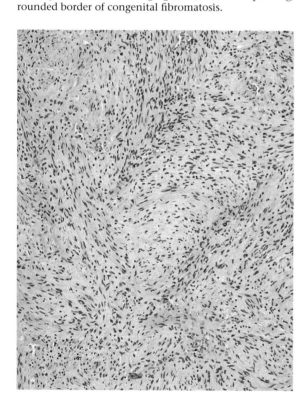
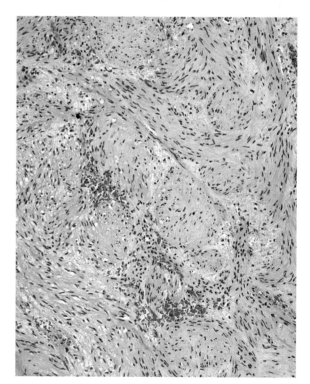

Figure 15-3

CONGENITAL FIBROMATOSIS

Left: Spindled cells are arranged in a loose, nodular pattern. The cells have pink, eosinophilic cytoplasm.
Right: Congenital fibromatosis often shows a nodular pattern.

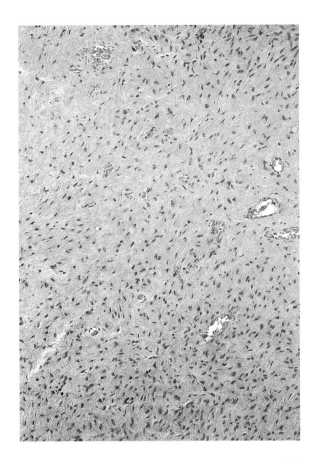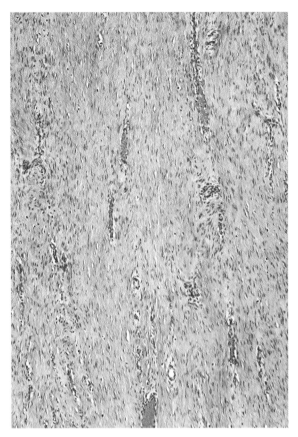

Figure 15-4

DESMOPLASTIC FIBROMA

Left: Small, curvilinear nuclei are set in a dense collagenous stroma.
Right: Dense collagen contains nearly parallel arrangements of spindled cells with small elongated nuclei.

recurrence. It is the osseous counterpart of soft tissue fibromatosis (desmoid tumor).

General Features. The osseous counterpart of extraosseous fibromatosis, desmoplastic fibroma is most commonly noted in the long bones and the mandible (13,14). First reported in the jaws in 1965, this neoplasm is rare (15). Less than 80 jaw cases were noted in a literature review by Schneider in 2009 (16).

The gender distribution is essentially equal. Age distribution ranges from the first to the sixth decades but most patients present before the end of the third decade (17,18).

Clinical Features. At least 75 percent of the jaw tumors involve the mandible (13,19). Whether in the mandible or maxilla, most tumors are posterior but an anterior location can be seen (20). Pain is an unusual symptom, and most patients report a mass effect of swelling.

Radiographic Features. Radiographically, the tumors are similar to their counterparts in the long bones and are seen as lytic and expansile lesions (21). They can be unilocular or multilocular, with or without a sclerotic margin. These findings are not specific for desmoplastic fibroma, however, and a large number of odontogenic lesions have a similar appearance (13).

Microscopic Findings. Desmoplastic fibroma is a densely collagenous spindle-cell lesion with variable cellularity (figs. 15-4, 15-5). The nuclei are usually spindle-shaped to elongated and lack pleomorphism or other signs of atypia. While the overall cellularity is low, occasional areas of higher cellularity can be seen. Mitoses may present but are rare and never atypical.

Cytogenetic Findings. Trisomy 8 and trisomy 20, considered to be nonrandom changes,

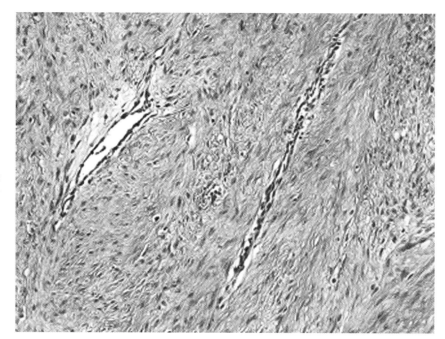

Figure 15-5

DESMOPLASTIC FIBROMA

Some slit-like vascular spaces are present in a dense, collagenous stroma.

have been noted in desmoplastic fibroma, similar to the findings in other histologically benign fibrous lesions such as desmoid tumors and fibrous dysplasia (22).

Differential Diagnosis. The differential diagnosis includes intraosseous low-grade fibrosarcoma, low-grade osteosarcoma, fibrous dysplasia, and in very young individuals, infantile myofibromatosis. Infantile myofibromatosis is generally seen in patients under 2 years of age. Paradoxically, infantile myofibromatosis is usually more cellular and mitotically active. Myofibromatosis is also often multifocal and thus the clinical findings are suggestive of the process. Low-grade sarcomas, such as fibrosarcoma and osteosarcoma, show atypical nuclear features. Osteosarcoma produces osteoid whereas desmoplastic fibroma does not; however, limited biopsies of osteosarcoma could sample areas with no osteoid. Fibrosarcoma, another rare tumor, may be extremely difficult to separate from desmoplastic fibroma but similar to osteosarcoma, it has nuclear atypia. The amount of osseous material in fibrous dysplasia is variable and the spindled component can be mistaken for desmoplastic fibroma.

Treatment and Prognosis. Complete excision is preferable for achieving control of the lesion rather than curettage (13). Some investigators have suggested that more cellular lesions are more likely to recur (23).

FIBROSARCOMA

Definition. *Fibrosarcoma* is a malignant mesenchymal tumor composed of collagen-producing spindle cells.

General Features. Fibrosarcoma of bone is an uncommon tumor and fibrosarcoma of the jaws is even rarer. Out of 271 fibrosarcomas originating in bone, 7.0 and 4.1 percent were found in the mandible and maxillary regions, respectively, in a Mayo Clinic series (24). Of 24 fibrosarcomas occurring in Sweden between the years 1958 and 1968, 2 were located in the jaws (25). The average age of patients is in the third decade but reported cases involve patients from the first through the sixth decades (25–29). The etiology of fibrosarcoma in the jaws is not clear but it has been reported to occur following radiation to the head (30,31).

Clinical and Radiographic Features. The mandible is more often affected than the maxilla. No specific gender is more likely to be affected. Some patients present with painless swelling, although pain or paresthesia may be encountered. Temporomandibular joint malfunction has been noted (32–34). Radiographs reveal a predominantly lytic process that can involve the cortex or break through into the soft tissues. Teeth overlying the tumor seem to float over the neoplasm when their apices are involved (26).

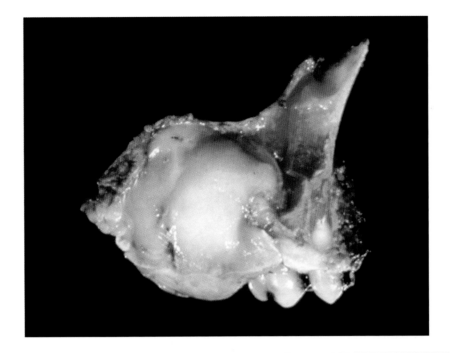

Figure 15-6

FIBROSARCOMA

Fibrosarcoma arising in the jaw.

Figure 15-7

FIBROSARCOMA

Low-power microscopy reveals the interlacing patterns in fibrosarcoma.

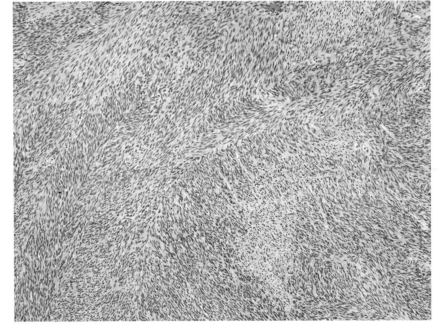

Gross and Microscopic Findings. Grossly, fibrosarcomas are fleshy tumors that often invade with a pushing border on gross observation (fig. 15-6). At the microscopic level, however, fingers of tumor cells infiltrate the surrounding tissues. The neoplasm is composed of spindle cells arranged in fascicles with a herringbone pattern (figs. 15-7, 15-8). Varying degrees of cellularity and collagen deposition are present (figs. 15-9, 15-10). The nuclei are elongated with rounded or tapered ends (fig. 15-11). Fibrosarcomas with an abundant myxoid component are termed *myxoid fibrosarcomas*. These tumors have been occasionally reported in the jaw (35).

Fibrosarcomas are graded by the degree of cellularity and nuclear atypia; usually these two findings move in concert with one another, with increasing cellularity paralleling an increase in

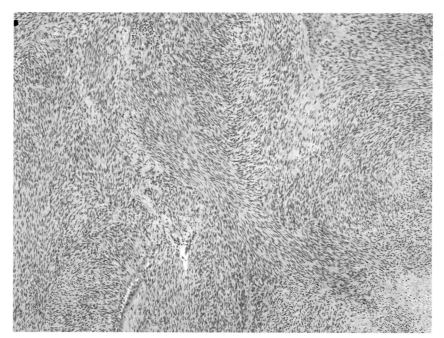

Figure 15-8

FIBROSARCOMA

Intersecting bundles of spindled cells are evident.

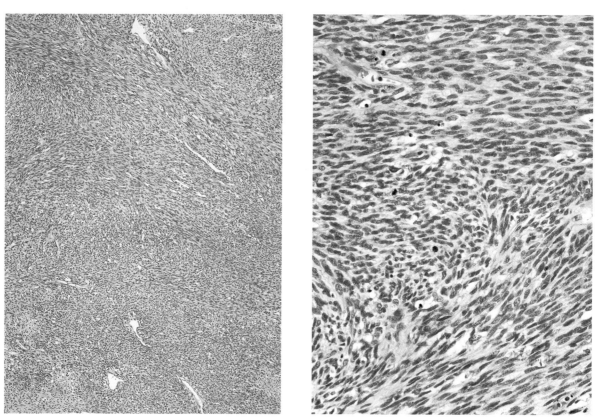

Figure 15-9

FIBROSARCOMA

Left: A herringbone arrangement of cells is present.
Right: Intersecting bundles of cells with hyperchromatic nuclei and dark pink cytoplasm are seen.

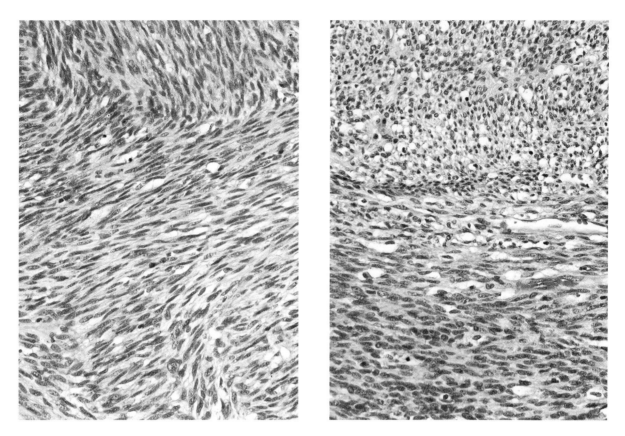

Figure 15-10

FIBROSARCOMA

Left: Nuclear atypia is evidenced by irregular nuclear chromatin and nuclear hyperchromasia.
Right: Bundles of atypical cells are arranged in alternating directions.

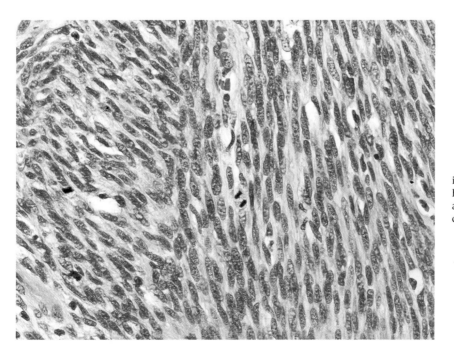

Figure 15-11

FIBROSARCOMA

Mitotic figures are present in this fibrosarcoma. The nuclei have blunt to rounded ends and the nuclear chromatin is clumped.

nuclear atypia. The nuclei of the lowest grade tumors, grade 1, have minimal atypia with little hyperchromasia or irregularity. These tumors are also of lower cellularity and only occasional mitotic figures are evident. Grade 2 tumors have more nuclear atypia, increased mitoses, and greater cellularity with less collagen production. Grade 3 tumors have much less collagen and are very cellular. Necrosis can be seen.

Fibrosarcomas are positive for vimentin by immunohistochemistry but essentially no other markers of differentiation are consistently positive (35,36).

Differential Diagnosis. Desmoplastic fibroma can mimic low-grade fibrosarcoma but, in general, desmoplastic fibroma is less cellular. High-grade fibrosarcoma must be differentiated from osteosarcoma but the latter has a mineralized matrix.

Odontogenic sarcomas could enter into the differential diagnosis although these lesions are uncommon. Reichart (37) reported the transformation of an ameloblastic fibroma to an ameloblastic fibrosarcoma.

Spread and Metastases. Fibrosarcomas of the jaws recur locally and metastases to visceral organs, including lung, kidney, and spleen, as well as bone metastases, have been reported (27,32).

Treatment and Prognosis. Complete excision of the tumor is required for adequate therapy and this may require a radical procedure. Insufficient evidence is present to clearly indicate whether or not adjuvant therapy should be administered, although there are numerous case reports where radiotherapy as well as chemotherapy have been used in addition to surgery (36). Because of the low number of cases of fibrosarcoma occurring in the jaws, the exact survival rate is difficult to ascertain. When fibrosarcoma of all bones is considered, the overall survival rate at 10 years has varied from 21.8 to 83.0 percent. As in all neoplasms, stage, histologic grade of malignancy, and local recurrences are critical prognostic indicators (36).

REFERENCES

Congenital Fibromatosis

1. Coffin CM, Dehner LP. Fibroblastic-myofibroblastic tumors in children and adolescents: a clinicopathologic study of 108 examples in 103 patients. Pediatr Pathol 1991;11:569-588.
2. Sugatani T, Inui M, Tagawa T, Seki Y, Mori A, Yoneda J. Myofibroma of the mandible. Clinicopathologic study and review of the literature. Oral Surg Oral Med Oral Pathol Oral Radiol Endod 1995;80:303-309.
3. Oliver RJ, Coulthard P, Carre C, Sloan P. Solitary adult myofibroma of the mandible simulating an odontogenic cyst. Oral Oncol 2003;39:626-629.
4. Allon I, Vered M, Buchner A, Dayan D. Central (intraosseous) myofibroma of the mandible: clinical, radiologic, and histopathologic features of a rare lesion. Oral Surg Oral Med Oral Pathol Oral Radiol Endod 2007;103:e45-53.
5. Alaggio R, Barisani D, Ninfo V, Rosolen A, Coffin CM. Morphologic overlap between infantile myofibromatosis and infantile fibrosarcoma: a pitfall in diagnosis. Pediatr Dev Pathol 2008;11:355-362.
6. Foss RD, Ellis GL. Myofibromas and myofibromatosis of the oral region: a clinicopathologic analysis of 79 cases. Oral Surg Oral Med Oral Pathol Oral Radiol Endod 2000;89:57-65.
7. Vigneswaran N, Boyd DL, Waldron CA. Solitary infantile myofibromatosis of the mandible. Report of three cases. Oral Surg Oral Med Oral Pathol 1992;73:84-88.
8. Sedghizadeh PP, Allen CM, Kalmar JR, Miloro M, Suster S. Solitary central myofibroma presenting in the gnathic region. Ann Diagn Pathol 2004;8:284-289.
9. Shibuya Y, Takeuchi J, Sakaguchi H, Yokoo S, Umeda M, Komori T. Myofibroma of the mandible. Kobe J Med Sci 2008;54:E169-173.
10. Unni KK, Inwards CY, Kindblom LG, Wold, LE. Tumors of the bones and joints. AFIP Atlas of Tumor Pathology, 4th Series, Fascicle 2. Washington, DC: American Registry of Pathology; 2005:345-346.
11. Zand DJ, Huff D, Everman D, et al. Autosomal dominant inheritance of infantile myofibromatosis. Am J Med Genet A 2004;126A:261-266.

12. Slootweg PJ, Müller H. Localized infantile myofibromatosis. Report of a case originating in the mandible. J Maxillofac Surg 1984;12:86-89.

Desmoplastic Fibroma

13. Said-Al-Naief N, Fernandes R, Louis P, Bell W, Siegal GP. Desmoplastic fibroma of the jaw: a case report and review of literature. Oral Surg Oral Med Oral Pathol Oral Radiol Endod 2006;101:82-94.

14. Inwards CY, Unni KK, Beabout JW, Sim FH. Desmoplastic fibroma of bone. Cancer 1991;68:1978-1983.

15. Griffith JG, Irby WB. Desmoplastic fibroma. Report of a rare tumor of the oral structures. Oral Surg Oral Med Oral Pathol 1965;20:269-275.

16. Schneider M, Zimmermann AC, Depprich RA, et al. Desmoplastic fibroma of the mandible—review of the literature and presentation of a rare case. Head Face Med 2009;5:25.

17. Vally IM, Altini M. Fibromatoses of the oral and paraoral soft tissues and jaws. Review of the literature and report of 12 new cases. Oral Surg Oral Med Oral Patholc 1990;69:191-198.

18. Templeton K, Glass N, Young SK. Desmoplastic fibroma of the mandible in a child: report of a case. Oral Surg Oral Med Oral Pathol Oral Radiol Endod 1997;84:620-623.

19. Hopkins KM, Huttula CS, Kahn MA, Albright JE. Desmoplastic fibroma of the mandible: review and report of two cases. J Oral Maxillofac Surg 1996;54:1249-1254.

20. Reid EN, Lawoyin DO, Suresh L, Longwe E. Desmoplastic fibroma of the anterior mandible. Case report and review of literature. N Y State Dent J 2009;75:32-33.

21. Young JW, Aisner SC, Levine AM, Resnik CS, Dorfman HD. Computed tomography of desmoid tumors of bone: desmoplastic fibroma. Skeletal Radiol 1988;17:333-337.

22. Bridge JA, Swarts SJ, Buresh C, et al. Trisomies 8 and 20 characterize a subgroup of benign fibrous lesions arising in both soft tissue and bone. Am J Pathol 1999;154:729-733.

23. Kwon PH, Horswell BB, Gatto DJ. Desmoplastic fibroma of the jaws: surgical management and review of the literature. Head Neck 1989;11:67-75.

Fibrosarcoma

24. Unni KK, Inwards CY, Kindblom LG, Wold, LE. Tumors of the bones and joints. AFIP Atlas of Tumor Pathology, 4th Series, Fascicle 2. Washington, DC: American Registry of Pathology; 2005:196-199.

25. Larsson SE, Lorentzon R, Boquist L. Fibrosarcoma of bone. A demographic, clinical and histopathological study of all cases recorded in the Swedish cancer registry from 1958 to 1968. J Bone Joint Surg Br 1976;58-B:412-417.

26. Taconis WK, van Rijssel TG. Fibrosarcoma of the jaws. Skeletal Radiol 1986;15:10-13.

27. Slootweg PJ, Müller H. Fibrosarcoma of the jaws. A study of 7 cases. J Maxillofac Surg 1984;12:157-162.

28. Gosau M, Draenert FG, Winter WA, Mueller-Hoecker J, Driemel O. Fibrosarcoma of the childhood mandible. Head Face Med 2008;4:21.

29. Bang G, Baardsen R, Gilhuus-Moe O. Infantile fibrosarcoma in the mandible: case report. J Oral Pathol Med 1989;18:339-343.

30. Ferlito A, Recher G, Tomazzoli L. Radiation-induced fibrosarcoma of the mandible following treatment for bilateral retinoblastoma. J Laryngol Otol 1979;93:1015-1020.

31. Moloy PJ, Kowal KA, Siegel WM. Fibrosarcoma of the mandible following supravoltage irradiation. Report of a case. Arch Otolaryngol Head Neck Surg 1989;115:1250-1252.

32. Soares AB, Lins LH, Macedo AP, Pereira-Neto JS, Vargas PA. Fibrosarcoma originating in the mandible. Med Oral Patol Oral Cir Bucal 2006;11: E243-246.

33. Orhan K, Orhan AI, Oz U, Pekiner FN, Delilbasi C. Misdiagnosed fibrosarcoma of the mandible mimicking temporomandibular disorder: a rare condition. Oral Surg Oral Med Oral Pathol Oral Radiol Endod 2007;104:e26-29.

34. Herrera AF, Mercuri LG, Petruzzelli G, Rajan P. Simultaneous occurrence of 2 different low-grade malignancies mimicking temporomandibular joint dysfunction. J Oral Maxillofac Surg 2007;65:1353-1358.

35. Angiero F, Rizzuti T, Crippa R, Stefani M. Fibrosarcoma of the jaws: two cases of primary tumors with intraosseous growth. Anticancer Res 2007;27:2573-2581.

36. Pereira CM, Jorge J Jr, Di Hipolito O Jr, Kowalski LP, Lopes MA. Primary intraosseous fibrosarcoma of jaw. Int J Oral Maxillofac Surg 2005;34:579-581.

37. Reichart PA, Zobl H. Transformation of ameloblastic fibroma to fibrosarcoma. Int J Oral Surg 1978;7:503-507.

16 HEMATOPOIETIC TUMORS

LANGERHANS CELL HISTIOCYTOSIS

Definition. *Langerhans cell histiocytosis* is a disease in which there is a proliferation of abnormal Langerhans cells.

General Features. Langerhans cells are specialized histiocytic cells that are defined, in part, by their specific ultrastructural features and antigenic determinants. Normal Langerhans cells are nonclonal dendritic cells with important immune regulating functions related to antigen presenting properties (1). In contrast, the Langerhans cells in Langerhans cell histiocytosis are clonal (2). Three clinically distinct disease processes comprise Langerhans cell histiocytosis: *eosinophilic granuloma, Hand-Schuller-Christian disease,* and *Letterer-Siwe disease.* Although the terminology for these diseases has changed over time, the clinical findings have been recognized for more than eight decades. It was not until the 1940s and 1950s that these three diseases were understood to be related and formed a spectrum. Initially grouped together under the name *histiocytosis X,* Langerhans cell histiocytosis has been the most recent appellation and serves as a good functional description.

Clinical Features. The clinical features depend on the form of Langerhans cell histiocytosis. Eosinophilic granuloma is the most common form and presents as a solitary bone lesion, usually involving the skull bones but also affecting the long bones and ribs. In Hand-Schuller-Christian disease, multiple lesions are present in a single tissue type, most often bone (so-called multifocal unisystem involvement). In Letterer-Siwe disease, many organ systems are involved with many lesions occurring in the organs involved (multifocal multisystem involvement). This disease is generally restricted to infants.

Another form of the disease, which does not affect the jaws, is the pulmonary-only disease. This disease, restricted to the lungs, is highly correlated to smoking tobacco and can regress when the patient stops smoking.

There is an equal gender distribution except in the pulmonary-only disease, which affects women twice as often as men. Langerhans cell histiocytosis is most often found in children, usually in the first several years of life and more than 50 percent are under 15 years of age (3). In children, the disease occurs most often in the bone, with bone pain one of the most common complaints. While adults can be affected, they less frequently have bone involvement.

When Langerhans cell histiocytosis occurs in the jaws, the mandible is more frequently affected than the maxilla. The teeth are frequently displaced. Radiographically, lesions in the jaws are radiolucent and unilocular and most have a well-demarcated border (4,5).

Microscopic Findings. Normal Langerhans cells occur in the basal layer of the epithelium and are 12 to 15 μm in diameter. The Langerhans cells in Langerhans cell histiocytosis are slightly larger but otherwise have a similar morphology. The cell cytoplasm is pale and eosinophilic. The nucleus is single (mononuclear) and appears to have a groove or fold. Biopsies of the lesion reveal non-Langerhans histiocytes, small lymphocytes, and eosinophils, in addition to the Langerhans cells (fig. 16-1). It is frequently the eosinophils admixed with the pale Langerhans cells that bring attention to the process as Langerhans cell histiocytosis. Eosinophils can be variable in number and are occasionally absent. Necrosis is common and a granulomatous appearance may be seen.

Despite finding the classic microscopic features of Langerhans cell histiocytosis by hematoxylin and eosin (H&E) staining, confirmation of the diagnosis requires immunohistochemical stains.

Immunohistochemical Findings. CD1a is the marker of choice for establishing the histologic diagnosis of Langerhans cell histiocytosis (fig. 16-2). Another marker, CD207, has become available, which binds to the langerin protein. Langerin, found on the surface of Langerhans

225

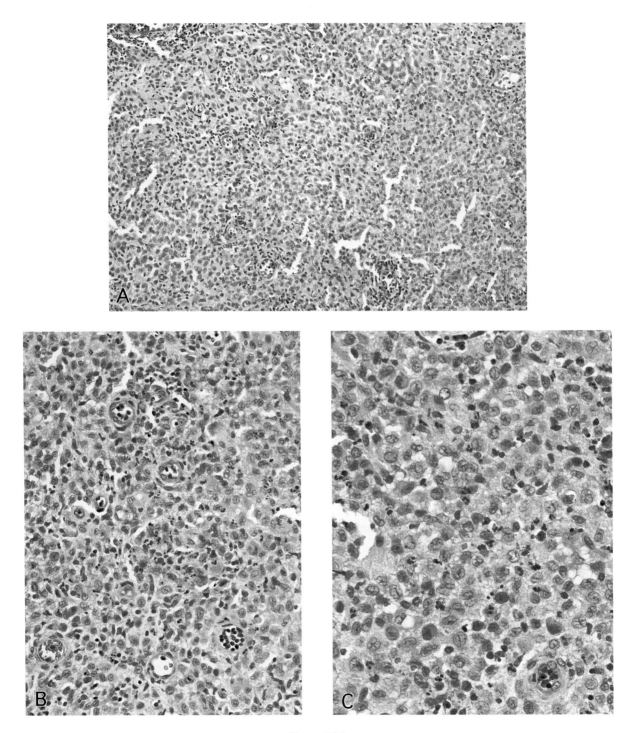

Figure 16-1

LANGERHANS CELL HISTIOCYTOSIS

A: A sheet of cells with indistinctly defined cytoplasmic borders contains scattered lymphocytes. The nuclei are pale and round to oval.

B: The nuclei are vesicular and the cytoplasm of the cells is pale pink. Scattered neutrophils and eosinophils are present in addition to lymphocytes.

C: Eosinophils and neutrophils are present. The nuclei of the Langerhans cells are irregular and many contain a groove. The nuclei display a small nucleolus.

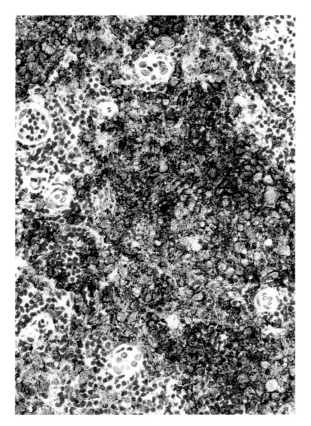

Figure 16-2

LANGERHANS CELL HISTIOCYTOSIS

CD1a staining is present in the Langerhans cells.

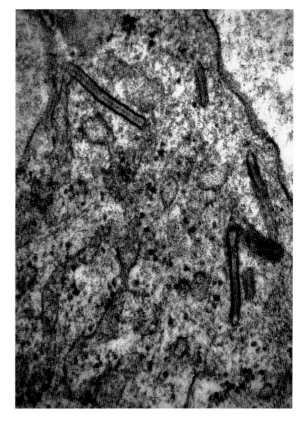

Figure 16-3

LANGERHANS CELL HISTIOCYTOSIS

Detail of a Birbeck granule shows a trilaminar structure and drumstick-shaped extremity.

cells, helps induce Birbeck granule formation (1). Nevertheless, CD1a is the only marker required for the confirmation of the histologic findings. As in the interpretation of any immunohistochemical stain, the expression of CD1a must occur in the correct histologic background of Langerhans cells, eosinophils, and lymphocytes that make up the lesion of Langerhans cell histiocytosis. S-100 protein is also positive in the Langerhans cells but is not specific, giving little practical reason for its use.

Ultrastructural Findings. The Birbeck granule is the characteristic and defining ultrastructural observation by electron microscopy. It is an intracytoplasmic, pentalaminar body that is 250- to 450-nm long with a zipper-like handle, best described as a "tennis racket" (fig. 16-3). Birbeck granules are fragile and often destroyed by usual formalin fixation with paraffin process-

ing although in some cases the organelles are present in electron microscopic preparations derived from deparaffinized tissue.

Differential Diagnosis. Because of the varying mixture of inflammatory cells, osteomyelitis is a consideration in the differential diagnosis. Small vessel proliferation is present in osteomyelitis, a finding absent in Langerhans cell histiocytosis. Acute osteomyelitis has more neutrophils and does not contain the mixture of eosinophils and numerous CD1a-positive Langerhans cells. Chronic osteomyelitis can more difficult to separate histologically, particularly if the tumor has few eosinophils. The radiographic appearance of a radiolucent lesion with well-demarcated borders favors Langerhans cell histiocytosis.

Treatment and Prognosis. In at least half of all cases involving the jaws, surgical curettage of the osseous lesion is often sufficient. Isolated

227

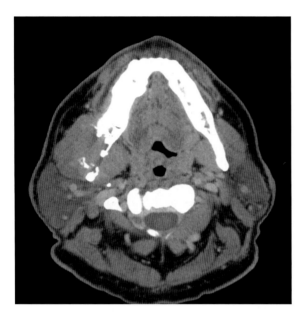

Figure 16-4

PLASMACYTOMA/MYELOMA

Computerized tomography (CT) image of a destructive lesion in the mandible as the result of involvement by multiple myeloma.

lesions are also treated by steroid injection. Single lesions of bone are usually eradicated with these limited treatments. Radiotherapy can be used if necessary in lesions that cannot be treated by excision or curettage. Those patients with multiple sites of involvement, particularly visceral involvement such as the liver, have a much worse prognosis.

PLASMACYTOMA/MULTIPLE MYELOMA

Definition. *Plasmacytoma* is a clonal proliferation of malignant plasma cells occurring in a single location. *Multiple myeloma* is a clonal proliferation of abnormal plasma cells occurring as a disseminated bone marrow disease with associated clinical and laboratory abnormalities.

General Features. Multiple myeloma usually presents in patients past 50 years of age and accounts for approximately 10 to 15 percent of all hematopoietic neoplasms (6) Witt et al. (7) found that 46.7 percent of 77 patients had involvement of the skull bones and 15.6 percent had jaw involvement. In a study of plasma cell neoplasia involving the jaws, Lae et al. (8) noted that two thirds were solitary plasmacytomas of

bone and the remainder represented involvement by multiple myeloma. Importantly, of the solitary lesions, nearly half converted to multiple myeloma in 20.7 months on average. To establish a diagnosis of multiple myeloma, some authorities require both a demonstration of at least 10 percent or more clonal plasma cells in the bone marrow or a biopsy-proven plasmacytoma in conjunction with other evidence of disease or end-organ damage such as other bone lesions or other findings such as anemia or renal insufficiency that are considered to be due to the plasma cell process. Clinical laboratory tests for myeloma include testing for abnormal M proteins with serum protein electrophoresis, serum free light chain assays, and serum immunofixation (6–8).

Clinical Features. There is some variance in the literature as to the most common site in the jaws for plasma cell neoplasia to occur. Most reports find the mandible to be the most common site but in some series the maxilla is more commonly affected (8–11). Clinical manifestations include pain, loose teeth, and occasionally numbness in the lip or chin (10). Some patients have exophytic lesions on the alveolar ridge. The clinical differential diagnosis is wide and includes metastatic carcinoma, odontogenic tumors, traumatic bone cyst, and infection. Radiographically, the lesions are often seen as punched-out osteolytic areas with or without a rim of sclerosis. The tumors can enlarge and be locally destructive (fig. 16-4).

Microscopic Findings. Solitary plasmacytoma and multiple myeloma show similar findings. An almost pure population of plasma cells is evident. These cells have the features of plasma cells, with an eccentrically placed nucleus that has clumped peripheral chromatin giving the characteristic clock-face nucleus. In H&E-stained sections of bone, however, the cytoplasm can shrink around the cell and the eccentricity of the nucleus is not pronounced or even evident (fig. 16-5).

The degree of nuclear atypia varies from minimal to marked. Amyloid production is seen in approximately 15 percent of cases. Immunohistochemistry shows light chain restriction.

Cytologic Findings. The cytologic diagnosis is often straightforward in patients with known multiple myeloma since the aspirate reveals a

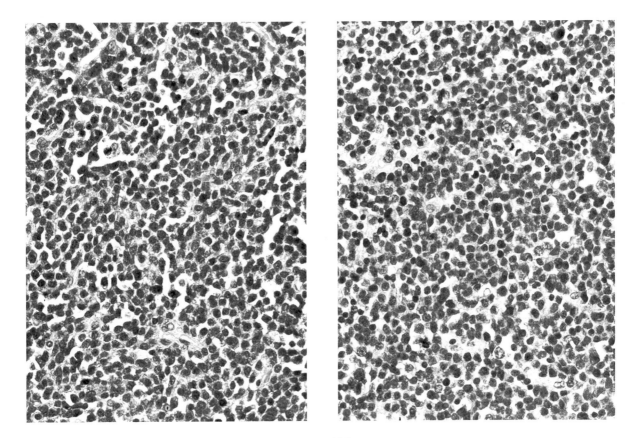

Figure 16-5

PLASMACYTOMA/MYELOMA

Left: The hematoxylin and eosin (H&E)-stained sections of decalcified bone involved by a plasma cell neoplasm can be initially deceptive. Although the appearance is that of a hematologic malignancy, the shrinkage of the cytoplasm and the nucleus makes initial recognition of a plasma cell neoplasm difficult. This image shows a monotonous population of small cells with round dark nuclei. Some of the nuclei exhibit a clock-face chromatin pattern. In some cells, the nucleus is in an eccentric location.

Right: The eccentrically placed nuclei in the amphophilic cytoplasm of the tumor cells is seen.

near pure population of plasma cells (fig. 16-6). The cytoplasm of the plasma cells is pale pink to gray using Giemsa-type stains. Binucleate forms are often easily found.

Even in cases of undiagnosed multiple myeloma or solitary plasmacytoma the diagnosis is usually not a significant dilemma because of the abundance of the almost pure population of plasma cells.

Cytogenic Findings. Multiple myeloma demonstrates numerous chromosomal abnormalities. Trisomies are common and involve chromosomes 3, 5, 7, 9, 11, 15, 19, and 21. Deletions in chromosome 13 are seen in over half of cases. While the individual chromosomal abnormalities are not specific, the disease can be separated into two groups based on whether the chromosomal gains or losses result in a hyperdiploid or nonhyperdiploid karyotype. A little over half (55 to 60 percent) of patients have a hyperdiploid karyotype. The other nonhyperdiploid group includes near-diploid, pseudodiploid, hypodiploid, and near tetraploid chromosomal numbers. The ploidy abnormalities rarely change even as the disease progresses. Patients with a hyperdiploid karyotype (chromosomes ranging from 48 to 74) have a better prognosis than those with a nonhyperdiploid karyotype (12,13). Patients whose tumors have deletions in chromosome 13 also have a worse outcome.

Nonrandom translocations involving the immunoglobulin heavy chain (IgH) locus (14q32.2) are seen in 20 to 40 percent of

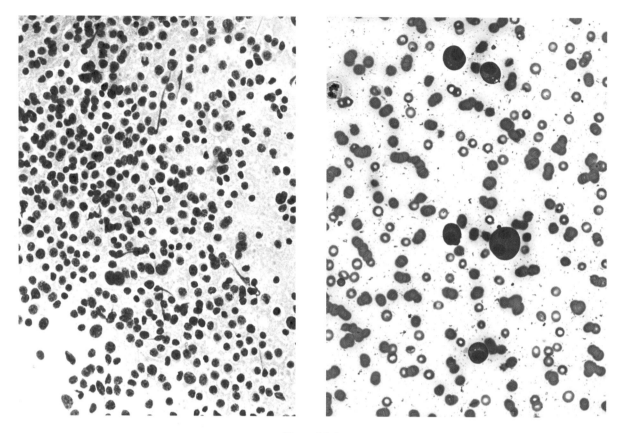

Figure 16-6

PLASMACYTOMA/MYELOMA

Left: This touch preparation of a bone biopsy of a plasmacytoma more readily reveals the classic appearance of cells with pale, delicate amphophilic cytoplasm and eccentrically placed nuclei.

Right: A fine needle aspirate of a lytic lesion of the mandible shows few plasma cells, but in this background of only a single neutrophil and accompanying red blood cells, the findings of nearly all plasma cells are suggestive of a plasma cell neoplasm and confirmatory studies such as flow cytometry or serum studies for abnormal proteins should be carried out. A binucleate form is present.

myeloma cells and some of these induce the expression of cyclins. Less frequently, the immunoglobulin light chain (IgL) locus (2p12 [kappa] or 22q11[lambda]) is involved (12).

Differential Diagnosis. In osteomyelitis, numerous plasma cells can be seen, and inflammatory lesions of the gingiva can also have sheets of plasma cells. In inflammatory processes, however, there is a mixture of lymphocytes and capillaries along with scattered neutrophils.

Treatment and Prognosis. Radiotherapy is advocated for solitary lesions (plasmacytoma) while chemotherapy is given for multiple myeloma. Chemotherapeutic regimens alone or combined with autologous stem cell transplantation are used (14,15). While chemotherapy

can result in a long-term favorable response, the overall prognosis of patients with multiple myeloma is poor.

MALIGNANT LYMPHOMA

Lymphoma is a neoplasm consisting of malignant lymphoid cells, either T or B type. In the bone it usually represents systemic disease but can represent a primary tumor.

When considering lymphomatous involvement of the jaws, endemic Burkitt lymphoma occurring in children of equatorial Africa usually is the classically associated subtype. In adults, the majority of lymphomas involving bone are diffuse large B-cell type. The non-Burkitt lymphomas and Burkitt lymphoma are considered separately.

Non-Burkitt Lymphoma

Clinical Features. When *non-Burkitt lymphoma* involves bone, it usually does so in the red bone marrow and affects sites such as the vertebrae, pelvis, and long bones of the extremities. The jaws are not often affected but when it is, the maxilla and mandible are the usual sites (16). In a Mayo Clinic series of lymphomas involving bone (17), 3.9 percent affected the mandible and 1.1 percent affected the maxilla. Although most adult lymphomas in bone are *diffuse large B-cell lymphoma*, other types are possible, including *follicular lymphoma, extranodal marginal zone lymphoma,* and *small lymphocytic lymphoma/small lymphocytic leukemia.* Patients with non-Burkitt lymphoma of the jaws are usually in the fifth to eighth decades. The gender predilection varies between studies, with some showing no pronounced gender differences while others showing more involvement in men (16,18–20). Patients most often present with swelling and some may experience pain. Occasionally there is numbness of the chin with localized swelling (16, 21).

Hodgkin lymphoma can involve bone but most cases are systemic manifestations of the disease. Hodgkin lymphoma of the jaw is rare and in the few cases reported, only several have represented primary involvement (22).

Radiographically, the findings of lymphomatous involvement of bone are not specific. They include sclerosis, lytic changes, or a mixture of sclerosis and lysis giving rise to a moth-eaten or permeative destructive pattern (fig. 16-7) (16,23–25).

Microscopic Findings. Diffuse large B-cell lymphoma in the bone has an infiltrative growth pattern that often does not destroy bone trabeculae but permeates in and around them. The trabeculae appear thinned or in some cases normal. Lymphomas in the bone rarely produce a mass. Under high microscopic power, the atypical lymphocytes in diffuse large B-cell lymphoma have a vesicular nucleus that is the same size as or slightly larger than a macrophage nucleus. There is prominent membrane-bound chromatin (fig. 16-8). The polymorphous cellular pattern includes numerous small and medium-sized lymphocytes. In some cases, lymphoma in bone has a markedly sclerotic appearance or even clearing of the cytoplasm (17).

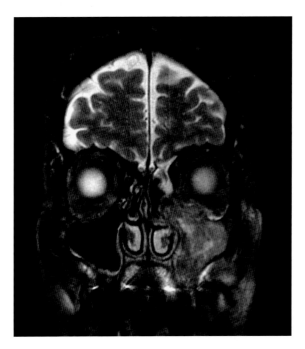

Figure 16-7

MALIGNANT LYMPHOMA

Magnetic resonance image (MRI) shows a large B-cell lymphoma arising in the maxilla. There is destruction of the maxillary bone and the tumor has spilled into the maxillary sinus.

Immunohistochemical and Cytogenetic Findings. Diffuse large B-cell lymphomas express CD45 and CD20 (fig. 16-9) (26). Genetic abnormalities are common in lymphomas of bone but none are specific enough to indicate a subtype of lymphoma. In diffuse large cell lymphoma, translocations (t3;14) involving the *BCL6* (3q27) and *IgH* genes (14q32) are common.

Differential Diagnosis. The histologic differential diagnosis includes small cell tumors of bone including small cell osteosarcoma, Langerhans cell histiocytosis, and leukemia (27). Lymphoblastic lymphoma can be difficult to differentiate from Ewing sarcoma (27).

Some lymphomas have molecular and immunohistochemical features of both Burkitt lymphoma and large B-cell lymphoma (so-called B-cell lymphoma, unclassifiable, with features intermediate between diffuse large B-cell lymphoma and Burkitt lymphoma) (28,29). While their occurrence in the jaws is not reported as yet, B-cell lymphoma, unclassifiable, should be considered for those tumors in which features

231

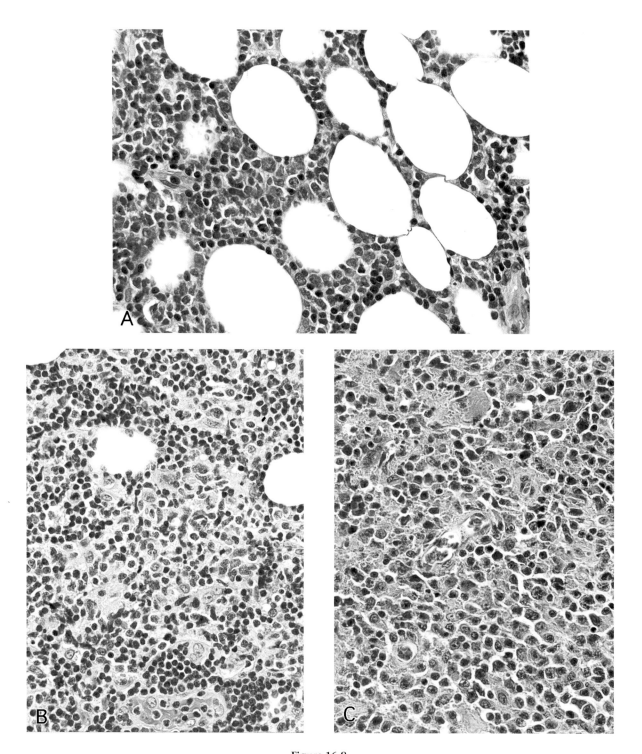

Figure 16-8

MALIGNANT LYMPHOMA

A: The bone marrow of this jaw large B-cell lymphoma is replaced by large lymphoid cells, many containing an enlarged nucleolus. As often is the case for hematopoietic neoplasms, the tumor cells push in and around surrounding mesenchymal tissues, in this case bone marrow fat, rather than completely replacing the tissue.

B: In this large B-cell lymphoma, the contrast of cell size in the large lymphocytes is apparent.

C: There are one to several prominent nucleoli in the cells of this large B-cell lymphoma.

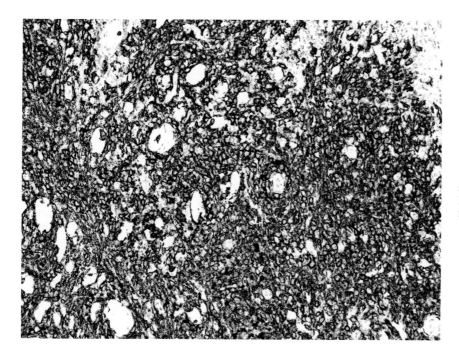

Figure 16-9

MALIGNANT LYMPHOMA

Intense membranous CD20 staining of the cells in the large B-cell lymphoma illustrated in figure 16-8.

of Burkitt lymphoma and diffuse large B-cell lymphoma are both present (30).

Treatment and Prognosis. Radiotherapy is used for localized disease in bone, as is chemotherapy (20). If a diagnosis of primary lymphoma of bone is established, the patient must undergo imaging studies for the evaluation of potential spread or multifocality of the disease. In a study involving lymphomas of the oral cavity by van der Waal et al. (21) in which nearly all the patients had diffuse large B-cell lymphoma, the mean survival time was 38 months, with a mean recurrence-free time of 31 months.

Burkitt Lymphoma

Clinical Features. Burkitt lymphoma presents as three clinicopathologic types: endemic, sporadic, and acquired immunodeficiency syndrome (AIDS) related. *Endemic Burkitt lymphoma* usually occurs in equatorial Africa, is associated with Epstein-Barr virus (EBV), and usually occurs in children. The jaws are affected, usually the mandible, in at least half the cases. There is involvement of the kidneys and gonads as well. *Sporadic Burkitt lymphoma* affects the terminal ileum and Waldeyer ring in children and young adults in the Western hemisphere. EBV is found in approximately a quarter of the cases. In sporadic Burkitt lymphoma, only about 15

percent of patients have mandibular involvement and there is an equal incidence in children and adults. When compared to endemic Burkitt lymphoma, usually only one quadrant of the jaw is involved (31–33).

Microscopic Findings. Burkitt lymphoma is defined by the World Health Organization (WHO) classification as a highly aggressive non-Hodgkin lymphoma consisting of monomorphic medium-sized B cells with basophilic cytoplasm containing vacuoles, best appreciated on smears. A starry-sky appearance is due to the numerous histiocytes engulfing the abundant apoptotic material present in this rapidly proliferating tumor (fig. 16-10) (34). The tumor cells have round nuclei with multiple nucleoli, clumped chromatin, and numerous mitotic figures (fig. 16-11).

Immunohistochemical Findings. Burkitt lymphoma cells have a germinal center phenotype and express CD10, CD19, CD20, CD22, CD79a, and BCL6 as well as surface IgM. They are negative for BCL2, Mum-1, and CD138. Ki-67 is positive in 95 to 100 percent of the cells (fig. 16-12).

Molecular Findings and Other Special Techniques. In endemic Burkitt lymphoma, EBV is positive in nearly all cases while for sporadic cases that number drops to 25 percent. Almost all cases have a translocation involving

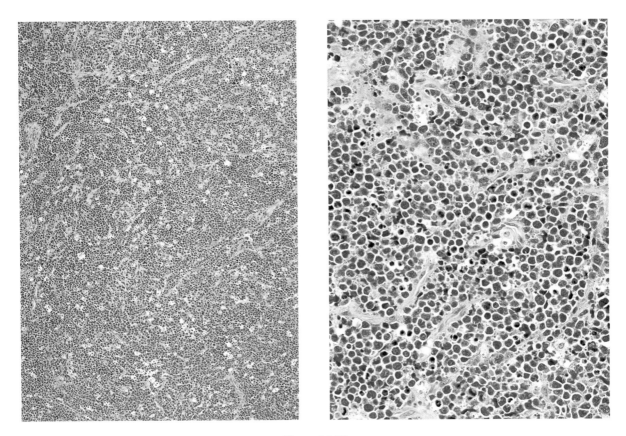

Figure 16-10

BURKITT LYMPHOMA

Left: A low-power microscopic view reveals a starry-sky pattern.
Right: The tingible body macrophages, giving the low-power starry-sky appearance, have engulfed cellular debris.

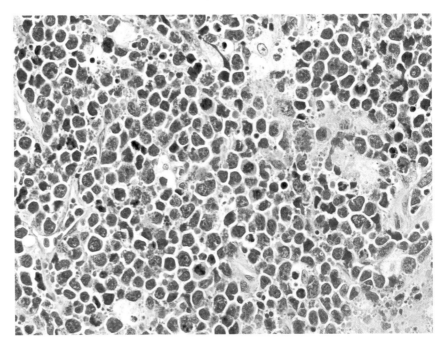

Figure 16-11

BURKITT LYMPHOMA

Burkitt lymphoma is characterized by a high mitotic rate.

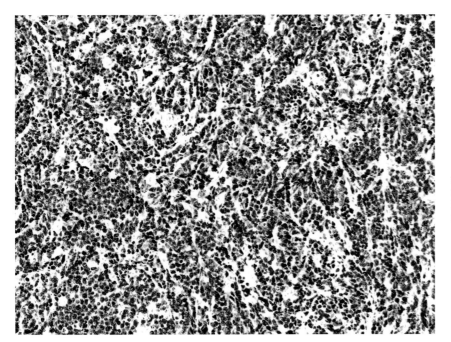

Figure 16-12

BURKITT LYMPHOMA

Nearly every cell is positive with the immunohistochemical stain for MIB-1, indicating the high cell proliferation rate of this neoplasm.

the *MYC* gene (8q24) and an immunoglobulin heavy chain, usually 14q32 or sometimes with a kappa (2q11) or lambda (22q11) locus. Cytogenetic amplifications or gains in 12q, 20q, and 22q and losses of 13q are seen (28).

Treatment and Prognosis. Endemic Burkitt lymphoma can be treated successfully but survival is stage dependent. Short-term chemotherapy is used for the highly chemosensitive endemic form. In a study by Koffi et al. (35), patients responded well to combination chemotherapy but those with high-stage tumors and bone marrow involvement died of disease.

REFERENCES

Langerhans Cell Histiocytosis

1. Hicks J, Flaitz CM. Langerhans cell histiocytosis: current insights in a molecular age with emphasis on clinical oral and maxillofacial pathology practice. Oral Surg Oral Med Oral Pathol Oral Radiol Endod 2005;100(Suppl):S42-66.
2. Willman CL. Detection of clonal histiocytes in Langerhans cell histiocytosis: biology and clinical significance. Br J Cancer Suppl 1994;23: S29-33.
3. Jones AV, Franklin CD. An analysis of oral and maxillofacial pathology found in children over a 30-year period. Int J Paediatr Dent 2006;16:19-30.
4. Li Z, Li ZB, Zhang W, et al. Eosinophilic granuloma of the jaws: an analysis of clinical and radiographic presentation. Oral Oncol 2006;42:574-580.

5. Nakamura S, Bessho K, Nakao K, Iizuka T, Scott RF. Langerhans' cell histiocytosis confined to the jaw. J Oral Maxillofac Surg 2005;63:989-995.

Plasmacytoma/Multiple Myeloma

6. Alexander DD, Mink PJ, Adami HO, et al. Multiple myeloma: a review of the epidemiologic literature. Int J Cancer 2007;120(Suppl 12):40-61.
7. Witt C, Borges AC, Klein K, Neumann HJ. Radiographic manifestations of multiple myeloma in the mandible: a retrospective study of 77 patients. J Oral Maxillofac Surg 1997;55:450, 453-455.
8. Lae ME, Vencio EF, Inwards CY, Unni KK, Nascimento AG. Myeloma of the jaw bones: a clinicopathologic study of 33 cases. Head Neck 2003;25:373-381.

9. Furutani M, Ohnishi M, Tanaka Y. Mandibular involvement in patients with multiple myeloma. J Oral Maxillofac Surg 1994;52:23-25.

10. Elias HG, Scott J, Metheny L, Quereshy FA. Multiple myeloma presenting as mandibular ill-defined radiolucent lesion with numb chin syndrome: a case report. J Oral Maxillofac Surg 2009;67:1991-1996.

11. Pisano JJ, Coupland R, Chen SY, Miller AS. Plasmacytoma of the oral cavity and jaws: a clinicopathologic study of 13 cases. Oral Surg Oral Med Oral Pathol Oral Radiol Endod 1997;83:265-271.

12. Hideshima T, Mitsiades C, Tonon G, Richardson PG, Anderson KC. Understanding multiple myeloma pathogenesis in the bone marrow to identify new therapeutic targets. Nat Rev Cancer 2007;7:585-598.

13. Mahindra A, Hideshima T, Anderson KC. Multiple myeloma: biology of the disease. Blood Rev 2010;24(Suppl 1):S5-11.

14. Rajkumar SV. Multiple myeloma: 2011 update on diagnosis, risk-stratification, and management. Am J Hematol 2011;86:57-65.

15. Fonseca R, San Miguel J. Prognostic factors and staging in multiple myeloma. Hematol Oncol Clin North Am 2007;21:1115-1140, ix.

Malignant Lymphoma and Burkitt Lymphoma

16. Kemp S, Gallagher G, Kabani S, Noonan V, O'Hara C. Oral non-Hodgkin's lymphoma: review of the literature and World Health Organization classification with reference to 40 cases. Oral Surg Oral Med Oral Pathol Oral Radiol Endod 2008;105:194-201.

17. Unni KK, Inwards CY, Kindblom LG, Wold LE. Tumors of the bones and joints. AFIP Atlas of Tumor Pathology, 4th Series, Fascicle 2. Washington, DC: American Registry of Pathology; 2005:231-240.

18. Pileri SA, Montanari M, Falini B, et al. Malignant lymphoma involving the mandible. clinical, morphologic, and immunohistochemical study of 17 cases. Am J Surg Pathol 1990;14:652-659.

19. Nocini P, Lo Muzio L, Fior A, Staibano S, Mignogna MD. Primary non-Hodgkin's lymphoma of the jaws: immunohistochemical and genetic review of 10 cases. J Oral Maxillofac Surg 2000;58:636-644.

20. Djavanmardi L, Oprean N, Alantar A, Bousetta K, Princ G. Malignant non-Hodgkin's lymphoma (NHL) of the jaws: A review of 16 cases. J Craniomaxillofac Surg 2008;36:410-414.

21. van der Waal RI, Huijgens PC, van der Valk P, van der Waal I. Characteristics of 40 primary extranodal non-Hodgkin lymphomas of the oral cavity in perspective of the new WHO classification and the international prognostic index. Int J Oral Maxillofac Surg 2005;34:391-395.

22. Ishimaru T, Hayatsu Y, Ueyama Y, Shinozaki F. Hodgkins lymphoma of the mandibular condyle: Report of a case. J Oral Maxillofac Surg 2005;63:144-147.

23. O'Neill J, Finlay K, Jurriaans E, Friedman L. Radiological manifestations of skeletal lymphoma. Curr Probl Diagn Radiol 2009;38:228-236.

24. Amano Y, Wakabayashi H, Kumazaki T. MR signal changes in bone marrow of mandible in hematologic disorders. J Comput Assist Tomogr 1995;19:552-554.

25. Weber AL, Rahemtullah A, Ferry JA. Hodgkin and non-Hodgkin lymphoma of the head and neck: Clinical, pathologic, and imaging evaluation. Neuroimaging Clin N Am 2003;13:371-392.

26. Said J. Diffuse aggressive B-cell lymphomas. Adv Anat Pathol 2009;16:216-235.

27. Li S, Siegal GP. Small cell tumors of bone. Adv Anat Pathol 2010;17:1-11.

28. Carbone A, Gloghini A, Aiello A, Testi A, Cabras A. B-cell lymphomas with features intermediate between distinct pathologic entities. From pathogenesis to pathology. Hum Pathol 2010;41:621-631.

29. Snuderl M, Kolman OK, Chen YB, et al. B-cell lymphomas with concurrent IGH-BCL2 and MYC rearrangements are aggressive neoplasms with clinical and pathologic features distinct from Burkitt lymphoma and diffuse large B-cell lymphoma. Am J Surg Pathol 2010;34:327-340.

30. Bellan C, Stefano L, Giulia de F, Rogena EA, Lorenzo L. Burkitt lymphoma versus diffuse large B-cell lymphoma: a practical approach. Hematol Oncol 2010;28:53-56.

31. Sariban E, Donahue A, Magrath IT. Jaw involvement in American Burkitt's lymphoma. Cancer 1984;53:1777-1782.

32. Ogwang MD, Bhatia K, Biggar RJ, Mbulaiteye SM. Incidence and geographic distribution of endemic Burkitt lymphoma in northern Uganda revisited. Int J Cancer 2008;123:2658-2663.

33. Orem J, Mbidde EK, Lambert B, de Sanjose S, Weiderpass E. Burkitt's lymphoma in Africa, a review of the epidemiology and etiology. Afr Health Sci 2007;7:166-175.

34. Leoncini L, Raphael M, Stein H, Harris NL, Jaffe ES, Kluin PM. Burkitt lymphoma. In: Swerdlow SH, Campo E, Harris NL, et al., eds. WHO classification of tumours of haematopoietic and lymphoid tissues. Lyon: IARC; 2008:262–264.

35. Koffi GK, Tolo A, Nanho DC, et al. Results of treatment with CMA, a low intermediate regimen, in endemic Burkitt lymphomas in sub-Saharian Africa: Experience of Cote d'Ivoire. Int J Hematol 2010;91:838-843.

17 VASCULAR LESIONS

HEMANGIOMA/VASCULAR MALFORMATIONS

Definition. *Hemangioma* of bone is a benign proliferation of small blood vessels, generally occurring in the medullary cavity. *Vascular malformation* is a related lesion but is composed not only of small vessels with a thin endothelial lining but also larger vessels, some with complete or partial muscular coats. Synonyms for vascular malformation include *arteriovenous malformation* and *high-flow angioma.*

General Features. Hemangiomas of bone are unusual, with the skull the most frequently affected osseous site, followed by the vertebrae and the jaws. Vascular malformations are histologically similar but have more smooth muscle in their walls and are associated with more blood flow. Some consider these entities as representing a spectrum. The exact histologic differentiation of hemangioma from vascular malformation is less critical than whether the lesion has a high blood flow. The propensity for high-flow tumors to bleed excessively during treatment or inadvertently during tooth extraction is of prime importance, as discussed below (1–5). Vascular malformations are associated with the Sturge-Weber syndrome.

Clinical Features. Vascular lesions of the bone are unusual, and only 10 percent of bone hemangiomas occur in the jaws. In the Mayo Clinic experience (9), 6.8 percent of hemangiomas occurred in the maxilla and 3.8 percent in the maxilla. They are most commonly found in the premolar and molar regions. Most are found incidentally on radiographs and the radiographic findings are not specific. They often present as a unilocular radiolucency, with a well-corticated border (5). Although many lesions are asymptomatic and found incidentally on radiographs, hemangiomas can cause swelling and loosened teeth. Life-threatening hemorrhage may result if they are surgically entered inadvertently or are associated with a tooth that is extracted.

Radiographic Features. Magnetic resonance imaging (MRI) helps in determining the vascularity of the lesion, as does arteriography. In cases where rapid blood flow is anticipated, arteriography can be supplemented by embolization of feeder vessels in order to decrease the chances of uncontrolled hemorrhage.

Microscopic Findings. Hemangiomas are composed of thin-walled vessels that are lined by a single layer of endothelial cells. They may be of cavernous or capillary type (figs. 17-1, 17-2). The *capillary type* is composed of collections of very small diameter vessels while the

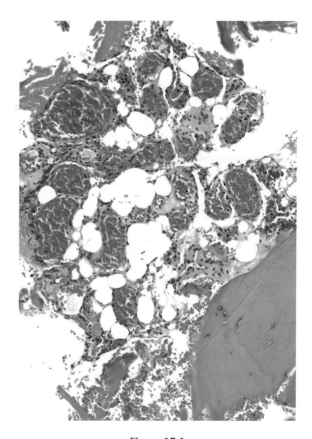

Figure 17-1

HEMANGIOMA

Numerous small caliber vessels are seen in this hemangioma of bone.

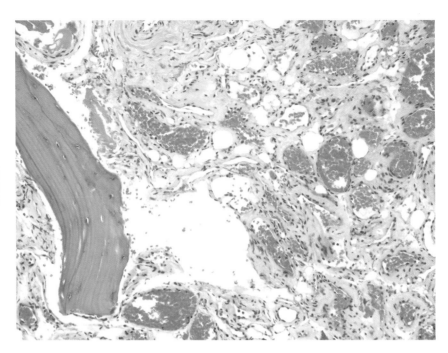

Figure 17-2

HEMANGIOMA

Stromal collagen is increased in the bone marrow space. The vessels have a thin endothelial lining.

cavernous type has large nearly macroscopic vascular spaces. Frequently, both types are observed in the same lesion. Vascular malformations contain vessels with variable amounts of smooth muscle in their walls (figs. 17-3–17-5).

Differential Diagnosis. In the clinical differential diagnosis, the plain film radiographs do not always suggest a vascular lesion. Hemangiomas or vascular malformations can present as a benign unilocular radiolucency with a well-corticated border, similar to benign nonvascular mandibular cysts.

In the histologic differential diagnosis, Gorham disease, also known as phantom bone disease or disappearing bone disease, should be considered (7). This rare disease is manifest radiologically by radiolucencies and eventual shrinkage of the bone. It usually affects the bones of the shoulder girdle. Biopsies of this process sometimes reveal a vascular proliferation similar to hemangioma or lymphangioma.

Treatment and Prognosis. Although hemangiomas occurring in bones other than the jaws are sometimes not treated and only observed clinically, hemangiomas or vascular malformations of the jaw are considered by some to require therapy especially for larger or symptomatic lesions, in order to prevent uncontrolled hemorrhage, particularly in dental procedures (8). Before biopsy or curettage of vascular le-

sions in the jaw, some authors advocate needle aspiration (8). Abundant blood return suggests that the lesion may have a high blood-flow rate. These lesions are best treated preoperatively by selective embolization and segmental resection rather than curettage.

MALIGNANT VASCULAR TUMORS

Definition. A number of different, but similarly sounding names have been appended to *malignant vascular tumors*, including *angiosarcoma*, *hemangioendothelioma*, and *hemangioendothelioma sarcoma*, which causes some confusion. Many of these different appellations are related to the level of atypia or aggressiveness of the tumor. For example, the term hemangioendothelioma refers to a low histologic grade malignant vascular neoplasm while the term angiosarcoma refers to a high-grade malignant tumor for many authorities. Angiosarcoma is defined as a malignant neoplasm with endothelial differentiation and vasoformative features. It is most often seen in the skin and superficial soft tissues where it behaves in an aggressive fashion. It is uncommonly seen in the jaw. Some authors support the concept that most malignant vascular tumors of bone should be designated as angiosarcoma and then histologically graded as to low or high (9). Some important exceptions exist in an all inclusive

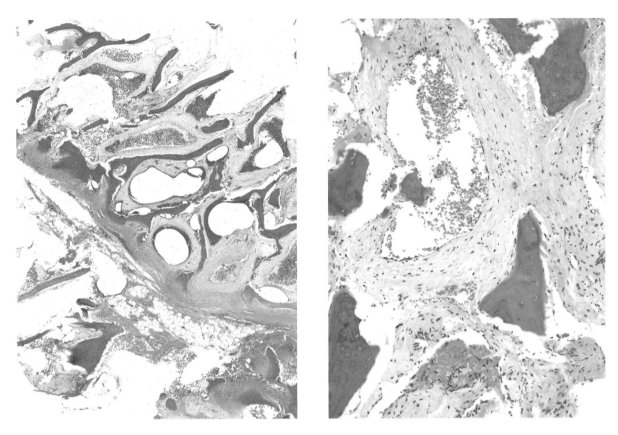

Figure 17-3

ARTERIOVENOUS MALFORMATION

Left: Large vascular spaces are present in this arteriovenous malformation. It is easy to imagine that this lesion could bleed excessively if surgically entered inadvertently.

Right: Higher microscopic view reveals that some of the vessel walls have variable thickness.

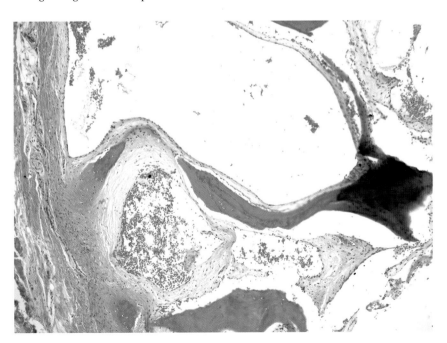

Figure 17-4

ARTERIOVENOUS MALFORMATION

The thick vessel walls separate and push apart the cancellous bone trabeculae.

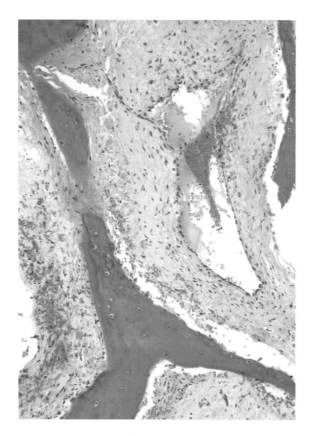

Figure 17-5

ARTERIOVENOUS MALFORMATION

A vessel with a muscular wall is present in this arteriovenous malformation.

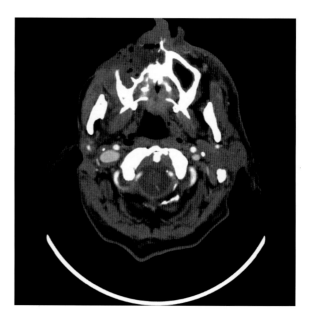

Figure 17-6

ANGIOSARCOMA

Computerized tomography (CT) image of an angiosarcoma that arose in the maxilla.

terminology such as in the case of epithelioid hemangioendothelioma, a low-grade vascular tumor with epithelioid cellular features, which should be separated for the diagnostic reasons discussed below (10,11).

General Features. While angiosarcoma is most common in the head and neck region, angiosarcoma of any bone is rare and involvement of the jaws is exceptional (12–14). In a Mayo Clinic series, fewer than 100 cases of angiosarcoma of bone were reported (9). Of these, 2 percent were reported in the maxilla and none in the mandible. Epithelioid hemangioendothelioma involving the jaws is also rare (15,16). Mohtasham et al. (17) found 26 cases of intraoral hemangioendothelioma in a review in 2008.

Clinical Features. The age range of patients with angiosarcoma of bone is nearly equal from the first to the eighth decades (18). The literature

is variable in the reports of gender distribution, with some authors suggesting a near equal distribution and others suggesting that these tumors are more common in men (9). Patients present with pain and swelling of the affected jaw and some teeth can be loosened. The tumors are described as having a red to blue coloration.

Radiographic Features. Radiographically, angiosarcomas are usually lytic and extend into the soft tissues (fig. 17-6) (14). As noted by Unni et al. (9), high-grade tumors are often poorly marginated while lower-grade tumors are well demarcated.

Microscopic Findings. Angiosarcomas have a wide range of appearances. Some tumors have small, ectatic, anastomosing blood-filled vessels of varying caliber while others are solidly packed with tumor cells with only slit-like vascular spaces or essentially no spaces at all (fig. 17-7). Any vascular spaces are lined by atypical endothelial cells. Some tumor cells have small intracytoplasmic lumens. This feature is useful in poorly differentiated angiosarcomas as these lumens often contain red blood cells or red blood cell fragments. Other features of angiosarcoma, apart from the atypia of the endothelial cells, are multiple layers of endothelial cells and

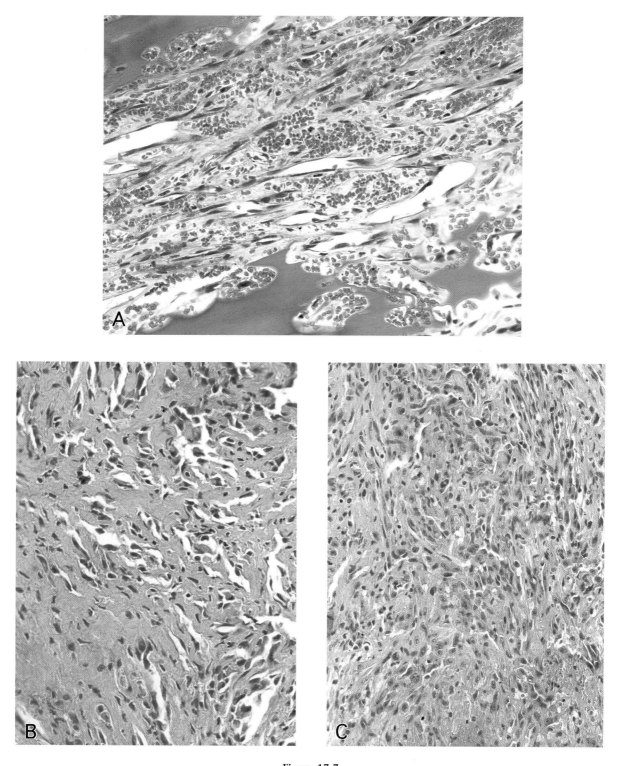

Figure 17-7

ANGIOSARCOMA

A: This angiosarcoma shows a minimal degree of cellularity with hyperchromatic endothelial cell nuclei.
B: The vascular spaces are slit-like.
C: A solid pattern is present in this angiosarcoma. Occasional red blood cells are seen in some of the narrowed spaces.

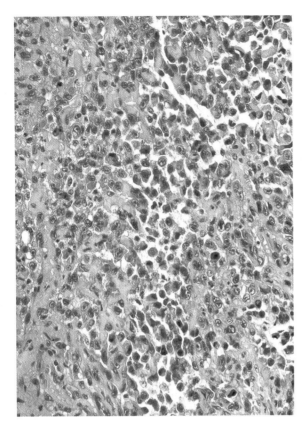

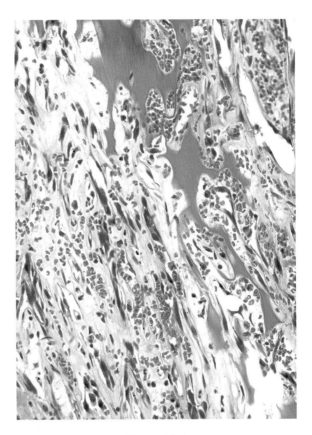

Figure 17-8

ANGIOSARCOMA

A high-grade angiosarcoma shows spaces between the highly atypical cells. There is some resemblance to an epithelial malignancy.

Figure 17-9

ANGIOSARCOMA

Reactive osteoid is present in this angiosarcoma of bone.

infiltrative growth. High-grade angiosarcomas appear as sheets of cells, and have a spindled morphology or aggregates of cells with intervening vascular spaces (fig. 17-8). Osteoid can be seen as a reaction to the angiosarcoma (fig. 17-9). Some angiosarcomas can have densely eosinophilic stroma that resembles osteoid (fig. 17-10).

Epithelioid hemangioendotheliomas are composed of endothelial cells that are round and contain eosinophilic cytoplasm that is often vacuolated. The cells are often arranged in trabeculae, cords, or nests, with minimal vascular space formation (fig. 17-11). The mitotic activity is usually low but when there is significant atypia, high mitotic rates, and necrosis, the tumor's behavior is more aggressive. Epithelioid hemangioendotheliomas are notable because their appearance can be similar to carcinomas,

which leads to an expanded differential diagnosis. They mark immunohistochemically as vascular neoplasms (fig. 17-12). Occasional erythrocytes within intracytoplasmic lumens are seen in the tumor cells. Inflammatory cells, particularly eosinophils, can be common. These tumors are usually found in the extremities, liver, lung, and bone. They are rarely reported in the oral cavity or jaw.

While many angiosarcomas have cells with more abundant cytoplasm, only those in which this finding is widespread should be designated as epithelioid. As opposed to epithelioid hemangioendothelioma, *epithelioid angiosarcomas* are always high grade. Unni et al. (9) suggest the following scheme for grading angiosarcomas: grade 1 tumors have minimally atypical endothelial cells and easily identified vascular space formation; grade 2 tumors are still recognizable

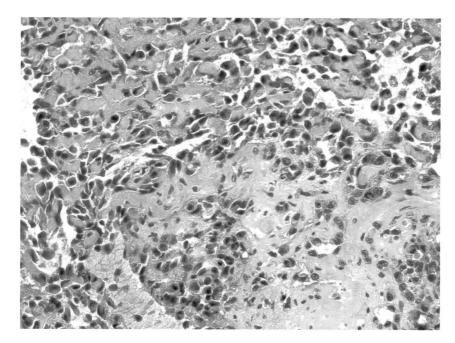

Figure 17-10

ANGIOSARCOMA

The tumor cells have produced a dense collagenous stroma that superficially resembles osteoid.

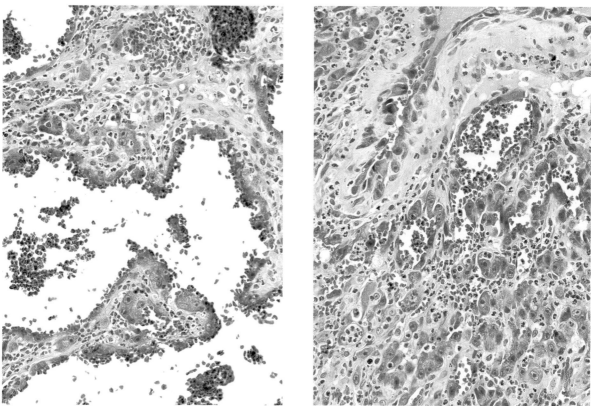

Figure 17-11

EPITHELIOID ANGIOSARCOMA

Left: Epithelioid angiosarcoma has vascular spaces lined by large epithelial-like cells.

Right: The vascular spaces are lined by atypical endothelial cells. Red blood cells are in direct contact with the atypical cells, a characteristic of angiosarcoma.

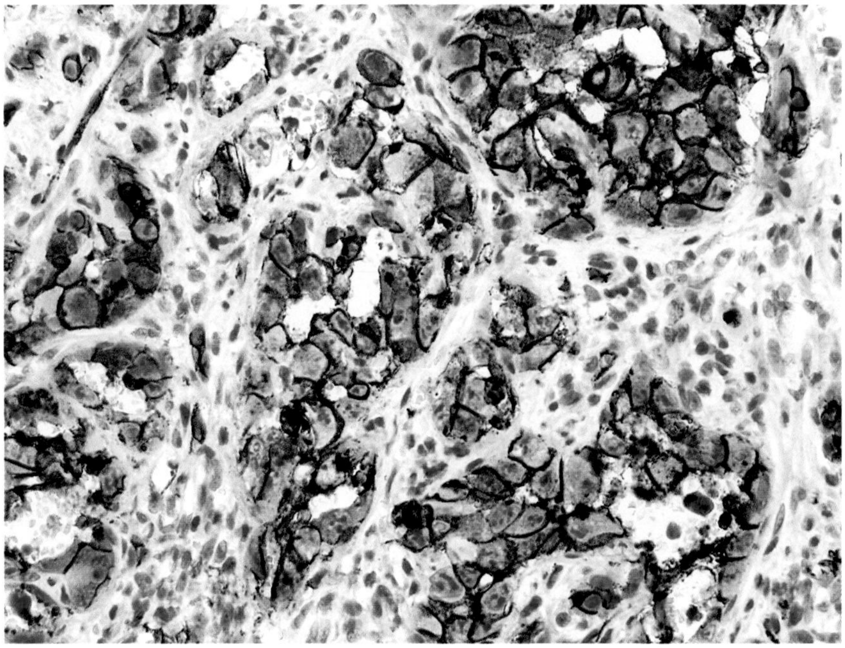

Figure 17-12

EPITHELIOID ANGIOSARCOMA

Anti-CD31 staining is present in this epithelioid angiosarcoma.

as vasoformative but more nuclear atypia is present; and grade 3 tumors have much more cytologic atypia and it may be difficult to recognize that the tumor is a vascular neoplasm.

Immunohistochemical Findings. Angiosarcomas show vascular differentiation by the expression of antigens to CD31, CD34, and factor VIII. Epithelioid vascular tumors can exhibit keratin positivity for pankeratin cocktails, in addition to endothelial markers.

Molecular Findings. Angiosarcomas overexpress vascular endothelial growth factor (VEGF) protein as well as VEGF receptor (VEGF-R). VEGF-A is overexpressed in angiosarcomas compared to normal tissues or benign vascular tumors. The overexpression of the receptor proteins includes VEGF-R1, VEGF-R2, and VEGF-R3. (19) Upstream regulators of VEGF expression, including hypoxia inducible factor (HIF)-1 alpha and HIF-2 alpha, are also expressed in angiosarcomas (9).

Differential Diagnosis. Angiosarcomas that exhibit the histologic features of well-defined vessels lined by atypical endothelial cells are not problematic in the histologic differential diagnosis. However, benign and nonvascular malignant lesions can mimic the findings of angiosarcoma. Hemangiomas form vascular channels but the endothelial cells show no atypia.

Granulation tissue and pyogenic granulomas also form small vessels, often in dense clusters with nuclear hyperchromasia (fig. 17-13) (20). The nuclei of these hyperchromatic cells are bland, however, and lack the size variability and irregularity of the nuclei in angiosarcomas. As spindled areas can be seen in angiosarcoma, other sarcomas are considered in the differential diagnosis. High-grade angiosarcomas have solid areas with minimal vascular space formation, and therefore metastases from melanoma or undifferentiated carcinomas must be considered and separated with immunohistochemical studies as well as a pertinent clinical history. An important caveat, as mentioned above, is that some epithelioid angiosarcomas can react with antikeratin antibodies.

Some malignant vascular tumors have cells that exhibit epithelial features that potentially lead to a mistaken diagnosis of an epithelial neoplasm. These include epithelioid hemangioendothelioma and epithelioid angiosarcoma. Although low-grade angiosarcoma and hemangioendothelioma have identical clinical appearances and behavior, they are distinct histologically.

Treatment and Prognosis. The outcome is dependent on the stage and grade of the tumor, with lower-stage and -grade neoplasms confirming a better outcome. Death is usually due to

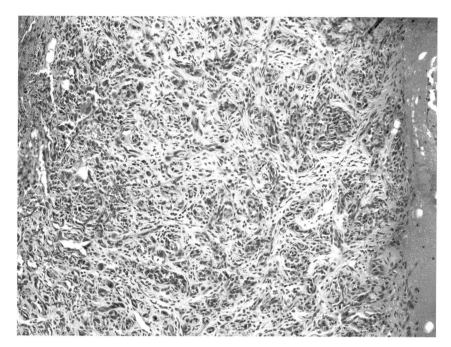

Figure 17-13

ANGIOSARCOMA

This angiosarcoma super-ficially resembles granulation tissue. On careful examination, there is marked nuclear atypia.

recurrent or persistent local disease but also to distant metastases to the lungs and liver. Surgery is the mainstay of therapy in most patients, but radiation and neoadjuvant or adjuvant chemo-therapy are usually used. Chemotherapy is used for unresectable tumors, such as hemangioen-dothelioma. Complete surgical excision may be sufficient for lower-grade neoplasms (9).

REFERENCES

Hemangioma/Arteriovenous Malformation

1. Mulliken JB, Glowacki J. Hemangioma and vascular malformation in infants and children: a classification based on endothelial character-istics. Plast Reconstr Surg 1982;69:412–420.
2. Yih WY, Ma GS, Merrill RG, Sperry DW. Central hemangioma of the jaws. J Oral Maxillofac Surg 1989;47:1154-1160.
3. Ozdemir R, Alagoz S, Uysal AC, Unlu RE, Ortak T, Sensoz O. Intraosseous hemangioma of the mandible: a case report and review of the litera-ture. J Craniofac Surg 2002;13:38-43.
4. Alves S, Junqueira JL, de Oliveira EM, et al. Con-dylar hemangioma: report of a case and review of the literature. Oral Surg Oral Med Oral Pathol Oral Radiol Endod 2006;102:e23-27.
5. Drage NA, Whaites EJ, Hussain K. Haemangioma of the body of the mandible: a case report. Br J Oral Maxillofac Surg 2003;41:112-114.
6. Unni KK, Inwards CY, Kindblom LG, Wold LE. Tumors of the bones and joints. AFIP Atlas of Tumor Pathology, 4th Series, Fascicle 2. Wash-ington, DC: American Registry of Pathology; 2005:262-264.
7. Escande C, Schouman T, Francoise G, et al. Histological features and management of a mandibular Gorham disease: a case report and review of maxillofacial cases in the literature. Oral Surg Oral Med Oral Pathol Oral Radiol En-dod 2008;106:e30-37.
8. Giaoui L, Princ G, Chiras J, Guilbert F, Bertrand JC. Treatment of vascular malformations of the mandible: a description of 12 cases. Int J Oral Maxillofac Surg 2003;32:132-136.

Malignant Vascular Tumors

9. Unni KK, Inwards CY, Kindblom LG, Wold LE. Tumors of the bones and joints. AFIP Atlas of Tumor Pathology, 4th Series, Fascicle 2. Washington, DC: American Registry of Pathology; 2005:266-273

10. Freedman PD, Kerpel SM. Epithelioid angiosarcoma of the maxilla. A case report and review of the literature. Oral Surg Oral Med Oral Pathol 1992;74:319-325.

11. Hamakawa H, Omori T, Sumida T, Tanioka H. Intraosseous epithelioid hemangioendothelioma of the mandible: a case report with an immunohistochemical study. J Oral Pathol Med 1999;28:233-237.

12. Lanigan DT, Hey JH, Lee L. Angiosarcoma of the maxilla and maxillary sinus: report of a case and review of the literature. J Oral Maxillofac Surg 1989;47:747-753.

13. Karmody CS, Kim CH. Angiosarcoma of the premaxilla. Laryngoscope 1974;84:560-564.

14. Zakrzewska JM. Angiosarcoma of the maxilla—a case report and review of the literature including angiosarcoma of maxillary sinus. Br J Oral Maxillofac Surg 1986;24:286-292.

15. Flaitz CM, McDaniel RK, Mackay B, Kennady MC, Luna MA, Hicks MJ. Primary intraoral epithelioid hemangioendothelioma presenting in childhood: review of the literature and case report. Ultrastruct Pathol 1995;19:275-279.

16. Chi AC, Weathers DR, Folpe AL, Dunlap DT, Rasenberger K, Neville BW. Epithelioid hemangioendothelioma of the oral cavity: report of two cases and review of the literature. Oral Surg Oral Med Oral Pathol Oral Radiol Endod 2005;100:717-724.

17. Mohtasham N, Kharrazi AA, Jamshidi S, Jafarzadeh H. Epithelioid hemangioendothelioma of the oral cavity: a case report. J Oral Sci 2008;50:219-223.

18. Loudon JA, Billy ML, DeYoung BR, Allen CM. Angiosarcoma of the mandible: a case report and review of the literature. Oral Surg Oral Med Oral Pathol Oral Radiol Endod 2000;89:471-476.

19. Park MS, Ravi V, Araujo DM. Inhibiting the VEGF-VEGFR pathway in angiosarcoma, epithelioid hemangioendothelioma, and hemangiopericytoma/solitary fibrous tumor. Curr Opin Oncol 2010;22:351-355.

20. Muñoz M, Monje F, Alonso del Hoyo JR, Martin-Granizo R. Oral angiosarcoma misdiagnosed as a pyogenic granuloma. J Oral Maxillofac Surg 1998;56:488-491.

18 SYNOVIAL AND TEMPOROMANDIBULAR JOINT LESIONS

SYNOVIAL CHONDROMATOSIS

Definition. *Synovial chondromatosis* is a proliferative process involving synovial tissues. In the jaw, the temporomandibular joint is affected.

General Features. The etiology of synovial chondromatosis is not understood. Although long considered a metaplastic process, chromosomal abnormalities are found that suggest a neoplastic origin (1,2). There is proliferation of osteochondromatous tissue which forms small nodules in the synovium. These gradually enlarge and many eventually break free to float in the joint space. These nodules survive by being bathed by nutrients present in the synovial fluid. Synovial chondromatosis most often occurs in the large joints of the body such as the hip and knee. It is estimated that only a few percent of all cases affect the temporomandibular joint (3).

Clinical Features. Most patients present in mid-life but the age range varies from late teens to the eighth decade. There is a female predominance (4). A variety of symptoms bring the patient to attention including pain, swelling, and limitation of motion of the jaw. As loose bodies are formed, locking and clicking of the joint occur. Because the symptoms are nonspecific, the diagnosis is usually late, with patients often having joint pain or swelling for several years before therapy is instituted. If left unchecked, the process can erode into the auditory canal or even the cranium and brain (5).

Radiographic Features. Many cases show no abnormalities on plain films. With computerized tomography (CT) and magnetic resonance imaging (MRI), the nodules of cartilaginous tissue can be seen as small densities surrounding the joint (fig. 18-1). Most authors suggest that MRI is superior to CT (6–8).

Gross Findings. Tissues removed for synovial chondromatosis reveal nodules of cartilage (9). These are usually firm and can have some mineralization.

Microscopic Findings. Microscopically, the lesion is characterized by rounded aggregates of hyaline cartilage which have a thin overlying cover of synovial cells (fig. 18-2). The nodules are single or aggregated (fig. 18-3). Hyaline cartilage comprises the tumors and generally there is a nodular configuration (fig. 18-4). The most cellular portions of the nodules are located peripherally (fig.18-5). Since the cartilaginous nodules are often cellular and show nuclear enlargement as well as binucleation, features seen in malignancy, this should be ruled out (fig. 18-6). An important finding to help in the separation from malignancy is the clustered

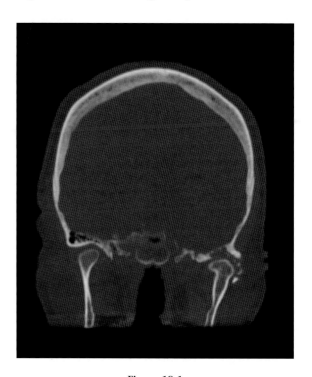

Figure 18-1

SYNOVIAL CHONDROMATOSIS

The computerized tomography (CT) image shows small separated nodules of chondroid islands outlining the joint capsule at the periphery of the left temporomandibular joint.

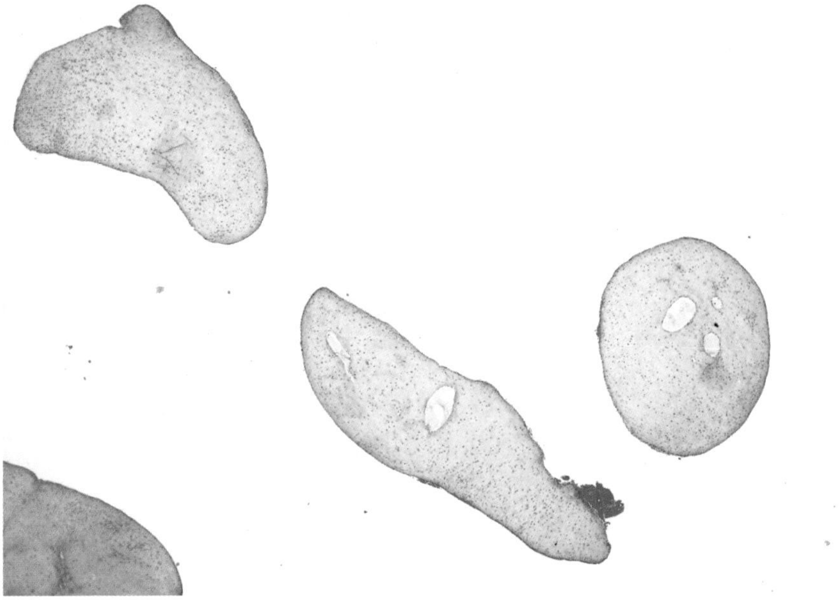

Figure 18-2

SYNOVIAL CHONDROMATOSIS

Small, free-floating chondroid islands are present in the temporomandibular joint space.

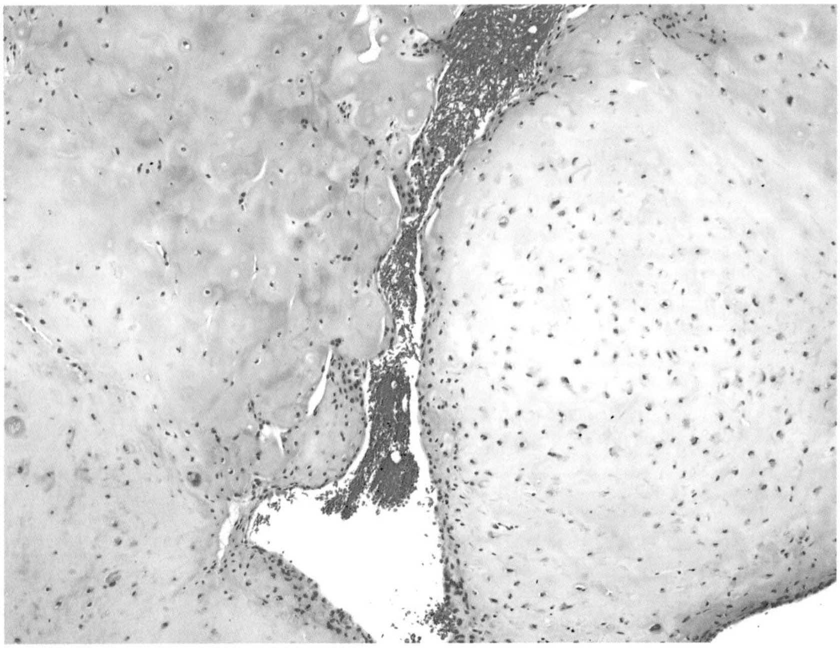

Figure 18-3

SYNOVIAL CHONDROMATOSIS

The chondroid nodules aggregate and small spaces are formed between them.

arrangement of the cartilage cells in synovial chondromatosis.

Fine needle aspiration of the synovial nodule shows cartilaginous tissue fragments, but this finding is not specific. The correlation with the clinical and radiographic findings is critical since aspiration of other cartilaginous lesions such as chondrosarcoma or osteochondroma could give similar findings.

Molecular Findings. In the few cases studied, abnormalities are found in chromosome 6. Rearrangements of this chromosome have been noted as well as loss of some to nearly the entire chromosome (1). Rearrangements of 1p22 and 1p13 have also been reported (1).

Differential Diagnosis. With no clinical or radiographic information to guide the pathologist, the histologic or cytologic appearance

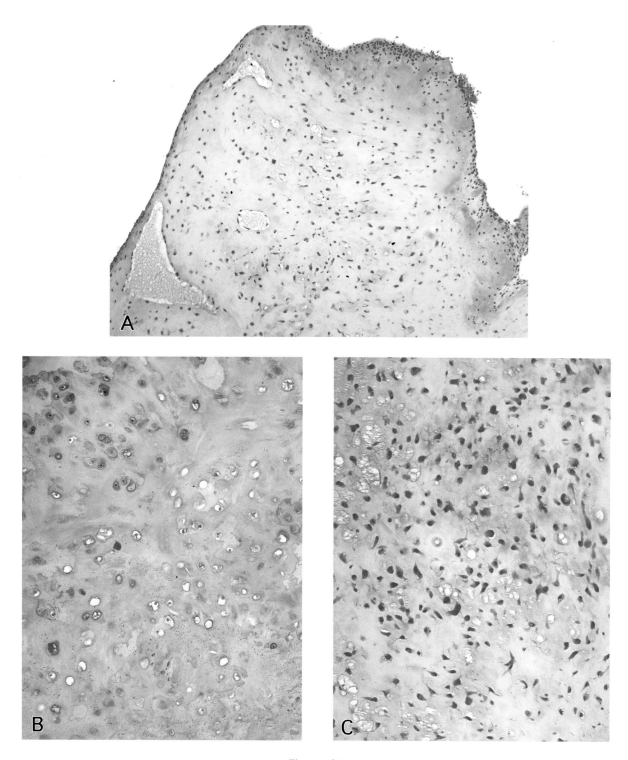

Figure 18-4

SYNOVIAL CHONDROMATOSIS

A: A small space filled with mucinous material is present in this chondroid fragment of synovial chondromatosis. There is a slight yet discernable aggregation of cells at the periphery, similar to normal cartilage as it interfaces with a joint space.

B: Hyaline cartilage with lacunae is present. There is mild to moderate cellularity.

C: This example of synovial chondromatosis shows marked cellularity that is initially alarming for malignancy.

Figure 18-5

SYNOVIAL CHONDROMATOSIS

The cells in synovial chondromatosis are often more numerous peripherally in the nodules. The nuclei show nuclear hyperchromasia and irregularity.

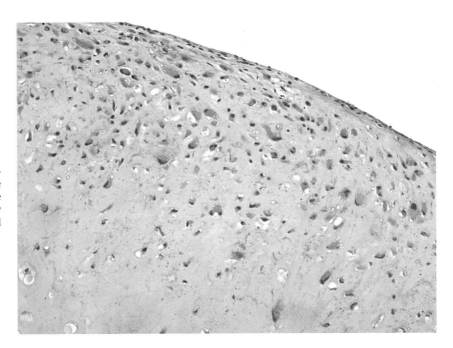

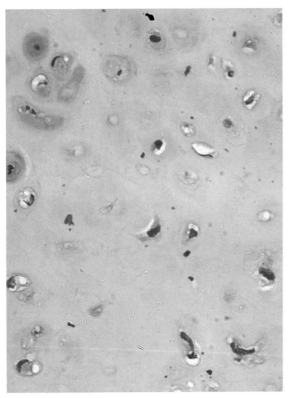
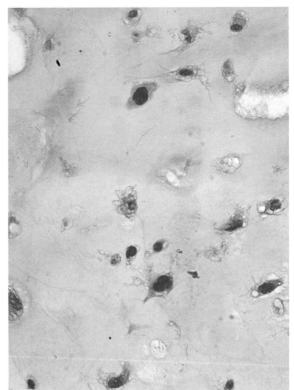

Figure 18-6

SYNOVIAL CHONDROMATOSIS

Left: Nuclear hyperchromasia and irregularity are seen.

Right: The nuclear atypia in this synovial chondromatosis could easily be mistaken for a malignant process if only the histologic features were considered. This demonstrates the importance of the correlation of the clinical, radiologic, and gross pathology for interpretation of many lesions, particularly those of the bones and joints.

alone could be mistaken for chondrosarcoma on limited material. Chondrosarcoma can involve joints and appears as nodular proliferations in the joint space. Synovial chondromatosis, however, has no myxoid change and the clustering of the chondrocytes points to a benign process. Also, the radiographic images demonstrate an osseous neoplasm as opposed to one centered in the synovium or joint space.

Treatment and Prognosis. Open temporomandibular joint surgery is the treatment of choice, with synovectomy and diskectomy (4). Condylectomy has been used in some cases. Arthroscopy to remove the loose bodies is usually less successful in removing all the cartilaginous nodules. When most of the loose bodies are removed along with the synovium, the recurrence rate is lower.

PIGMENTED VILLONODULAR SYNOVITIS

Definition. *Pigmented villonodular synovitis* is an uncommon inflammatory lesion affecting the joints and characterized grossly by brown, shaggy synovial tissue that microscopically is composed of a proliferation of villous synovium containing hemosiderin-laden histiocytic cells. Once considered a reactive process, recurrent chromosomal abnormalities in some cases suggest that the process may be neoplastic.

General Features. Pigmented villonodular synovitis is an uncommon process and most often affects large joints such as the hip and knee. It rarely affects the temporomandibular joint. In a 2009 review, only 27 cases were reported in the temporomandibular joint (10). Although pigmented villonodular synovitis is usually diffuse, it occasionally is localized as a sessile or polypoid nodule growing from the synovium.

Clinical Features. Patient age ranges from the third to the seventh decade. A review of reported patients by Herman et al. (10) revealed an equal gender distribution although the mean age of onset was younger in men (38.8 years) than women (49.5 years). Patients complain of pain and swelling in the joint and nearly three fourths of patients have erosive bone changes (10). Although usually localized to the joint, cranial extension has been reported (10,11).

Radiographic Features. Plain radiographs may show no lesion or erosion of the articular

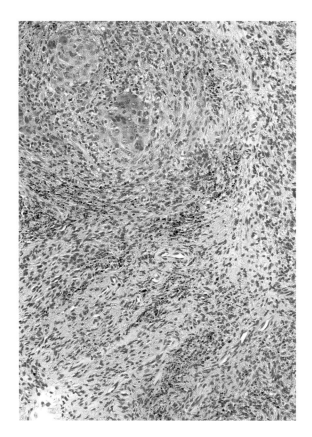

Figure 18-7

PIGMENTED VILLONODULAR SYNOVITIS

A composite of cells, including giant cells, mononuclear cells, and cells whose cytoplasm is filled with hemosiderin, is characteristic of pigmented villonodular synovitis.

surface and increased soft tissue densities within the joint. MRI shows the characteristic picture of a heterogeneous synovial lesion extending peripherally away from the joint as well as low signal intensity on both the T1- and T2-weighted images (12).

Gross and Microscopic Findings. On direct visual observation, the process is brown and has a shaggy appearance. On microscopic examination, synovial villi are expanded by histiocytes with foamy cytoplasm containing hemosiderin, imparting the brown coloration observed grossly (figs. 18-7–18-9). There is often a pseudoglandular pattern of cells (fig. 18-10). Spindled stromal cells and multinucleated giant cells are present (fig. 18-11). Increased collagen is present in some areas, separating the more cellular components (fig. 18-12). The

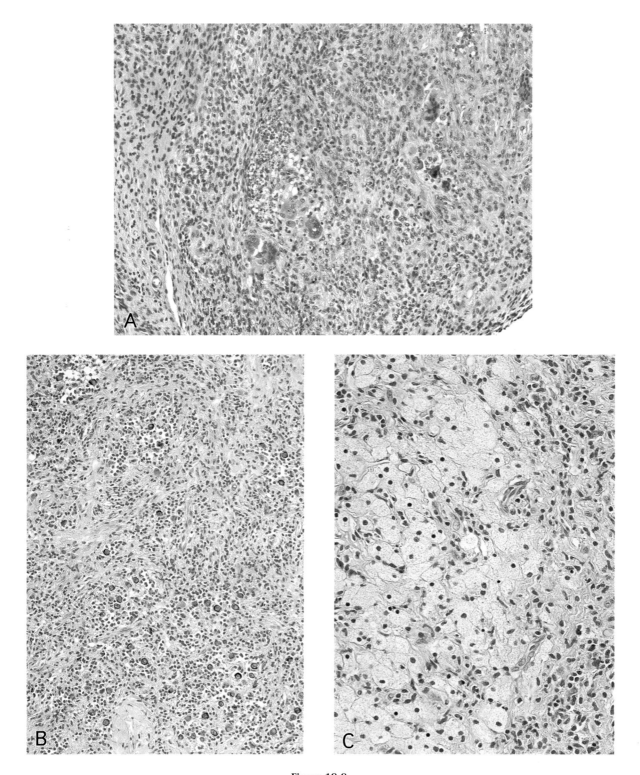

Figure 18-8

PIGMENTED VILLONODULAR SYNOVITIS

A: Hemosiderin-laden cells are not always present in all areas of pigmented villonodular synovitis.
B: Scattered large hemosiderin-laden cells populate the background.
C: Foam cells are commonly seen in pigmented villonodular synovitis.

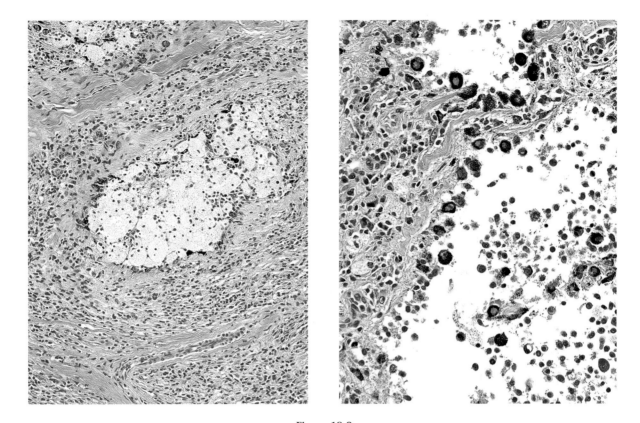

Figure 18-9

PIGMENTED VILLONODULAR SYNOVITIS

Left: Dense collagen bundles separate the cellular portions. A large area of foam cells with clear cytoplasm is ringed by hemosiderin-laden cells.

Right: The cells in the center of the nodule have undergone degeneration. Pigmented cells are seen.

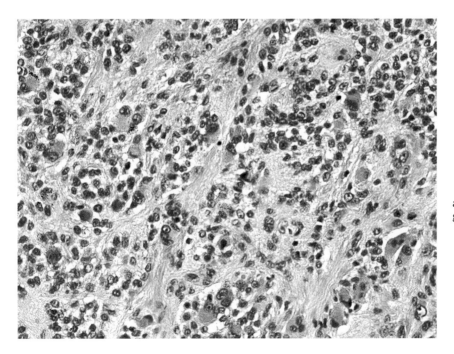

Figure 18-10

PIGMENTED VILLONODULAR SYNOVITIS

A mixture of lymphocytes and histiocytes exhibits a pseudo-glandular growth pattern.

253

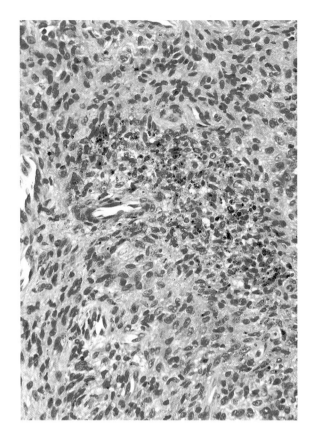

Figure 18-11

PIGMENTED VILLONODULAR SYNOVITIS

Spindling of the cells is commonly seen in pigmented villonodular synovitis.

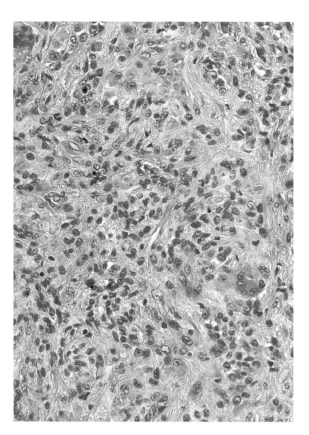

Figure 18-12

PIGMENTED VILLONODULAR SYNOVITIS

Some foci in pigmented villonodular synovitis show increased collagen production.

multinucleated giant cells, similar to the single nucleated histiocytes, have foamy cytoplasm and contain hemosiderin. Mitotic figures may be common but are never atypical. Atypical mitoses should cause consideration of a malignant process. Osseous and chondroid metaplasia should not be interpreted as signs of malignancy (13). Although usually not needed for diagnosis, immunohistochemical staining shows the cells to be positive for CD68, HAM56, and other histiocytic markers. The cytologic findings are similar to the histologic findings: histiocytes and giant cells, both containing hemosiderin, are in a milieu of lymphocytes and scattered connective tissue fragments (14).

Molecular Findings. Chromosomal translocations have been found in many cases of pigmented villonodular synovitis or its extraarticular counterpart, giant cell tumor of tendon sheath. The gene for CSF1, an inflammatory mediator,

has been found at the chromosomal 1p13 breakpoint (15,16). While this suggests a link between this inflammatory mediator and a recurrent molecular abnormality, approximately 40 percent of the cases of pigmented villonodular synovitis reported by Cupp et al. (16) had no translocation identified in spite of elevated CSF1 levels, suggesting other mechanisms for the upregulation of this inflammatory mediator in this disease.

Differential Diagnosis. Inflammatory arthropathies such as rheumatoid arthritis or degenerative joint disease can cause the synovium to take on a villous appearance. In these processes, however, there is no proliferation of histiocytic cells to the degree seen in pigmented villonodular synovitis.

Treatment and Prognosis. Synovectomy, with removal of as much of the affected synovium as possible, is the treatment of choice (17). Recurrences are frequent.

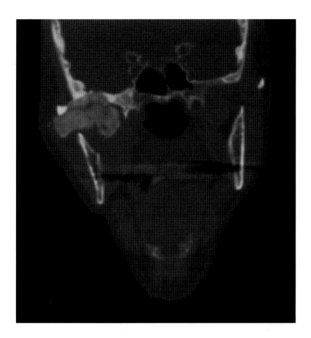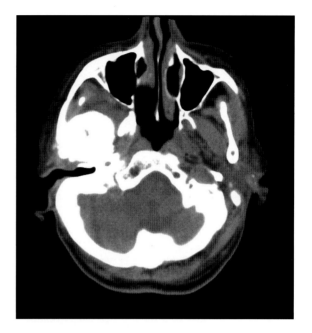

Figure 18-13

TOPHACEOUS PSEUDOGOUT

Left: Magnetic resonance imaging (MRI) of the temporomandibular joint involved with tophaceous pseudogout.
Right: In the CT image, the ear canal is partially obstructed and there is temporal bone destruction.

TOPHACEOUS PSEUDOGOUT

Definition. *Tophaceous pseudogout* is caused by the deposition of calcium dihydrate pyrophosphate in the joint, but rarely affects the temporomandibular joint. *Calcium pyrophosphate dihydrate crystal deposition disease* (CPPD) is another term for this disease.

General Features. Tophaceous pseudogout of the temporomandibular joint is rare, with less than 50 cases reported (18). The pathogenesis of pseudogout is not clearly understood (19). Most cases present in the knee, wrist, or hand. While larger joints, such as the knee, more frequently have an acute presentation with an associated effusion, pseudogout of the temporomandibular joint is generally chronic, with few reports of an acute presentation (18).

Calcium pyrophosphate crystals are mainly formed in cartilage but can be seen in the synovium as well as supporting structures of the joint. Tophaceous pseudogout is generally associated with older age and is thought to be due to trauma to the cartilage. It has also been linked with a number of metabolic disorders, including hyperparathyroidism. It is most commonly found in women greater than 50 years

of age, but it is unknown if there is a link to a decrease in sex hormones.

Clinical Features. In the review by Reynolds et al. (18), the mean age of the patients was 58 years and the ratio of women to men was 2 to 1. While in larger joints there is diffuse involvement of the joint space, the temporomandibular joint is more often affected with a tumoral deposition. Pain, trismus, and malocclusion are common complaints (20). Besides the deposition of calcium pyrophosphate, there is often calcification in the joint space as well as the disc, with destruction or erosion of the condyle in some cases. The clinical findings often cause concern for a malignant process. The process can expand out of the joint to involve cranial structures in some cases (21). Radiographic studies can reveal often large masses that strongly resemble neoplasms (fig. 18-13).

Gross and Microscopic Findings. On gross examination, the material has a white, chalk-like appearance. The microscopic appearance on hematoxylin and eosin (H&E)-stained slides is that of amorphous masses of crystalline material with a histiocytic and granulomatous response (fig. 18-14). Calcium pyrophosphate dihydrate

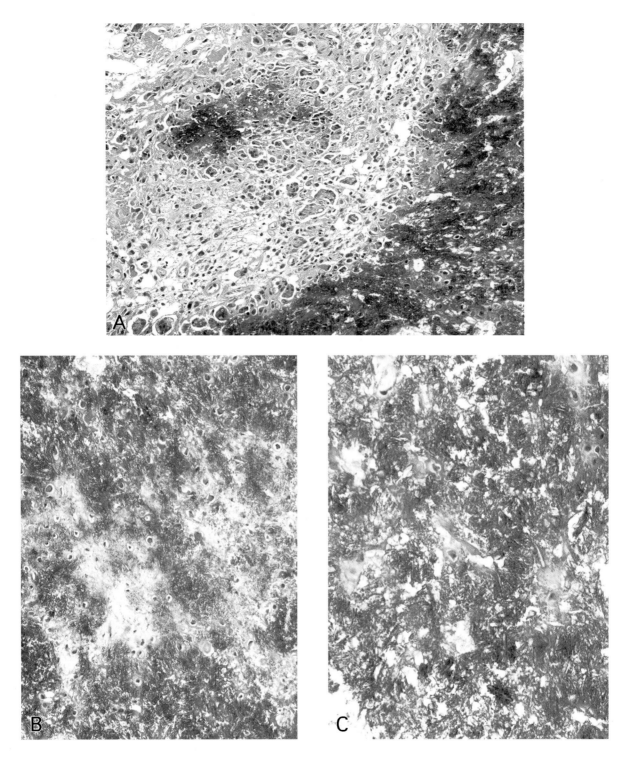

Figure 18-14

TOPHACEOUS PSEUDOGOUT

A: A mixture of amorphous purple-staining material along with a granulomatous response composed of histiocytes and giant cells is seen in this example of tophaceous pseudogout.

B: Some areas have no granulomatous response and are composed of only crystalline material and cartilaginous cells.

C: Crystalline shapes can be discerned in tophaceous pseudogout, often as "negative" images.

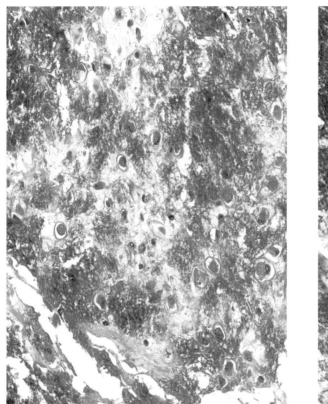 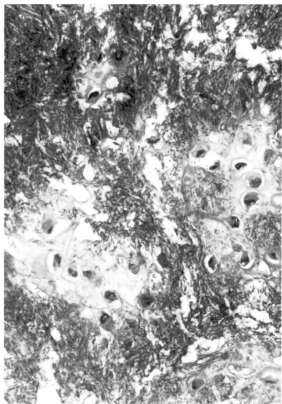

Figure 18-15

TOPHACEOUS PSEUDOGOUT

Left: Cartilaginous atypia, characterized by nuclear enlargement and hyperchromasia, is common in tophaceous pseudogout.

Right: Cartilaginous atypia is seen.

crystals are somewhat rhomboid and display weakly positive birefringence. They are seen both in an intracellular and extracellular location and when intracellular, are often seen in histiocytes and multinucleated giant cells, but also in stromal cells. Chondroid metaplasia and a chronic inflammatory infiltrate are present. The cartilaginous cells can exhibit marked cytologic atypia (fig. 18-15).

Fine needle aspiration cytology is useful in the diagnosis when aspirates reveal the birefringent crystals of rhomboid shape. These are best be observed with Giemsa or similar stains such as Diff-Quik (figs. 18-16, 18-17) (22).

Differential Diagnosis. Although the clinical and radiographic findings may suggest chondroma or synovial chondromatosis, the crystalline material in masses points to pseudogout. The inflammatory reaction can be associated with reactive atypia of the chondrocytes in the joint and this could be misinterpreted as a neoplasm such as chondroma, chondrosarcoma, or synovial chondromatosis (23).

Treatment and Prognosis. Some authors have advocated reconstruction of the joint after removal of the tophaceous material, although treatment in the majority of reports is only removal of the deposits (24). Recurrence is possible. If arthroplasty is not carried out, patients may still have complaints of malocclusion.

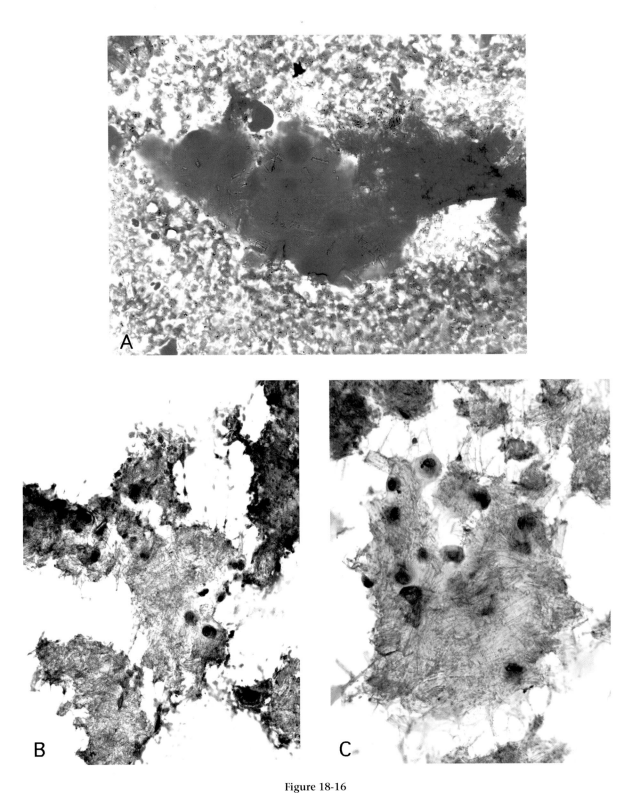

Figure 18-16

TOPHACEOUS PSEUDOGOUT

A: Metachromatic-stained fine needle aspirate material shows a giant cell with engulfed crystals.
B: Papanicolaou-stained aspirate shows crystalline material and chondrocytes with enlarged nuclei.
C: The nuclear atypia of the chondrocytes is apparent in the fine needle aspirate from the temporomandibular joint.

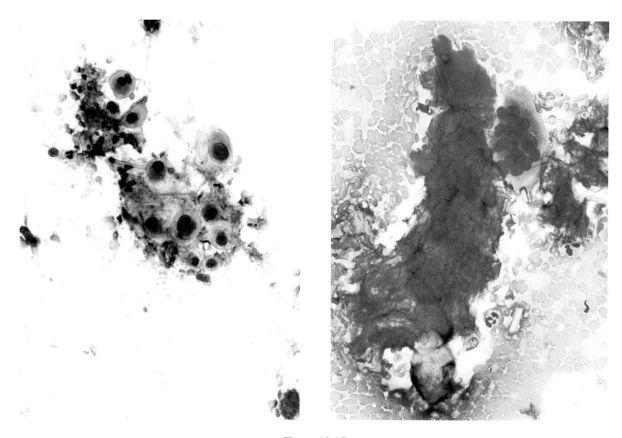

Figure 18-17

TOPHACEOUS PSEUDOGOUT

Left: The nuclear atypia of the chondrocytes can suggest a cartilaginous neoplasm in fine needle aspirates.
Right: Crystals are seen adjacent to a multinucleated giant cell in the metachromatic-stained aspirate of pseudogout.

REFERENCES

Synovial Chondromatosis

1. Buddingh EP, Krallman P, Neff JR, Nelson M, Liu J, Bridge JA. Chromosome 6 abnormalities are recurrent in synovial chondromatosis. Cancer Genet Cytogenet 2003;140:18-22.
2. Boffano P, Viterbo S, Bosco GF. Diagnosis and surgical management of synovial chondromatosis of the temporomandibular joint. J Craniofac Surg 2010;21:157-159.
3. Hohlweg-Majert B, Metzger MC, Bohm J, Muecke T, Schulze D. Advanced imaging findings and computer-assisted surgery of suspected synovial chondromatosis in the temporomandibular joint. J Magn Reson Imaging 2008;28:1251-1257.
4. Guarda-Nardini L, Piccotti F, Ferronato G, Manfredini D. Synovial chondromatosis of the tem-poromandibular joint: a case description with systematic literature review. Int J Oral Maxillofac Surg 2010;39:745-755.
5. Mercuri LG. Synovial chondromatosis of the temporomandibular joint with middle cranial fossa extension. Int J Oral Maxillofac Surg 2008;37:684.
6. Ardekian L, Faquin W, Troulis MJ, Kaban LB, August M. Synovial chondromatosis of the temporomandibular joint: report and analysis of eleven cases. J Oral Maxillofac Surg 2005;63:941-947.
7. Holmlund AB, Eriksson L, Reinholt FP. Synovial chondromatosis of the temporomandibular joint: Clinical, surgical and histological aspects. Int J Oral Maxillofac Surg 2003;32:143-147.

8. Yu Q, Yang J, Wang P, Shi H, Luo J. CT features of synovial chondromatosis in the temporomandibular joint. Oral Surg Oral Med Oral Pathol Oral Radiol Endod 2004;97:524-528.

9. Unni KK, Inwards CY, Kindblom LG, Wold LE. Tumors of the bones and joints. AFIP Atlas of Tumor Pathology, 4th Series, Fascicle 2. Washington, DC: American Registry of Pathology; 2005:386-389.

Pigmented Villonodular Synovitis

10. Herman CR, Swift JQ, Schiffman EL. Pigmented villonodular synovitis of the temporomandibular joint with intracranial extension: a case and literature review. Int J Oral Maxillofac Surg 2009;38:795-801.

11. Eisig S, Dorfman HD, Cusamano RJ, Kantrowitz AB. Pigmented villonodular synovitis of the temporomandibular joint. Case report and review of the literature. Oral Surg Oral Med Oral Pathol 1992;73:328-333.

12. Kim KW, Han MH, Park SW, et al. Pigmented villonodular synovitis of the temporomandibular joint: MR findings in four cases. Eur J Radiol 2004;49:229-234.

13. Oda Y, Izumi T, Harimaya K, et al. Pigmented villonodular synovitis with chondroid metaplasia, resembling chondroblastoma of the bone: a report of three cases. Mod Pathol 2007;20:545-551.

14. Shapiro SL, McMenomey SO, Alexander P, Schmidt WA. Fine-needle aspiration biopsy diagnosis of "invasive" temporomandibular joint pigmented villonodular synovitis. Arch Pathol Lab Med 2002;126:195-198.

15. West RB, Rubin BP, Miller MA, et al. A landscape effect in tenosynovial giant-cell tumor from activation of CSF1 expression by a translocation in a minority of tumor cells. Proc Natl Acad Sci U S A 2006;103:690-695.

16. Cupp JS, Miller MA, Montgomery KD, et al. Translocation and expression of CSF1 in pigmented villonodular synovitis, tenosynovial giant cell tumor, rheumatoid arthritis and other reactive synovitides. Am J Surg Pathol 2007;31:970-976.

17. Day JD, Yoo A, Muckle R. Pigmented villonodular synovitis of the temporomandibular joint: A rare tumor of the temporal skull base. J Neurosurg 2008;109:140-143.

Tophaceous Pseudogout

18. Reynolds JL, Matthew IR, Chalmers A. Tophaceous calcium pyrophosphate dihydrate deposition disease of the temporomandibular joint. J Rheumatol 2008;35:717-721.

19. Ishida T, Dorfman HD, Bullough PG. Tophaceous pseudogout (tumoral calcium pyrophosphate dihydrate crystal deposition disease). Hum Pathol 1995;26:587-593.

20. Marsot-Dupuch K, Smoker WR, Gentry LR, Cooper KA. Massive calcium pyrophosphate dihydrate crystal deposition disease: a cause of pain of the temporomandibular joint. AJNR Am J Neuroradiol 2004;25:876-879.

21. Kalish LH, Ng T, Kalnins I, Da Cruz MJ. Pseudogout mimicking an infratemporal fossa tumor. Head Neck 2010;32:127-132.

22. Naqvi AH, Abraham JL, Kellman RM, Khurana KK. Calcium pyrophosphate dihydrate deposition disease (CPPD)/Pseudogout of the temporomandibular joint—FNA findings and microanalysis. Cytojournal 2008;5:8.

23. Lambrecht N, Nelson SD, Seeger L, Bose S. Tophaceous pseudogout: a pitfall in the diagnosis of chondrosarcoma. Diagn Cytopathol 2001;25:258-261.

24. Kathju S, Cohen R, Lasko LA, Aynechi M, Dattilo DJ. Pseudogout of the temporomandibular joint: Immediate reconstruction with total joint

19 MISCELLANEOUS LESIONS

MELANOTIC NEUROECTODERMAL TUMOR OF INFANCY

Definition. *Melanotic neuroectodermal tumors of infancy* (MNTI) are rare neoplasms of neural crest origin most often identified in the anterior maxilla of infants. A synonym is *melanotic progonoma*. The lesion was first described by Krompecher in 1918 (1), and the currently used terminology was proposed by Borello and Gorlin in 1966 (2). MNTI probably represents a neoplasm that recapitulates the retina at 5 weeks of gestation (3).

Clinical Features. As indicated above, most lesions occur in infants and involve the anterior maxilla (4–7). Other craniofacial sites include the mandible, orbit, and flat bones of the skull. Rarely, the long bones are involved (8). Although many tumors are nonfunctional, some elevate serum levels of adrenalin, noradrenalin, vanillymandelic acid, and neuron-specific enolase (9).

Radiographic Features. Radiographically, the lesion appears as a radiolucency (fig. 19-1). Displaced, developing primary teeth are often seen within or at the peripheral margins of the radiolucency.

Microscopic Findings. Nests and cords of epithelial cells are surrounded by cellular fibrous connective tissue (fig. 19-2). Closer examination reveals two cell types: large polygonal cells with pale eosinophilic cytoplasm, often containing melanin pigment, and small round cells with scant cytoplasm characteristic of neuroblasts (fig. 19-3). Ultrastructural analysis has revealed melanosomes in the large polygonal cells and neurosecretory granules within the cytoplasm of the small cells (3,10).

Immunohistochemical and Molecular Findings. Immunohistochemical studies show staining for cytokeratin, HMB45, vimentin, epithelial membrane antigen, neuron-specific

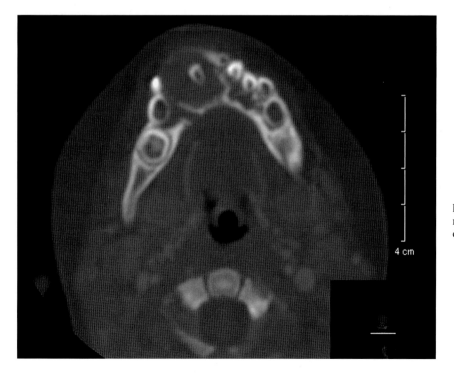

4 cm

Figure 19-1

MELANOTIC NEUROECTODERMAL TUMOR OF INFANCY

A well-demarcated radio-lucency is located in the anterior maxilla. A forming, primary tooth crown is seen within the lesion.

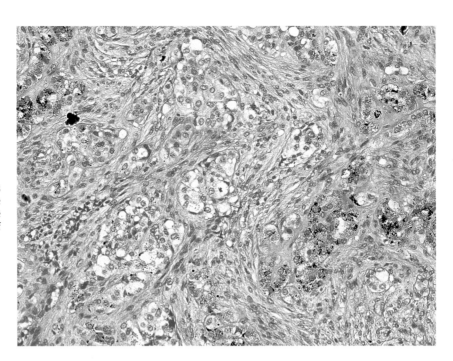

Figure 19-2

MELANOTIC NEUROECTODERMAL TUMOR OF INFANCY

Islands of ovoid epithelial cells with lightly staining cytoplasm are in nests within a fibrous connective tissue background. Granules of melanin are also seen.

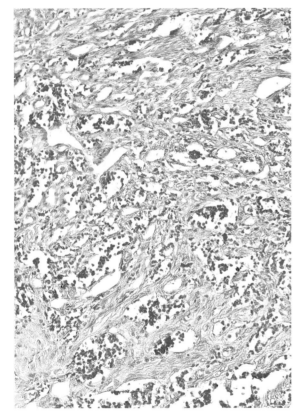

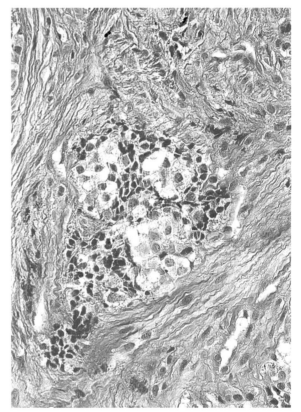

Figure 19-3

MELANOTIC NEUROECTODERMAL TUMOR OF INFANCY

Left: Groups of ovoid cells with scant cytoplasm similar to neuroblasts are seen.
Right: There are large cells with melanin granules and small round cells with scant cytoplasm.

enolase, leu7, synaptophysin, glial fibrillary acidic protein (GFAP), S-100 protein, desmin, and chromogranin (11). There is no staining for carcinoembryonic antigen, retinol-binding protein, or alpha-fetoprotein (3,11). These staining features are similar to those of the pigmented epithelium of the retina (3). Expression of melanotransferrin mRNA is an additional indicator of neural crest origin (10). Loss of heterozygosity of chromosome 1p and gain of chromosome 7q, analogous to neuroblastomas, has been shown in these tumors (12).

Flow cytometry of eight tumors revealed four to be diploid, three aneuploid, and one diploid with a prominent shoulder (3). Aneuploidy may be an important predictor of recurrence.

Differential Diagnosis. The differential diagnosis of these lesions usually includes neuroblastoma and rarely malignant melanoma.

Treatment and Prognosis. Most lesions are managed with simple excision although more aggressive surgery may be necessary (3,12–15). In an evaluation of 12 cases, 5 tumors recurred within 4 months of initial treatment, but none metastasized (11).

In a review of 195 cases, 13 were clearly malignant with evidence of metastasis (3). In an evaluation of 378 previously published cases by Fowler et al. (16), the local recurrence rate was 36 percent and the metastatic rate was 7 percent. There were no histologic or molecular features to predict aggressive behavior.

EWING SARCOMA/PERIPHERAL NEUROECTODERMAL TUMOR

Definition. *Ewing sarcoma/peripheral neuroectodermal tumor* (PNET) is one of the tumors that is classified under the rubric of small blue cell tumor. It is usually a primary tumor of bone but may arise in the soft tissues. This tumor is characterized in most cases by a chromosomal translocation that results in a fusion between the *EWS* gene and an *ETS* type gene. It belongs to a family of closely related tumors sometimes known as the Ewing sarcoma family of tumors (ESFT), which share genetic abnormalities but differ slightly in their pathway of differentiation or location. In the past, when this neoplasm showed light microscopic neural differentiation, such as prominent rosettes, it was designated as peripheral neuroectodermal tumor (PNET);

when it occurred in the bone and had no neural differentiation, it was termed Ewing sarcoma; and when it occurred in the thoracolumbar area it was termed Askin tumor (17). Now the neoplasm is most commonly referred to as Ewing sarcoma/PNET regardless of site.

General Features. Ewing sarcoma/PNET can affect any age group but is rare in newborns and those over 40 years of age. It is most common in the first and second decades. It comprises up to 10 percent of all primary malignant bone lesions (18). While it is not a common tumor, if myeloma is excluded, it is the third most common primary tumor of bone in adults and is the second most common primary bone sarcoma in children. When considering primary neoplasms of bones in adults, only myeloma, osteosarcoma, and chondrosarcoma are more common and in children only osteosarcoma is more common (18,19). In the jaws Ewing sarcoma/PNET is rare, and only 1 to 2 percent of all cases of Ewing sarcoma/PNET present in this location. In a series of Unni et al. (18), only 1 percent of their total cases of Ewing sarcoma/PNET occurred in the jaws. Arafat et al. (20) found only 17 cases in the files of the Armed Forces Institute of Pathology (AFIP) in 1983. Other authors also find that this neoplasm rarely involves the jaws (21–24).

Clinical Features. The overwhelming majority of patients with Ewing sarcoma/PNET are in the first two decades of life and there is a male predominance. In the jaws, the mandible is more often affected than the maxilla. The complaints of pain and swelling are common (20,25). "Numb chin" has been described when the tumor impinges on nerves. In a study of Ewing sarcoma/PNET sarcoma presenting in the bones of the head and neck, Siegal et al. (25) found that the skull was the most frequently affected site, followed by the mandible and maxilla. In general, most tumors are primary but 10 percent are metastases from other sites (21,26).

Radiographic Features. Plain films can show a periosteal reaction or none at all. The classic radiographic appearance of Ewing sarcoma/PNET is cortical bone formation due to stimulation by infiltrative tumor cells. In this manner new bone grows in layers and produces an "onionskin" appearance. In a study of Ewing sarcoma/PNET involving the bones of the

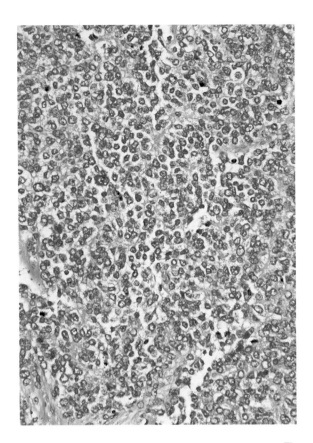 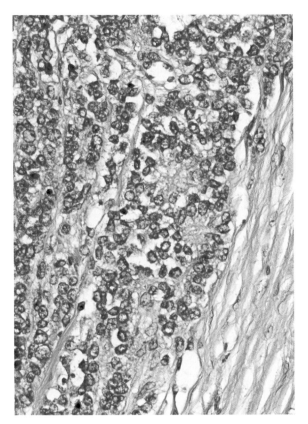

Figure 19-4

EWING SARCOMA/PERIPHERAL NEUROECTODERMAL TUMOR (PNET)

Left: This tumor is characterized as a small blue cell tumor. Similar to all small blue cell tumors, the nucleus is prominent and shows marked hyperchromasia. These neoplasms have a high nuclear to cytoplasmic ratio.

Right: The nuclei have finely distributed chromatin and some nuclei are minimally vesicular. There are essentially no nucleoli but small chromocenters are present. The cytoplasm is pale with indistinct borders.

head and neck, however, only 8 percent of the patients had a cortical reaction and a permeative pattern throughout the bone was seen in slightly over half of the patients, a number much lower than seen in long bones (25). Sclerotic bone changes and involvement of the soft tissue were also much less common, while pure lytic changes and honeycomb patterns were much more common in these head and neck lesions.

Magnetic resonance imaging (MRI) is extremely useful since it evaluates the extent of the tumor in the bone and marrow as well as its extension into the soft tissues better than other methods. MRI has become the most useful method for imaging the primary tumor. It is also useful for monitoring therapeutic response (27,28).

Regardless of the radiographic findings, the imaging features of Ewing sarcoma/PNET are not specific and osteosarcoma is almost always a clinical consideration.

Gross Findings. Ewing sarcoma/PNET often has a liquid consistency and is associated with necrosis and cyst formation.

Microscopic Findings. Ewing sarcoma/PNET is a small round blue cell tumor. Sheets of small cells with round nuclei surrounded by clear but often minimal cytoplasm characterize the tumor (fig. 19-4). The nuclei have finely dispersed chromatin and nucleoli are small and often poorly visualized. Mitoses are present but are quite variable in degree from tumor to tumor. Historically, the presence of rosettes or other features of neural differentiation led to the diagnosis of PNET, and some authorities required neural differentiation as evidenced by immunohistochemical studies. The knowledge

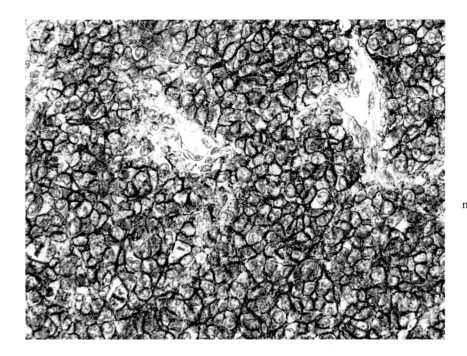

Figure 19-5

EWING SARCOMA/PNET

CD99 antibody stains the cell membrane.

of the same chromosomal abnormalities in Ewing sarcoma and PNET has made this point of academic interest only. Importantly, patients with either designation, Ewing sarcoma or PNET, have similar outcomes when treated similarly.

The absence of an eosinophilic tumor matrix is an important negative finding in the diagnosis of Ewing sarcoma/PNET, helping separate this neoplasm from osteosarcoma. The tumor cells can be arrayed in diffuse sheets, in lobular arrangements separated by fibrous septa, and by fine connecting strands of tumor, termed filigree (18,29). This third pattern is associated with a worse prognosis. The cytoplasm usually contains sufficient glycogen to be positive for periodic acid-Schiff (PAS) which is diastase sensitive. As most patients undergo preoperative chemotherapy, resected specimens may only show fibrosis and necrosis. Ewing sarcoma/PNET sarcoma is not graded, as all tumors are considered as high grade.

Histologic Types. Approximately 10 percent of Ewing sarcoma/PNET tumors are composed of larger, more atypical cells with increased mitoses and irregular nuclei. These tumors have been described as *atypical Ewing sarcoma* or as *large cell Ewing sarcoma* (30) There is no difference in the clinical behavior of these tumors.

Immunohistochemical Findings. Antibodies often employed in the immunohistochemical work-up of Ewing sarcoma/PNET include CD

99, Fli-1, and HNK1 (fig. 19-5). While CD99 is widely used in the diagnosis of this tumor, it is expressed in a large number of other tumors as well. Fli-1 is thought to be more specific since it represents the gene product of the chromosomal translocation seen in the vast majority of Ewing sarcoma/PNET lesions. Ewing sarcoma/PNET may also at times express keratins.

As in histologic sections, cytologic preparations show dispersed cells with poorly demarcated clear cytoplasm, yet with round and uniform nuclei containing diffuse nuclear chromatin and only small nucleoli. Cytology can be useful for abrogating the need for an open biopsy since molecular testing can be performed on aspirated material (31).

Molecular Findings and Other Special Techniques. The 11;22 translocation results in a fusion product that is thought to act as an aberrant transcription factor, upregulating genes responsible for tumor growth (32). Using cytogenetic techniques, Ewing sarcoma/PNET shows the t(11;22) (q24;q12) in approximately 95 percent of cases producing a EWS-Fli-1 transcript. Other translocations are seen as well: the t(21;22) (q22;q12), which produces a EWS-ERG transcript, makes up close to 5 percent of the other cases; other translocations involving 2;22 (producing a EWS-FEV transcript), 17;22 (EWS-E1AF transcript), 16;21, and 7;22 also can be found (18). Recently, a 2;16 translocation has been noted (33). Rarely, a third chromosome is involved in a complex translocation. It is important to note that the 11;22 translocation can be cryptic, requiring fluorescence in situ hybridization (FISH) or reverse transcriptase polymerase chain reaction (RT-PCR) to detect the abnormality (18,34).

Differential Diagnosis. The differential diagnosis of small blue cell tumors includes a large number of entities such as metastatic neuroblastoma, rhabdomyosarcoma (both alveolar and embryonal), monophasic synovial sarcoma, lymphoma, and synovial sarcoma. Neuroblastoma is often suspected on routine stains since it exhibits a prominent crush artifact, similar to that of small cell carcinoma of the lung. Although the tumor cells seen in Ewing sarcoma/PNET can appear similar, they are much more resistant to crush artifact. Neuroblastoma has rosettes similar to those of peripheral neuroectodermal tumor, a tumor in the same family as Ewing sarcoma/PNET. Neuroblastomas are negative for CD99 but positive for CD56 as well as other neural markers.

Embryonal rhabdomyosarcoma is composed of small blue cells but these often show some elongation or spindling of the cytoplasm, not a feature seen in Ewing sarcoma/PNET sarcoma. Alveolar rhabdomyosarcoma cells and their nuclei are larger than those of Ewing sarcoma/PNET. Importantly, rhabdomyosarcomas are positive for desmin and Myo-D1.

Lymphomas in the differential diagnosis include lymphoblastic lymphoma in children and small lymphocytic lymphoma in adults. Immunohistochemical stains in most instances readily separate these tumors. Lymphomas are positive for lymphoid markers such as CD45 and in the case of lymphoblastic lymphoma, terminal deoxynucleotidyltransferase (TdT). Lymphoblastic lymphoma is another malignancy that can be positive for CD99.

The small cell variant of osteosarcoma can be very difficult to separate from Ewing sarcoma/PNET. The production of matrix material should point to the diagnosis of osteosarcoma. Poorly differentiated synovial sarcoma can have identical histologic and immunohistochemical features to Ewing sarcoma/PNET. Molecular diagnostic tests for establishing the presence of the X;18 translocation seen in synovial sarcoma are useful in this setting.

Treatment and Prognosis. The overall survival rate for patients with Ewing sarcoma/PNET has improved markedly in the last decades. Treatment consists of chemotherapy followed by radiotherapy and/or surgery in most sites (35). In the head and neck region in children, radiotherapy is often avoided, if possible, to prevent potential growth arrest of developing facial structures (36). Although the few patients affected make statistical evaluation difficult, the filigree pattern of tumor appears to be associated with a worse prognosis than that of the diffuse pattern. When considering tumors at all anatomic sites in the body, the disease-free survival rate is over 65 percent (35). Interestingly, in a study of 29 patients with Ewing sarcoma/PNET involving the head and neck bones by Siegal et al. (25), none of the patients with mandibular involvement had evidence of disease after more than 2 years of follow-up.

SMOOTH MUSCLE TUMORS

Definition. Smooth muscle tumors, *leiomyomas* and *leiomyosarcomas* can arise in the jaws but are rare. Leiomyosarcomas are much more common than leiomyomas (37,38). Liang et al. (38) found only 12 well-documented patients with intraosseous leiomyoma of the jaws.

General Features. In 2007, Ethunandan et al. (39) reported 68 cases of oral leiomyosarcoma in a review of the literature including 4 of their cases. As in other studies, leiomyosarcomas in the oral cavity can involve the jaw bones (40–45). The etiology or inciting factors of these rare tumors are unknown although Sedghizadeh et al. (46) reported a leiomyosarcoma arising in the maxilla of a patient who had received radiation therapy for retinoblastoma 28 years previously. Martin-Hirsch et al. (47) also reported a case of leiomyosarcoma arising in the maxilla in a patient who had received prior radiotherapy. Although these numbers of reported cases is small, the overall rarity of leiomyosarcoma may suggest that prior radiotherapy is an important contributing cause. Some have suggested that they arise from the smooth muscle in blood vessels.

Clinical Features. In the study of leiomyomas of the jaws, Liang et al. (38) found the age range was 8 months to 71 years, with a mean of 36 years. Five patients were women and seven were men. Most had no symptoms

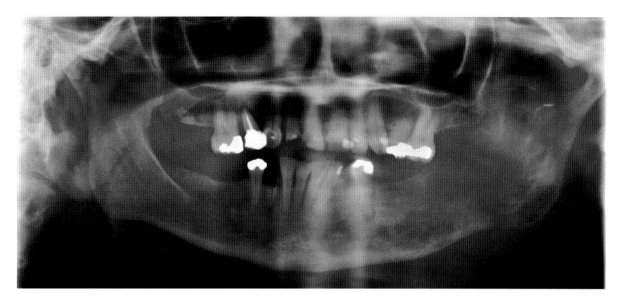

Figure 19-6

LEIOMYOSARCOMA

A radiolucency representing a leiomyosarcoma involves much of the left body of the mandible, ramus, and coronoid. A pathologic tracture is seen at the inferior border of the mandible.

or had asymptomatic swelling. Almost all tumors presented in the mandible, usually in the posterior aspect. Radiographically, the tumors were unilocular or multilocular radiolucencies. Even though the lesions were benign, some had ill-defined borders and many had cortical involvement.

Similarly, leiomyosarcomas of the jaws present as swelling and may not always be associated with pain early in their course. The gender distribution is almost equal in most studies (39,44,45). The age range of patients is wide, 6 to 91 years, with a mean of 41 years. Several studies have shown that the disease has a bimodal distribution when considering age at onset. The first is in the third decade and the second in the fifth to sixth (44,45). Similar to leiomyomas, the tumors have a unilocular or multilocular radiolucent appearance on radiographs (fig. 19-6).

Microscopic Findings. The tumor cells in leiomyoma and lower-grade leiomyosarcoma have spindled elongated cytoplasm that is eosinophilic in hematoxylin and eosin (H&E)-stained sections; the cells are arranged in a fascicular pattern (fig. 19-7). As in other smooth muscle tumors, the nuclei, also elongated and cigar shaped, have rounded blunt ends. High-

grade leiomyosarcomas also have a spindled morphology but the nuclei show marked variability in size (fig. 19-8). Mitotic figures vary from tumor to tumor and most are related directly to the degree of differentiation.

Immunohistochemical Findings. Immunohistochemical stains reveal differentiated smooth muscle tumors to be positive for smooth muscle actin and muscle-specific actin. Desmin is also found in a large percentage of tumors. Epithelial markers, including keratins and epithelial membrane antigen (EMA), may be positive in the lesions; S-100 protein can also be expressed (42).

Molecular Findings. Nikitakis et al. (42) found two cases of leiomyosarcoma to express cyclin-dependent kinase 4 (CDK4) and murine double minute (MDM)2. Using quantitative real-time PCR analysis of the genomic DNA, they did not detect any amplification of MDM2 or CDK4 in one case, while another exhibited amplification of MDM2 but not CDK4.

Differential Diagnosis. The differential diagnosis includes all spindle cell tumors. It is critical that other sources of smooth muscle tumor metastases to the jaws are excluded. This is particularly true in women over 40 years of age in which leiomyosarcomas of the uterus

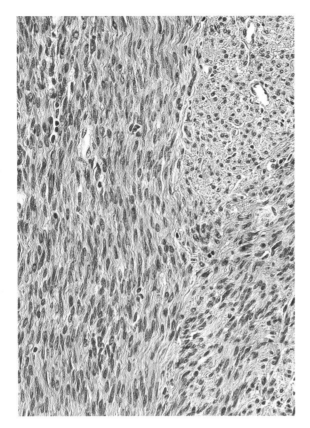

Figure 19-7

LEIOMYOMA

Spindle cells with elongated and slightly curved nuclei with blunt ends are present. No nuclear hyperchromasia or mitotic figures are seen.

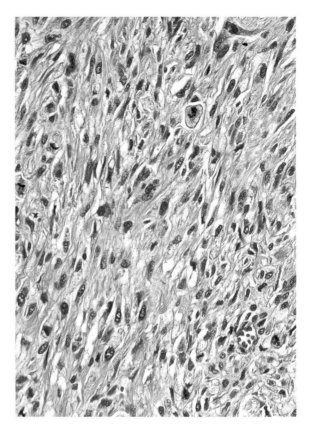

Figure 19-8

LEIOMYOSARCOMA

Spindle cells with indistinct cell borders contain hyperchromatic nuclei.

are common. It is recommended that patients undergo chest, abdomen, and pelvis CT examination prior to starting primary therapy.

Treatment and Prognosis. Complete surgical excision of the lesion is the treatment of choice. For leiomyosarcoma, radiotherapy and chemotherapy, when applied in recurrent tumors, have variable effects and chemotherapy is generally reserved for palliative control of distant metastatic disease.

The overall survival rates of patients with leiomyosarcoma are variable. The overall 5-year survival rate was 62 percent in a study by Vilos et al. (44) while Ethunadan et al. (39) found overall survival at 43 percent in their study of oral leiomyosarcomas that involved the bone. In a review, however, Schenberg et al. (43) found that 69 percent of the patients with oral leiomyosarcomas were dead of disease at 5 years.

A poor prognosis is associated with posterior anatomic locations in the vicinity of the infratemporal fossa, such as the posterior maxillary sinus, the pterygoid plates, and the mandibular condyle as well as positive surgical margins (44).

PERIPHERAL NERVE SHEATH TUMORS

Definition. *Peripheral nerve sheath tumors* are neoplasms arising within the peripheral nerves. In the jaws they comprise primarily two benign lesions, *neurofibroma* and *schwannoma*, the latter synonymous with *neurilemmoma*.

The malignant counterpart of neurofibroma is known as *malignant peripheral nerve sheath tumor* and synonyms include *neurofibrosarcoma* and *malignant schwannoma*.

General Features. Peripheral nerve sheath tumors are unusual in the jaws with only case reports and small series of patients in the literature (48–59). In a review in 2006, Che et al.

(48) found only 33 cases of central neurofibroma in this location. While both neurofibromas and schwannomas are composed of neural tissue, neurofibromas are composed of a greater mixture of cell types, including Schwann cells and fibroblasts. Neurofibromas can be solitary or part of neurofibromatosis 1 (NF1). In patients with neurofibromatosis, the lesions can be multiple in the jaws and have a plexiform pattern of growth.

As opposed to neurofibromas, schwannomas are differentiated toward Schwann cells. These neoplasms are slow growing. They are encapsulated, in contrast to neurofibroma (52,53).

Even rarer in the jaws are malignant peripheral nerve sheath tumors. The exact incidence of these neoplasms is difficult to know as many do not show obvious neural differentiation and could be misdiagnosed as fibrosarcoma or another malignant spindle cell neoplasm (54,55).

Clinical Features. Benign peripheral nerve sheath tumors most usually present as a painless swelling in most patients. The teeth can be loosened or even resorbed. Pain and paresthesia have also been reported. Many series suggest that neural tumors are more common in the mandible than the maxilla. This predilection is thought to be due to the fact that the trigeminal nerve branch in the mandible is the longest intraosseous nerve pathway in the skeleton. The posterior mandible is most affected and there is a slight female predominance (50).

Neurofibromas are uncommon in the jaws. They are multiple or solitary lesions. In the oral cavity, tumors arising in the soft tissues are more likely to be associated with neurofibromatosis. Central bony lesions, which are usually solitary, are usually not associated with neurofibromatosis. Besides the displacement of teeth, other radiographic abnormalities are present. The tumors can produce a variety of radiolucent lesions including ones that are unilocular or multilocular. They have been described as having discrete margins as well as ill-defined margins. In the mandible, the common radiographic findings of neurofibroma include an enlarged mandibular foramen which correlates with tumor involvement of this branch of the trigeminal nerve, an increase in bone density, lateral bowing of the mandibular ramus, increase in dimensions of the coronoid notch, and a decrease in the mandibular angle (56,57).

Schwannomas are also rare in the jaws as well as in skeletal bones in general (59). Chi et al. (52) found 43 acceptable cases of intraosseous schwannoma in a review in 2003. Of these 43, only 5 were located in the maxilla. In their study, the radiographic features of schwannomas in the jaws revealed a well-demarcated radiolucency that was unilocular. They generally had the appearance of a benign lesion and had thin sclerotic borders. Occasional cases were multilocular and some tumors were associated with root resorption. In only three cases were there features of mandibular canal expansion.

Malignant peripheral nerve sheath tumors are uncommon in the jaws although in the oral cavity, the mandible is one of the sites most often involved (54). Radiographically, these malignant neoplasms appear similar to benign peripheral nerve sheath tumors with enlargement of the mandibular canal. Grossly, they present as fleshy masses with pushing borders, although on microscopic sections, small fingers of tumor infiltrate the surrounding tissues (fig. 19-9).

Microscopic Findings. The cellularity of neurofibromas is highly variable. Neurofibromas are composed of fibroblasts, collagen, and Schwann cells in a myxoid background (fig. 19-10). The nuclei of some cells are described as "wavy" and in others they are curvilinear to oval. Lymphocytes can be present and mast cells are common.

Schwannomas are characterized by Antoni A (organized) and B (poorly organized) tissue. Antoni A areas contain Verocay bodies, which are composed of cells arranged in distinct parallel structures (fig. 19-11). Antoni B areas have spindle cells with random organization admixed with fibroblasts in mildly to moderately edematous stroma. A near constant finding in both Antoni A and Antoni B areas is the presence of vessels with very thick, hyalinized walls. Although variants of schwannoma exist, including epithelioid, plexiform, cellular, melanotic, and ancient, they are uncommonly seen in the jaws. Chi et al. (52) found rare examples of cellular and melanotic schwannomas in their review. In a patient reported by Vincent and Williams (58), biopsy of one of the lesions in the mandible revealed variably dense fibrous connective tissue containing infiltrates of lymphocytes, plasma cells, and neutrophils.

Figure 19-9

MALIGNANT PERIPHERAL NERVE SHEATH TUMOR

This large fleshy mass has a pushing border. Although it appears circumscribed, it revealed infiltrative growth microscopically.

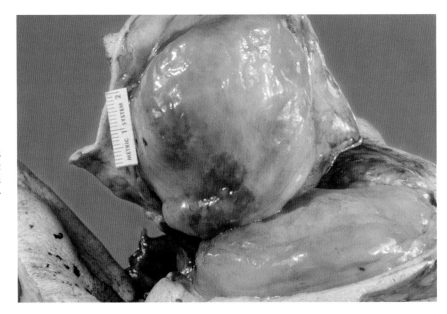

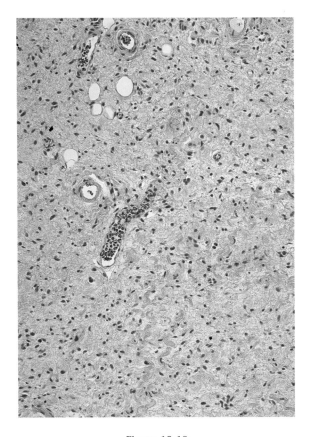

Figure 19-10

NEUROFIBROMA

A myxoid to collagenous background characterizes many neurofibromas. Cellularity is not marked and no distinct structural patterns are present. No mitotic figures are seen and the nuclei are small.

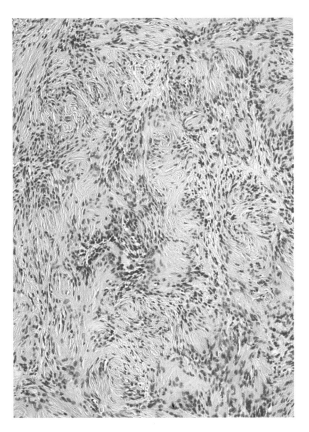

Figure 19-11

SCHWANNOMA

This area of a schwannoma shows the organized Antoni type A pattern of cells. Numerous Verocay bodies with palisading are evident.

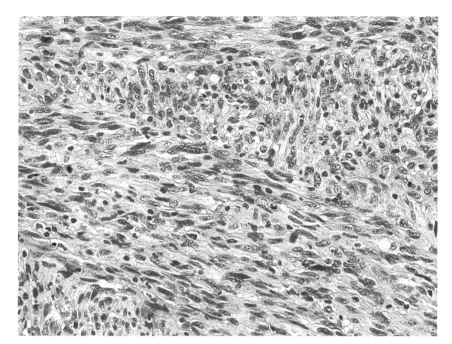

Figure 19-12

MALIGNANT PERIPHERAL NERVE SHEATH TUMOR

This is a hypercellular neoplasm with a spindled pattern. There is striking nuclear hyperchromasia with chromatin clumping and the presence of nucleoli.

No nerve fibers were evident on histochemical stains. The authors noted that these findings were those of the fibrous intrabony lesions seen in neurofibromatosis.

Malignant peripheral nerve sheath tumors may be difficult to classify as such since they have a spindled appearance but may not always show distinct neural features (fig. 19-12). Direct continuity with a nerve or a tumor arising in a preexisting neurofibroma is a helpful finding. Otherwise, malignant peripheral nerve sheath tumors have features of spindle cell sarcomas and exhibit a range of differentiation. Some rare tumors have an epithelioid appearance. Often the spindled cells have the herringbone pattern often associated with fibrosarcoma. Atypical nuclei and necrosis are seen in only some tumors.

Both neurofibromas and schwannomas are positive for S-100 protein. Usually, schwannomas are more strongly and diffusely positive than neurofibromas. Malignant peripheral nerve sheath tumors may not always be positive for S-100 protein, or at best, only focally positive.

Differential Diagnosis. Benign peripheral nerve sheath tumors are usually not a differential diagnostic problem. Similarly, low-grade malignant peripheral nerve sheath tumors show a spindled arrangement and features similar to neurofibroma. High-grade malignant peripheral nerve sheath tumors are frequently difficult to diagnose in almost any site. Any spindle cell tumor with "wavy" nuclei should be suspected of being of peripheral nerve sheath origin. Many if not most high-grade malignant peripheral nerve sheath tumors do not express S-100 protein immunohistochemically. High-grade sarcomas arising in patients with neurofibromatosis are likely malignant peripheral nerve sheath tumors.

Treatment and Prognosis. The treatment of neurofibroma and schwannoma is conservative but complete excision. Recurrences of solitary neurofibroma or schwannoma should not be expected if there is complete excision. In patients with neurofibromatosis, however, recurrences may be in fact new primary tumors developing in any residual nerve. In the series of Chi et al. (52), recurrence was seen in five mandibular schwannomas and in no maxillary cases; recurrence was associated with incomplete excision in some cases.

For malignant peripheral nerve sheath tumor, radical resection is indicated. Radiotherapy and chemotherapy can be utilized in the appropriate clinical settings (54). Malignant peripheral nerve sheath tumors recur locally and spread by perineural extension. They can also metastasize hematogenously to the lung and liver.

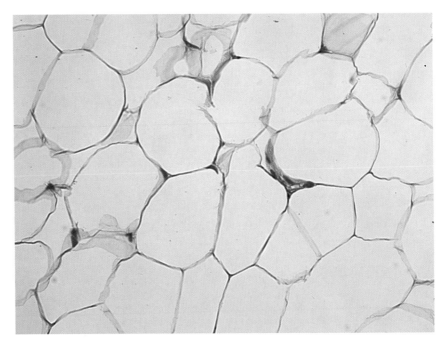

Figure 19-13

LIPOMA

The mature adipocytes have small nuclei.

FAT-PRODUCING TUMORS

Definition. *Lipomas* and *liposarcomas* represent the benign and malignant neoplasms, respectively, of fat-producing tumors.

General Features. Lipomas are common tumors throughout the soft tissues, usually affecting the trunk and proximal extremities, but they are exceedingly uncommon in the skeleton, despite the fact that the bone marrow in adults is richly supplied in fat. In the bone, lipomas represent less than 1 percent of all tumors (60). When intraosseous, lipomas are most commonly seen in the metaphyses of long bones as well as the calcaneus (61,62). Darling and Daley (63) reported a single case of lipoma in the mandible. Their review of the literature from 1948 to 2005 found an additional 15 cases.

While intraosseous lipomas of the jaws are rare, liposarcomas in this location are even more infrequently reported. Unni et al. (62) reported that only one liposarcoma was found in an intraosseous location in the experience of the Mayo Clinic. In a review in 1992, McCulloch et al. (64) found 77 liposarcomas in the head and neck and only 2 were located in the jaws. Some authors have noted that liposarcomas in the skeleton are more frequently pleomorphic (62).

Clinical and Radiographic Features. Usually patients with lipomas present with few or no symptoms. Radiographic images of the jawbones generally show a unilocular or multilocular radiolucent image, sometimes with a honeycomb or soap bubble appearance. Opacities are occasional (61). Radiographically, the differential diagnosis includes ameloblastoma, keratocystic odontogenic tumor, central giant cell granuloma, odontogenic myxoma, or early cemento-osseous lesions (63).

Microscopic Findings. Lipomas and liposarcomas are characterized by cells producing lipid-filled cytoplasm. The fat is removed in most routine processing by organic compounds such as alcohol and xylene with only the cell membrane remaining.

Microscopically, lipomas are characterized by mature adipose tissue. Intraosseous lipomas often show central calcification with small bony spicules (fig. 19-13). Liposarcomas may show minimal atypia with only slight enlargement of the nuclei and scattered lipoblasts (fig. 19-14). Some report a highly cellular tumor with minimal lipomatous differentiation making the diagnosis of a lipomatous tumor difficult. In order to diagnose liposarcoma, there should be at least some distinct lipoblast formation.

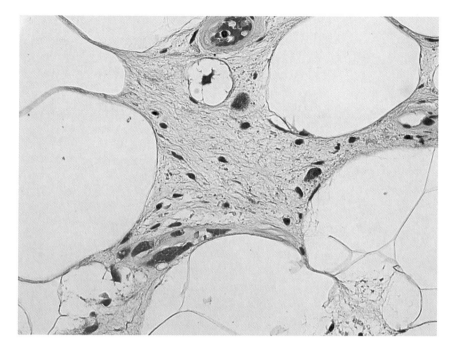

Figure 19-14

LIPOSARCOMA

This well-differentiated liposarcoma has a myxoid stroma focally and mild nuclear enlargement. A vacuolated lipoblast is present.

Differential Diagnosis. The histologic differential diagnosis of lipoma includes fatty bone marrow in an osteoporotic bone marrow defect. A distinct radiolucent lesion with calcifications or bony spicules in the center points to lipoma.

Treatment and Prognosis. Lipomas are conservatively excised with little chance of recurrence. There is very little literature to support the best treatment of liposarcoma of the jaw although complete excision would be required.

CONGENITAL EPULIS OF THE NEWBORN

Definition. *Congenital epulis,* also termed *Neumann tumor,* is a very rare tumor that arises from the gingiva of newborns.

General Features. Congenital epulis presents at birth. There is a marked predominance for female infants of 8 to 1–9 to 1. The etiology is still uncertain (65,66). Attesting to the rarity of the tumor, Zuker and Buenecha (67) found 163 acceptable cases reported prior to 1993.

Clinical Features. The tumor is noted clinically shortly after birth when it can interfere with feeding (67,68). Multiple tumors are found in 10 percent of patients. While the tumors are found in either the maxillary or mandibular gingiva, there is a maxillary predominance. The most common site is the area of the maxillary canine or incisor. MRI evaluation shows that the lesion does not extend deep into the gingiva or cause bony abnormalities.

Microscopic Findings. Congenital epulis is composed of large, rounded cells with granular cytoplasm. The rete are flattened in the overlying epithelium (fig. 19-15). There is no nuclear atypia and the nuclei are small. The capillaries may be in a plexiform arrangement within the tumor.

Immunohistochemical Findings. Congenital epulis is negative for S-100 protein, an important distinguishing characteristic to separate it from granular cell tumor. In addition to positivity for S-100 protein, granular cell tumors are positive for nerve growth factor receptor (NGFR) which is negative in congenital epulis.

Differential Diagnosis. The primary entity in the histologic differential diagnosis is granular cell tumor. Granular cell tumors arise in multiple sites in the oral cavity as well as elsewhere but are uncommon in the gingiva. Granular cell tumors are known for their ability to incite a pseudoepitheliomatous hyperplastic reaction whereas this does not occur in congenital epulis. The immunohistochemical markers of S-100 protein, NGFR, and alpha-inhibin are positive in granular cell tumors but not in congenital epulis.

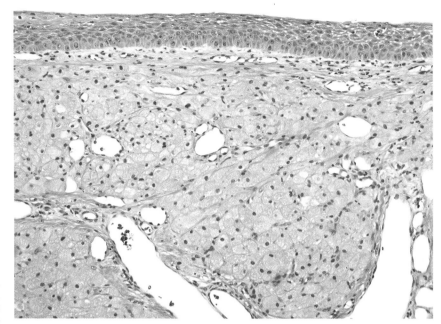

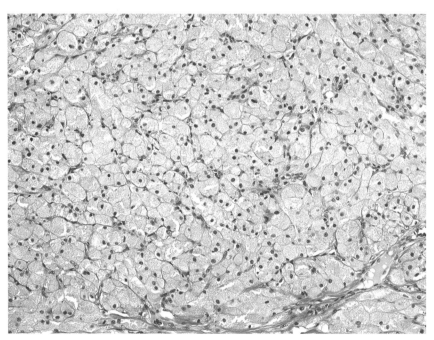

Figure 19-15

CONGENITAL EPULIS

Top: A thin squamous cell epithelium covers a proliferation of cells with granular gray-pink cytoplasm. There is no pseudo-epitheliomatous hyperplasia as seen in granular cell tumor.

Bottom: The nuclei of the cells are round and slightly vesicular and appear to be haphazardly placed in the voluminous cytoplasm.

Treatment and Prognosis. Most of these lesions are treated with conservative excision. Once the tumor is removed, there is no recurrence. There are reports of spontaneous regression (68). If the lesion does not interfere with respiration or feeding, some advocate only observation, with the expectation of tumor regression.

TUMORS METASTATIC TO THE JAWS

Definition. Malignant tumors metastatic from other organs can present in the jaws. Primarily these include *carcinomas* and *melanomas*.

General Features. Red bone marrow is associated with a large blood flow. Thus, it is not surprising that jaw metastases occur since many tumors spread hematogenously and the

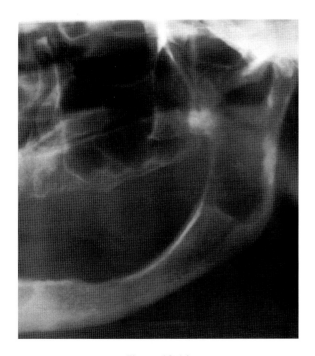

Figure 19-16

METASTATIC BREAST CARCINOMA

A lytic lesion of the mandibular ramus with a slightly irregular border was found to be a metastasis from ductal breast carcinoma.

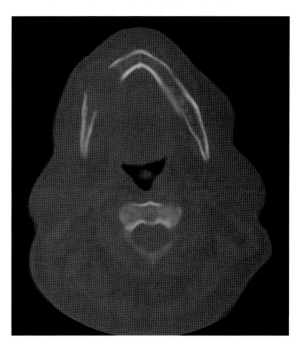

Figure 19-17

METASTATIC RENAL CELL CARCINOMA TO THE MANDIBLE

A large tumor has destroyed the bony aspects of the mandible.

jaws maintain a significant amount of red bone marrow throughout adult life (69). Overall, metastatic carcinoma accounts for most malignancies involving the jawbones. As in other sites, carcinomas of the breast, lung, kidney, and prostate are the most frequent to metastasize to the jaws (70–72). Importantly, metastatic tumors can mimic primary jaw tumors, and some primary tumors of the jaw suggest metastatic disease (73).

Clinical Features. Most patients with jaw metastases are in the fifth to seventh decades, an age range in which malignancies are particularly common in adults. In the jaws, the mandible is more frequently affected than the maxilla. Some authors note that women are more likely to present with metastases to the jaws than men, probably because breast cancer is the most common tumor to metastasize to this site (70). The frequency of any given tumor to metastasize to the jaws is also a factor of demographics. For example, in the study by Lim et al. (74) of Korean patients, men were more likely to present with metastases in the jaws, in a ratio of 2.3 to 1 compared to women, with lung, liver, and thyroid carcinomas reported

in the 23 patients in the series. Those authors noted that hepatocellular carcinoma is much more common in this population than in many Western populations, possibly accounting for the gender difference. Interestingly, breast carcinomas were not found in their series. In a review of the literature of metastases to the jawbone, Hirshberg et al. (72) found the most common metastases, in decreasing order, were from breast, lung, kidney, adrenal gland, bone, colon, prostate gland, and liver. Other sites in other series include thyroid gland, female gynecologic tract, male urogenital tract, salivary gland, and liver, as well as from melanoma (70,71,75,76).

When metastases affect the jaws, patients have numerous signs and symptoms including loose teeth, paresthesias, localized swelling, and pain (77). On radiographic examination, most metastatic lesions are radiolucent and have ill-defined borders, although on occasion the borders are circumscribed, mimicking a benign process (figs. 19-16–19-18). In a significant number of patients, the metastatic tumor in the oral region is the first sign of a malignancy that is

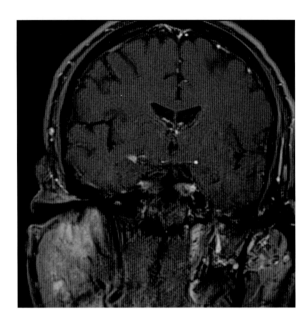

Figure 19-18

METASTATIC PULMONARY ADENOCARCINOMA

Magnetic resonance imaging (MRI) shows a large neoplasm in the right temporomandibular joint that has destroyed the joint space and much of the condyle.

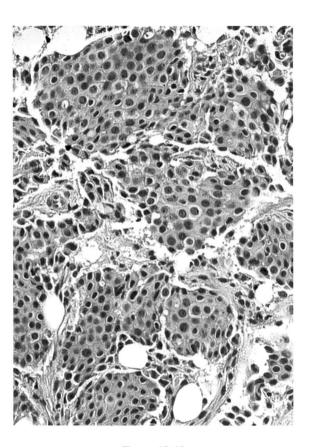

Figure 19-19

METASTATIC DUCTAL BREAST CARCINOMA

Nests of epithelial cells with large, round nuclei containing a single nucleolus are seen. Breast carcinoma often has distinct cell borders with an amphophilic cytoplasm.

primary elsewhere (70,72). Some authors point out that when aggressive clinical or radiographic lesions present in the jaws of older patients, consideration should be given to metastatic disease (78).

Immunohistochemical Findings and Differential Diagnosis. The immunohistochemical stains of most use in the work-up of a metastatic malignancy depend, in part, on the patient history available and the appearance of the neoplasm on hematoxylin and eosin (H&E)-stained sections (fig. 19-19). At times, it is possible to have a reasonable idea of the source of the metastasis given the appearance of the tumor on H&E-stained slides. Often, however, it is not possible to determine the source of the metastasis in routinely stained sections.

The presence of clear cells suggests several tumors. The most common metastatic clear cell tumor to the jaws is clear cell renal cell carcinoma, conventional type (fig. 19-20), followed by melanoma and malignant clear cell tumors of the prostate, bowel, thyroid gland, and liver (80). For metastatic clear cell renal cell carcinoma, PAX-8 and PAX-2 have been shown to be useful (81).

If no historical information is available to point to a likely source of metastasis, such as lung, then an initial limited panel of immunohistochemical markers are applied. The markers of most use are a pankeratin cocktail mix (pankeratin), thyroid transcription factor -1 (TTF-1; to mark lung adenocarcinoma as well as thyroid carcinoma), and CD45 to exclude a hematologic malignancy (fig. 19-21). In men, adding prostate-specific antigen (PSA) is of value. Other markers are S-100 protein and/or melanin A (Mart-1) for melanoma (fig. 19-22). This panel may then be followed by a more focussed subsequent panel.

Treatment. Metastatic disease to the jaws is usually an indication of advanced-stage disease. For local control of metastases, radiotherapy can be of benefit.

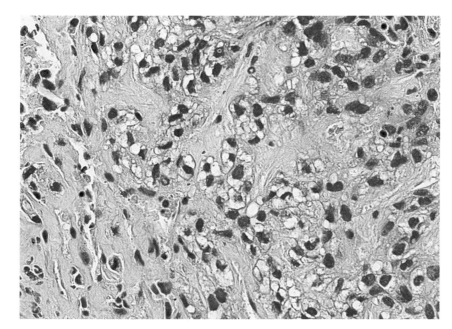

Figure 19-20

METASTATIC CLEAR CELL RENAL CELL CARCINOMA

The cell cytoplasm is cleared and the nucleus is often in an eccentric location.

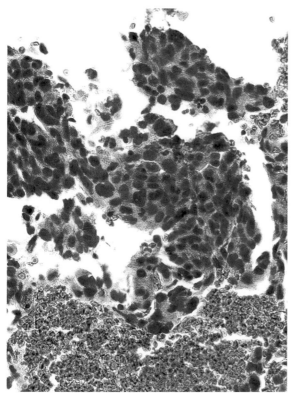
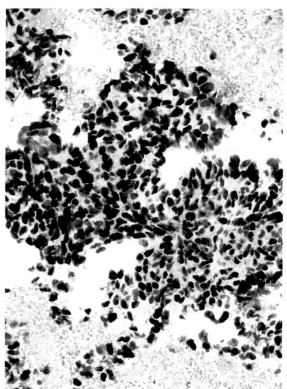

Figure 19-21

METASTATIC POORLY DIFFERENTIATED PULMONARY ADENOCARCINOMA

Left: The tumor cells show minimal differentiation but the clustering and cohesion are indicative of an epithelial-derived neoplasm. Immunohistochemical determination of a site of origin is required if no clinical information or prior histologic material is available.

Right: This immunohistochemical stain for thyroid transcription factor (TTF)-1 was performed on the tumor cells seen in the left figure. The tumor cell nuclei are strongly positive. The patient had a large lung mass and a clinical history of smoking.

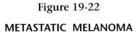

Figure 19-22

METASTATIC MELANOMA

Epithelioid cells with partially cleared cytoplasm have large round to oval nuclei that contain one or more prominent nucleoli. A distinct nesting pattern is seen.

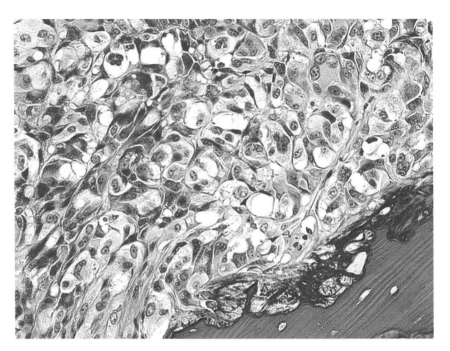

REFERENCES

Melanotic Neuroectodermal Tumor of Infancy

1. Krompecher E. Zur histogenese und morphologie der adamantinome und sonstiger kiefergeschwulste. Beitr Pathol Anat 1918;64:165-197.
2. Borello ED, Gorlin RJ. Melanotic neuroectodermal tumor of infancy—a neoplasm of neural crese origin. Report of a case associated with high urinary excretion of vanilmandelic acid. Cancer 1966;19:196-206.
3. Pettinato G, Manivel JC, d'Amore ES, Jaszcz W, Gorlin RJ. Melanotic neuroectodermal tumor of infancy. A reexamination of a histogenetic problem based on immunohistochemical, flow cytometric, and ultrastructural study of 10 cases. Am J Surg Pathol 1991;15:233-245.
4. Agarwal P, Saxena S, Kumar S, Gupta R. Melanotic neuroectodermal tumor of infancy: Presentation of a case affecting the maxilla. J Oral Maxillofac Pathol 2010;14:29-32.
5. Agoumi M, Al Dhaybi R, Powell J, Brochu P, Lapointe A, Kokta V. Rapidly growing gingival mass in an infant—quiz case. Melanotic neuroectodermal tumor of infancy (MNTI). Arch Dermatol 2010;146:337-342.
6. Jain P, Garg RK, Kapoor A. Melanotic neuroectodermal tumor of infancy in oral cavity at unusual age. Fetal Pediatr Pathol 2010;29:344-352.
7. Madrid C, Aziza J, Hlali A, Bouferrache K, Abarca M. Melanotic neuroectodermal tumour of infancy: a case report and review of the aetiopathogenic hypotheses. Med Oral Patol Oral Cir Bucal 2010;15:e739-42.
8. Choi IS, Kook H, Han DK, et al. Melanotic neuroectodermal tumor of infancy in the femur: a case report and review of the literature. J Pediatr Hematol Oncol 2007;29:854-857.
9. Hoshino S, Takahashi H, Shimura T, Nakazawa S, Naito Z, Asano G. Melanotic neuroectodermal tumor of infancy in the skull associated with high serum levels of catecholamine. Case report. J Neurosurg 1994;80:919-924.
10. Nitta T, Endo T, Tsunoda A, Kadota Y, Matsumoto T, Sato K. Melanotic neuroectodermal tumor of infancy: a molecular approach to diagnosis. Case report. J Neurosurg 1995;83:145-148.
11. Kapadia SB, Frisman DM, Hitchcock CL, Ellis GL, Popek EJ. Melanotic neuroectodermal tumor of infancy. Clinicopathological, immunohistochemical, and flow cytometric study. Am J Surg Pathol 1993;17:566-573.

12. Neven J, Hulsbergen-van der Kaa C, Groot-Loonen J, de Wilde PC, Merkx MA. Recurrent melanotic neuroectodermal tumor of infancy: a proposal for treatment protocol with surgery and adjuvant chemotherapy. Oral Surg Oral Med Oral Pathol Oral Radiol Endod 2008;106:493-496.

13. Butt FM, Guthua SW, Chindia ML, Rana F, Osundwa TM. Early outcome of three cases of melanotic neuroectodermal tumour of infancy. J Craniomaxillofac Surg 2009;37:434-437.

14. Hamilton S, Macrae D, Agrawal S, Matic D. Melanotic neuroectodermal tumour of infancy. Can J Plast Surg 2008;16:41-44.

15. Lambropoulos V, Neofytou A, Sfougaris D, Mouravas V, Petropoulos A. Melanotic neuroectodermal tumor of infancy (MNT1) arising in the skull. Short review of two cases. Acta Neurochir (Wien) 2010;152:869-875.

16. Fowler DJ, Chisholm J, Roebuck D, Newman L, Malone M, Sebire NJ. Melanotic neuroectodermal tumor of infancy: clinical, radiological, and pathological features. Fetal Pediatr Pathol 2006;25:59-72.

Ewing Sarcoma/PNET

17. Askin FB, Rosai J, Sibley RK, Dehner LP, McAlister WH. Malignant small cell tumor of the thoracopulmonary region in childhood: A distinctive clinicopathologic entity of uncertain histogenesis. Cancer 1979;43:2438-2451.

18. Unni KK, Inwards CY, Kindblom LG, Wold LE. Tumors of the bones and joints. AFIP Atlas of Tumor Pathology, 4th Series, Fascicle 2. Washington, DC: American Registry of Pathology; 2005:209-222.

19. Maheshwari AV, Cheng EY. Ewing sarcoma family of tumors. J Am Acad Orthop Surg 2010;18:94-107.

20. Arafat A, Ellis GL, Adrian JC. Ewing's sarcoma of the jaws. Oral Surg Oral Med Oral Pathol 1983;55:589-596.

21. Berk R, Heller A, Heller D, Schwartz S, Klein EA. Ewing's sarcoma of the mandible: a case report. Oral Surg Oral Med Oral Pathol Oral Radiol Endod 1995;79:159-162.

22. Li S, Siegal GP. Small cell tumors of bone. Adv Anat Pathol 2010;17:1-11.

23. Whaley JT, Indelicato DJ, Morris CG, et al. Ewing tumors of the head and neck. Am J Clin Oncol 2010;33:321-326.

24. Pitak-Arnnop P, Bellefqih S, Bertolus C, et al. Ewing's sarcoma of jaw bones in adult patients: 10-year experiences in a Paris university hospital. J Craniomaxillofac Surg 2008;36:450-455.

25. Siegal GP, Oliver WR, Reinus WR, et al. Primary Ewing's sarcoma involving the bones of the head and neck. Cancer 1987;60:2829-2840.

26. Wang CL, Yacobi R, Pharoah M, Thorner P. Ewing's sarcoma: metastatic tumor to the jaw. Oral Surg Oral Med Oral Pathol 1991;71:597-602.

27. Gorospe L, Fernandez-Gil MA, Garcia-Raya P, Royo A, Lopez-Barea F, Garcia-Miguel P. Ewing's sarcoma of the mandible: radiologic features with emphasis on magnetic resonance appearance. Oral Surg Oral Med Oral Pathol Oral Radiol Endod 2001;91:728-734.

28. Lopes SL, Almeida SM, Costa AL, Zanardi VA, Cendes F. Imaging findings of Ewing's sarcoma in the mandible. J Oral Sci 2007;49:167-171.

29. Kissane JM, Askin FB, Foulkes M, Stratton LB, Shirley SF. Ewing's sarcoma of bone: Clinicopathologic aspects of 303 cases from the Intergroup Ewing's Sarcoma Study. Hum Pathol 1983;14:773-779.

30. Nascimento AG, Unni KK, Pritchard DJ, Cooper KL, Dahlin DC. A clinicopathologic study of 20 cases of large-cell (atypical) Ewing's sarcoma of bone. Am J Surg Pathol 1980;4:29-36.

31. Sanati S, Lu DW, Schmidt E, Perry A, Dehner LP, Pfeifer JD. Cytologic diagnosis of Ewing sarcoma/peripheral neuroectodermal tumor with paired prospective molecular genetic analysis. Cancer 2007;111:192-199.

32. Bovee JV, Hogendoorn PC. Molecular pathology of sarcomas: concepts and clinical implications. Virchows Arch 2010;456:193-9.

33. Ng TL, O'Sullivan MJ, Pallen CJ, et al. Ewing sarcoma with novel translocation t(2;16) producing an in-frame fusion of FUS and FEV. J Mol Diagn 2007;9:459-463.

34. Bridge RS, Rajaram V, Dehner LP, Pfeifer JD, Perry A. Molecular diagnosis of Ewing sarcoma/primitive neuroectodermal tumor in routinely processed tissue: a comparison of two FISH strategies and RT-PCR in malignant round cell tumors. Mod Pathol 2006;19:1-8.

35. Bernstein M, Kovar H, Paulussen M, et al. Ewing's sarcoma family of tumors: current management. Oncologist 2006;11:503-519.

36. Solomon LW, Frustino JL, Loree TR, Brecher ML, Alberico RA, Sullivan M. Ewing sarcoma of the mandibular condyle: multidisciplinary management optimizes outcome. Head Neck 2008;30:405-410.

Smooth Muscle Tumors

37. Mechlin DC, Hamasaki CK, Moore JR, Davis WE, Templer J. Leiomyoma of the maxilla—report of a case. Laryngoscope 1980;90(Pt 1):1230-1233.

38. Liang H, Frederiksen NL, Binnie WH, Cheng YS. Intraosseous oral leiomyoma: systematic review and report of one case. Dentomaxillofac Radiol 2003;32:285-290.

39. Ethunandan M, Stokes C, Higgins B, Spedding A, Way C, Brennan P. Primary oral leiomyosarcoma: a clinico-pathologic study and analysis of prognostic factors. Int J Oral Maxillofac Surg 2007;36:409-416.

40. Izumi K, Maeda T, Cheng J, Saku T. Primary leiomyosarcoma of the maxilla with regional lymph node metastasis. Report of a case and review of the literature. Oral Surg Oral Med Oral Pathol Oral Radiol Endod 1995;80:310-319.

41. Kratochvil FJ 3rd, MacGregor SD, Budnick SD, Hewan-Lowe K, Allsup HW. Leiomyosarcoma of the maxilla. Report of a case and review of the literature. Oral Surg Oral Med Oral Pathol 1982;54:647-655.

42. Nikitakis NG, Lopes MA, Bailey JS, Blanchaert RH Jr, Ord RA, Sauk JJ. Oral leiomyosarcoma: review of the literature and report of two cases with assessment of the prognostic and diagnostic significance of immunohistochemical and molecular markers. Oral Oncol 2002;38:201-208.

43. Schenberg ME, Slootweg PJ, Koole R. Leiomyosarcomas of the oral cavity. Report of four cases and review of the literature. J Craniomaxillofac Surg 1993;21:342-347.

44. Vilos GA, Rapidis AD, Lagogiannis GD, Apostolidis C. Leiomyosarcomas of the oral tissues: clinicopathologic analysis of 50 cases. J Oral Maxillofac Surg 2005;63:1461-1477.

45. Yan B, Li Y, Pan J, Xia H, Li LJ. Primary oral leiomyosarcoma: a retrospective clinical analysis of 20 cases. Oral Dis 2010;16:198-203.

46. Sedghizadeh PP, Angiero F, Allen CM, Kalmar JR, Rawal Y, Albright EA. Post-irradiation leiomyosarcoma of the maxilla: report of a case in a patient with prior radiation treatment for retinoblastoma. Oral Surg Oral Med Oral Pathol Oral Radiol Endod 2004;97:726-731.

47. Martin-Hirsch DP, Habashi S, Benbow EW, Farrington WT. Post-irradiation leiomyosarcoma of the maxilla. J Laryngol Otol 1991;105:1068-1071.

Peripheral Nerve Tumors

48. Che Z, Nam W, Park WS, et al. Intraosseous nerve sheath tumors in the jaws. Yonsei Med J 2006;47:264-270.

49. Cherrick HM, Eversole LR. Benign neural sheath neoplasm of the oral cavity. Report of thirty-seven cases. Oral Surg Oral Med Oral Pathol 1971;32:900-909.

50. Ellis GL, Abrams AM, Melrose RJ. Intraosseous benign neural sheath neoplasms of the jaws. Report of seven new cases and review of the literature. Oral Surg Oral Med Oral Pathol 1977;44:731-743.

51. Polak M, Polak G, Brocheriou C, Vigneul J. Solitary neurofibroma of the mandible: case report

and review of the literature. J Oral Maxillofac Surg 1989;47:65-68.

52. Chi AC, Carey J, Muller S. Intraosseous schwannoma of the mandible: a case report and review of the literature. Oral Surg Oral Med Oral Pathol Oral Radiol Endod 2003;96:54-65.

53. Villanueva J, Gigoux C, Sole F. Central neurilemmoma of maxilla. A case report. Oral Surg Oral Med Oral Pathol Oral Radiol Endod 1995;79:41-43.

54. Chao JC, Ho HC, Huang CC, Tzeng JE. Malignant schwannoma of the mandible: a case report. Auris Nasus Larynx 2007;34:287-291.

55. Shirasuna K, Fukuda Y, Kitamura R, et al. Malignant schwannoma of the mandible. Int J Oral Maxillofac Surg 1986;15:772-776.

56. Lee L, Yan YH, Pharoah MJ. Radiographic features of the mandible in neurofibromatosis: a report of 10 cases and review of the literature. Oral Surg Oral Med Oral Pathol Oral Radiol Endod 1996;81:361-367.

57. Friedrich RE, Giese M, Schmelzle R, Mautner VF, Scheuer HA. Jaw malformations plus displacement and numerical aberrations of teeth in neurofibromatosis type 1: a descriptive analysis of 48 patients based on panoramic radiographs and oral findings. J Craniomaxillofac Surg 2003;31:1-9.

58. Vincent SD, Williams TP. Mandibular abnormalities in neurofibromatosis. Case report and literature review. Oral Surg Oral Med Oral Pathol 1983;55:253-258.

59. Unni KK, Inwards CY, Kindblom LG, Wold LE. Tumors of the bones and joints. AFIP Atlas of Tumor Pathology, 4th Series, Fascicle 2. Washington, DC: American Registry of Pathology; 2005:309-311.

Fat-Producing Tumors

60. González-Pérez LM, Pérez-Ceballos JL, Carranza-Carranza A. Mandibular intraosseous lipoma: Clinical features of a condylar location. Int J Oral Maxillofac Surg 2010;39:617-620.

61. Cakarer S, Selvi F, Isler SC, Soluk M, Olgac V, Keskin C. Intraosseous lipoma of the mandible: a case report and review of the literature. Int J Oral Maxillofac Surg 2009;38:900-902.

62. Unni KK, Inwards CY, Kindblom LG, Wold LE. Tumors of the bones and joints. AFIP Atlas of Tumor Pathology, 4th Series, Fascicle 2. Washington, DC: American Registry of Pathology; 2005:311-313

63. Darling MR, Daley TD. Radiolucent lesion of the anterior mandible. Oral Surg Oral Med Oral Pathol Oral Radiol Endod 2005;99:529-531.

64. McCulloch TM, Makielski KH, McNutt MA. Head and neck liposarcoma. A histopathologic reevaluation of reported cases. Arch Otolaryngol Head Neck Surg 1992;118:1045-1049.

Congenital Epulis of Newborn

65. Bosanquet D, Roblin G. Congenital epulis: a case report and estimation of incidence. Int J Otolaryngol 2009;2009:508780.
66. Chiba T, Okayama G. Congenital epulis of the newborn: Report of a case with a review of the Japanese literature. Nihon Geka Hokan 1990;59:408-411.
67. Zuker RM, Buenechea R. Congenital epulis: Review of the literature and case report. J Oral Maxillofac Surg 1993;51:1040-1043.
68. Ritwik P, Brannon RB, Musselman RJ. Spontaneous regression of congenital epulis: a case report and review of the literature. J Med Case Reports 2010;4:331.

Tumors Metastatic to the Jaws

69. Raubenheimer EJ, Noffke CE. Pathogenesis of bone metastasis: a review. J Oral Pathol Med 2006;35:129-135.
70. D'Silva NJ, Summerlin DJ, Cordell KG, et al. Metastatic tumors in the jaws: a retrospective study of 114 cases. J Am Dent Assoc 2006;137:1667-1672.
71. Bodner L, Sion-Vardy N, Geffen DB, Nash M. Metastatic tumors to the jaws: a report of eight new cases. Med Oral Patol Oral Cir Bucal 2006;11:E132-135.
72. Hirshberg A, Shnaiderman-Shapiro A, Kaplan I, Berger R. Metastatic tumours to the oral cavity—pathogenesis and analysis of 673 cases. Oral Oncol 2008;44:743-752.
73. Eversole LR, Duffey DC, Powell NB. Clear cell odontogenic carcinoma. A clinicopathologic analysis. Arch Otolaryngol Head Neck Surg 1995;121:685-689.
74. Lim SY, Kim SA, Ahn SG, et al. Metastatic tumours to the jaws and oral soft tissues: a retrospective analysis of 41 korean patients. Int J Oral Maxillofac Surg 2006;35:412-415.
75. Huang JW, Luo HY, Li Q, Li TJ. Primary intraosseous squamous cell carcinoma of the jaws. Clinicopathologic presentation and prognostic factors. Arch Pathol Lab Med 2009;133:1834-1840.
76. Li R, Walvekar RR, Nalesnik MA, Gamblin TC. Unresectable hepatocellular carcinoma with a solitary metastasis to the mandible. Am Surg 2008;74:346-349.
77. Halachmi S, Madeb R, Madjar S, Wald M, River Y, Nativ O. Numb chin syndrome as the presenting symptom of metastatic prostate carcinoma. Urology 2000;55:286.
78. Miles BA, Schwartz-Dabney C, Sinn DP, Kessler HP. Bilateral metastatic breast adenocarcinoma within the temporomandibular joint: a case report. J Oral Maxillofac Surg 2006;64:712-718.
79. Jones GM, Telfer MR, Eveson JW. Metastatic renal clear cell carcinoma of the jaws. Two cases illustrating clinical and pathological diagnostic problems. Br J Oral Maxillofac Surg 1990;28:172-175.
80. Maiorano E, Altini M, Favia G. Clear cell tumors of the salivary glands, jaws, and oral mucosa. Semin Diagn Pathol 1997;14:203-212.
81. Sangoi AR, Karamchandani J, Kim J, Pai RK, McKenney JK. The use of immunohistochemistry in the diagnosis of metastatic clear cell renal cell carcinoma: a review of PAX-8, PAX-2, hKIM-1, RCCma, and CD10. Adv Anat Pathol 2010;17:377-393.

Index*

*In a series of numbers, those in boldface indicate the main discussion of the entity.

P